AF757964

Salivary Gland Cancer

Lisa Licitra • Laura D. Locati
Editors

Salivary Gland Cancer

From Diagnosis to Tailored Treatment

Springer

Editors
Lisa Licitra
Head and Neck Medical Oncology Unit,
Fondazione IRCCS Istituto Nazionale dei
Tumori Milan
Milan
Italy

Laura D. Locati
Head and Neck Medical Oncology Unit,
Fondazione IRCCS Istituto Nazionale dei
Tumori Milan
Milan
Italy

ISBN 978-3-030-02957-9 ISBN 978-3-030-02958-6 (eBook)
https://doi.org/10.1007/978-3-030-02958-6

Library of Congress Control Number: 2018965730

© Springer Nature Switzerland AG 2019
This work is subject to copyright. All rights are reserved by the Publisher, whether the whole or part of the material is concerned, specifically the rights of translation, reprinting, reuse of illustrations, recitation, broadcasting, reproduction on microfilms or in any other physical way, and transmission or information storage and retrieval, electronic adaptation, computer software, or by similar or dissimilar methodology now known or hereafter developed.
The use of general descriptive names, registered names, trademarks, service marks, etc. in this publication does not imply, even in the absence of a specific statement, that such names are exempt from the relevant protective laws and regulations and therefore free for general use.
The publisher, the authors, and the editors are safe to assume that the advice and information in this book are believed to be true and accurate at the date of publication. Neither the publisher nor the authors or the editors give a warranty, expressed or implied, with respect to the material contained herein or for any errors or omissions that may have been made. The publisher remains neutral with regard to jurisdictional claims in published maps and institutional affiliations.

This Springer imprint is published by the registered company Springer Nature Switzerland AG
The registered company address is: Gewerbestrasse 11, 6330 Cham, Switzerland

Contents

Management-Based Pathology Assessment of Salivary Gland Carcinomas

1

Adel K. El-Naggar

1.1 Introduction

Salivary gland neoplasms are the most morphologically and clinically diverse solid epithelial tumors. There are 25 distinct salivary gland tumor types in the current WHO classification [1]. Given the clinical and management focus of this text, descriptions of pathologic features will be limited to gross and histopathologic manifestations relevant to surgical and oncologic management. Similarly, brief lineage-related biomarkers and genetic findings are present. Although the main focus is on malignant entities, benign tumors with differential diagnostic importance and those with potential progression to malignancy are discussed.

1.2 Salivary Gland Development and Tumorigenesis

Salivary glands evolve from the stomatodial surface of embryo at 6–8 weeks through branching morphogenesis where progressive indentation and elongation of an epithelial cord through the underlying ectomesenchyme leads to the formation of the ductal acinar unit [2–4]. The inner cellular lining of the ductal segments is epithelial in lineage except for the terminal duct component in which both epithelial and basal/myoepithelial cells are present. This fundamental formation in large part linked to the putative segmental ductal derivation and diversity of salivary gland neoplasms [5]. In that context, the presence of myoepithelial cells plays a critical role in the structural polarity and stromal organization in tumors composed of both cell types. The mechanism for the dual epithelial-myoepithelial neoplastic participation in some tumors is uncertain. It is, however, possible that an event in

A. K. El-Naggar (✉)
Department of Pathology, University of Texas MD Anderson Cancer Center, Houston, TX, USA
e-mail: anaggar@mdanderson.org

© Springer Nature Switzerland AG 2019

L. Licitra, L. D. Locati (eds.), *Salivary Gland Cancer*,
https://doi.org/10.1007/978-3-030-02958-6_1

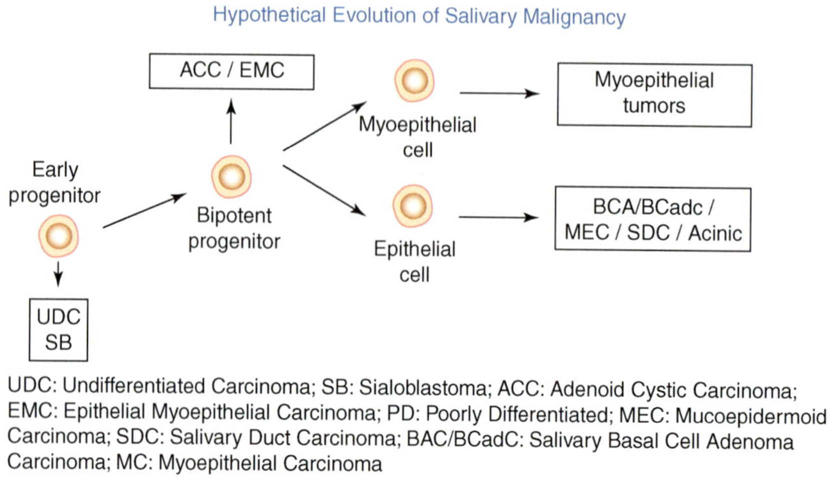

Fig. 1.1 Empirical diagram of the developmental pathway of the morphologic and cellular origins of salivary tumors

Table 1.1 Broad clinicopathologic categories of salivary gland carcinomas

Low/Indolent	Intermediate	Aggressive
• ACC, Tubular and Cribriform	• Predominantly Cribriform	• Salivary Duct Carcinoma
• Low grade MEC	• Intermediate MEC	• Solid—ACC
• EMC	• Adenocarcinoma, NOS	• High-grade MEC
• Basal Cell Adenocarcinoma	• Secretory Ca	• High grade transformation of different low and intermediate grade carcinomas
• Secretory Carcinoma	• Myoepithelial Ca	
• Acinic cell carcinoma	• Oncocytic Carcinoma	• Carcinosarcoma
• Myoepithelial Ca		• High-grade adenocarcinoma

uncommitted progenitor early in tumorigenesis gives rise to both epithelial and basal/myoepithelial cells (Fig. 1.1). In general, purely epithelial and majority of high-grade carcinoma arise from the main (nonterminal) ductal segments and those of low grade from the terminal duct-acinar unit.

1.3 Classification

Salivary gland tumors are broadly categorized into benign and malignant subtypes based on their histopathologic characteristics and the invasive nature of tumor at presentation. Grossly, benign tumors are well-circumscribed, thinly encapsulated, and soft to slightly firm in consistency. Histologically, generally these neoplasms display uniform epithelial and/or myoepithelial cell composition in variable manifestations. Malignant tumors, in contrast, present as firm, less mobile, ill-defined, and invariably infiltrative in nature. Histologically, tumors display heterogeneous neoplastic cellular and structural features (Table 1.1).

Table 1.2 Cytology in salivary gland mass evaluation

Indications	Limitations
• Confirm primary	• Differentiation between benign and malignant
• Exclusion of	• Basaloid, myoepithelial
– Metastasis	• Grade MEC
– Lymphoreticular disorders	• Dx of limited Ca EX PA
– Reactive	
– Inflammatory	

1.4 Pre-surgical Diagnosis of Salivary Gland Tumors

1.4.1 Fine Needle Aspirations (Table 1.2)

Initial assessment of salivary tumors commonly entails a fine needle aspiration cytology evaluation. The primary purpose of this procedure is to exclude metastasis, lymphoreticular disorders, infectious processes, and reactive lesions and to ascertain the primary salivary nature of mass. In general, the majority of primary and malignant tumors can be determined through this procedure. FNA, however, is limited in delineating benign and malignant nature of basaloid and oncocytic and myoepithelial and of carcinoma ex PA. The procedure is also valuable as a follow-up tool for harvesting cells for ancillary testing [6–11].

1.4.2 Core Biopsy

Occasionally, core biopsy is performed for salivary tumor diagnosis; however, this procedure should be limited to non-resectable, recurrent, and metastatic tumors.

1.4.3 Intraoperative Consultations

Although it is unnecessary, intraoperative frozen section can be requested where the nature of malignancy may alter the surgical plan and if surgical margins are of concern. In these instances, the surgeon and pathologist should be closely interacting during this process especially for minor salivary tumor resections. In these cases it is advisable that surgeons submit separate cavity-based margins.

1.5 Post Surgical Gross Assessment

Salivary tumor resections of major and minor glands should be inspected for gross infiltration of surrounding host tissue and processed to include tumor/host tissue interface and different regions of the tumor mass to assess invasion into periglandular soft tissue. Gross description of salivary resection should include size, appearance, and consistency, and the relation to surrounding host tissue is required.

1.5.1 Histopathologic Evaluation

Diagnosis for salivary gland tumors is based on the light-optic evaluation of well-prepared hematoxylin- and eosin-stained sections representing lesion and its boundaries. Certain immunomarkers may be used in certain instances for differential diagnosis and assessment of progression.

1.5.2 Pathologic Report

Pathology reports of salivary tumors must primarily include the following information: type of surgery, site, size, histologic diagnosis, presence or absence of perineural spaces, and margin status. Additional relevant findings may include grade if appropriate, and tumor diathesis, extraglandular extension margin status.

1.6 Common Benign Salivary Gland Tumors of Differential Diagnostic Significance

Benign salivary gland tumors are the most common in the parotid gland, and the vast majority pose no diagnostic difficulties. Certain subtypes may pose diagnostic challenges especially on the initial FNA evaluation. Generally, adenomas present as well-defined and encapsulated mass.

1.6.1 Pleomorphic Adenoma (PA)

PA is the most common benign salivary neoplasm and manifests a wide range of cellular and stromal component manifestations within and between tumors. Not uncommonly rare features such as squamous, sebaceous, and adipose tissue metaplasias are present, and this may lead to differential diagnostic challenges. PA generally presents as an ill-defined presentation and may manifest microscopic satellite formations that evade detection at the time of surgery leading to frequent recurrences. Histologically, tumors can be predominantly myoepithelial, epithelial, or paucicellular and can mostly be composed of chondroid, fibrotic, or myxoid elements. Occasionally, the delineation between myoepithelial dominant PA and myoepithelioma is difficult, but such distinction is of minimal clinical impact. Pleomorphic adenomas are also prone to recurrence and rarely distant dissemination. Metastasizing PA, in general, is histologically benign and typically presents in patients with multiple recurrence as a result of dislodgment of tumor in vascular spaces. These cases should be managed based on their presentation. Because of the not uncommon occurrence of carcinoma in long-standing PA, extensive sampling and careful examination of these tissues are critical especially in elderly patients with long-standing history of salivary swelling [12–15].

1.6.2 Myoepithelioma

Myoepithelial tumors are either entirely or largely composed of myoepithelial cells in spindle, plasmacytoid, and epithelioid features. The benign and malignant forms cannot be distinguished by FNA due to similar histologic features. Only on complete surgical excision the distinction of benign and malignant forms can be made. Immunohistochemistry may aid in confirming the diagnosis using SMA, p63, and calponin [16–18]. Their management is similar to pleomorphic adenoma.

1.6.3 Basal Cell Salivary Adenoma

Basal cell salivary tumors are composed of monotonous basal-like cells and classified into adenoma and adenocarcinoma based on the state of tumor invasion. Therefore, the initial assessment of these tumors by FNA is difficult if not impossible. Although the majority is cured by surgery, some adenomas may recur locally. Metastatic dermal basal cell carcinoma may lead to differential diagnostic difficulty especially in patients with remote history of skin primary. In these instances, immunostaining for keratin, p63, and SMA may confirm the dual cell formation of salivary basal neoplasms. Rarely, recurrence may develop due to multifocality. Not uncommonly, basaloid adenocarcinoma may evolve from adenoma [19–21].

1.6.4 Oncocytic Salivary Lesion

Oncocytic lesion/tumors are unique entities composed of mitochondrial-rich cells and are classified into hyperplastic and neoplastic lesions. The hyperplastic form is typically diagnosed as nodular oncocytic hyperplasia and may present unilaterally or bilaterally. These lesions regardless of their histologic classification are composed of monotonous epithelial cells with abundant eosinophilic cytoplasm and central nuclei. Histologic examination reveals the multinodular formation in variable sizes. The neoplastic types are classified into adenoma and carcinoma based on the status of the invasiveness [22–24].

1.6.5 Warthin's Tumor (WT)

Warthin's tumor can be presented bilaterally as single mass and rarely multifocally within intraparotid lymph nodes. The differential diagnosis of Warthin's tumors should be considered in oncocytic tumors and mucoepidermoid carcinoma, especially on FNA materials. Thorough examination of Warthin's tumors must be performed to exclude the latter possibility. Grossly, Warthin's tumor presents as a brown bulging and pliable soft mass. Histologically, lesions are formed of eosinophilic epithelial cell lining lymphoid nodules in distinct structural formation [25–27].

1.7 Malignant Salivary Tumors

1.7.1 Mucoepidermoid Carcinoma (MEC)

MEC is the most common salivary carcinoma of minor and major salivary glands in adults and children. MEC is also the only salivary cancer where histologic grading is associated with clinical behavior. Accurate diagnosis is difficult on FNA material and can be confused with cystic lesions and Warthin's tumor. Grossly, MEC presents as ill-defined cystic, partially cystic, or solid light tan and mucinous. Histologically, tumors are composed of mucinous, epidermoid (epithelial squamous-like), and transitioned (intermediate) cells in variable structural forms. Tumors are graded into low grade (grade 1), intermediate (grade 2), or poorly differentiated (grade 3) based on the extent of cystic and cellular manifestations. MEC may display oncocytic, clear, and transitional cell features of invariable proportion and patterns and display sclerotic. Mucoepidermoid carcinoma can rarely be associated with protracted radioactive iodine treatment in patients with papillary thyroid carcinoma. Low-grade cystic MEC is cured by complete surgery in major salivary gland. The most common grade is grade 2 where subjectivity plays a major role. Regardless of the reported grading systems, broadly speaking low-grade MECs are mainly cystic with limited foci of cellular proliferation, while intermediate grade displays more cellular formations with less cystic structure and the high-grade manifests markedly cellular with no cystic formation and focal intracellular mucin production [28–32].

Minor salivary gland MECs may pose surgical challenges if incompletely excised. Ancillary staining is rarely used in the diagnosis. Occasionally mucicarmine stain can be helpful in the diagnosis of poorly differentiated tumors. MEC is characterized by reciprocal translocations of chromosome 11p and 19q that lead to the formations of the CTRC1-MAML-2 fusion transcript [33–35]. Currently, there is no diagnostic, prognostic, and/or therapeutic validated evidence for this event. Mucoepidermoid carcinoma rarely shows keratin formation. Carcinoma with distinct keratin component and mucinous differentiation should be categorized as adenosquamous carcinoma. If metastasis is excluded, definitive distinction between these tumors should not influence the surgical management.

Complete surgical excision with free margins is the primary treatment for all grades of MEC. Post-operative XRT may be considered in case with close surgical margins and /or perineural invasion [32].

1.7.2 Adenoid Cystic Carcinoma (ACC)

ACC is the second most common and relentless salivary carcinoma subtype. ACC is assumed to develop from the terminal segment of the ductal-acinar unit and is formed of dual cell composition of outer myoepithelial and inner ductal cells [36]. The initial FNA diagnosis may not reliably be achieved, and definitive diagnosis can only be made on either excision biopsy, especially of minor salivary glands, or post-excision [37]. ACC is not graded due to the invariable presence of at least two histologic forms in any given tumor [38]. The tubular and the cribriform are composed of dual epithelial and myoepithelial cell. These forms retain the structural polarity, and pursue slow and progressive clinical course. Loss of myoepithelial component leads to epithelial solid form [39].

Solid epithelial development is typically associated with loss of myoepithelial cells and clinical progression. Solid myoepithelial transformation is typically of low-grade nature. ACC is characterized by translation between chromosomes (6;q) and (8;q) resulting in fusion genes of MY13 and MYBL1 genes with the NFIB genes in more than 60% of tumors. No definitive association between fusion and outcome has been established [40–45]. ACC of minor salivary glands, particularly the sin0-nasal sites, is difficult to eradicate unless clear margins are achieved intraoperatively.

1.7.3 Salivary Duct Carcinoma (De Novo and Ex-pleomorphic Adenoma)

Salivary duct carcinoma is one of the most aggressive malignancies of salivary glands and presents as de novo primary or as a malignant transformation of pleomorphic adenoma [46–49]. It is important that the carcinoma subtype be clearly stipulated in the diagnosis of this entity ex-PA. Generally, tumors histopathologically resemble high-grade mammary adenocarcinoma and share overlapping molecular and biomarker characteristics, an issue of differential diagnostic relevance in female patient. Multiple cytomorphologic features have been described including oncocytic, apocrine, rhabdoid, and squamoid. These morphologic forms have no clinical significance. SDC typically presents at high stage and wide surgical excision with neck lymph node dissection with radiotherapy and/or chemotherapy is the primary management [50–52].

Certain biomarkers may aid non-surgical therapy of these tumors including EGFR, AR and PTEN, and HER-2 [53, 54]. High AR nuclear expression is found in approximately 70% of males and 50% of female tumors. Recently, presence of AR isoform A7 has also been reported in AR-positive tumors of male and females [55–57]. Androgen deprivation treatment has been empirically used with variable and inconsistent results. PTEN expression is frequently lost in SDC and directly or indirectly is associated to PI3K pathway activation [58, 59].

1.7.4 Polymorphous Adenocarcinoma (PAC)

In the current WHO classification of head and neck tumors, the "low-grade" designation has been omitted due to the aggressive behaviors of some of these tumors. As the descriptive term implies, the tumor manifests variable neoplastic manifestation including lobular, trabecular, papillary, microcystic, and/or solid features. PAC is the second most common malignancy in the oral cavity, palate, and base of the tongue [60–63]. PAC has also been reported to occur in major salivary glands, the lacrimal gland, minor glands of the nasopharynx, and the nasal cavity. Grossly tumor presents as unencapsulated, light tan and soft with variable appearance and occasional hemorrhagic regions. A salient morphologic feature is the presence of distinctive cellular structures (eddy-like formation) along with the tubular, trabecular, and/or lobular structure. A reported subset with dominant cribriform and microcytic patterns has been reported as a separate entity but currently represents a variant of PAC [64]. Although a majority of these tumors pursue a good behavior with complete excision, not uncommonly recurrent and metastatic disease is encountered especially those of minor glands and base of tongue locations. This entity can be misclassified as adenoid cystic and epimyoepithelial carcinomas due to occasional overlapping features and definitive distinction may not be possible on small materials. Definitive diagnosis may not be achieved on biopsy materials and should not affect the surgical management. Rarely PAC may undergo high-grade undifferentiated transformation, and these cases typically pursue a more aggressive behavior [39, 65].

1.7.5 Acinic Cell Carcinoma

Acinic cell carcinoma is a distinctive entity composed of neoplastic cells of acinar cell features and coarse granules and afflicts a wide age range with no significant sex predilection. Acinic cell carcinoma is the second most common cancer in children and occurs mainly in the parotid and occasionally in mixed serious and mucinous glands. The tumor may rarely be encountered in mixed major and minor salivary glands [66–68]. Acinic cell carcinoma, as in Warthin's tumor and oncocytic and mucoepidermoid carcinoma, may develop in intraparotid lymph nodes and can be multifocal. Grossly acinic cell carcinoma is typically well-circumscribed with a brownish, mahogany color, soft, and can be cystic. Histopathologically, they are readily recognized by well-trained pathologists and may display variable phenotype patterns microcystic followed by macrocystic with papillary formation. In general, acinic cell carcinoma has a low to intermediate grade but occasionally displays solid transformation and poor differentiation. Patients with high grade transformation should be managed as other high salivary carcinomas [67, 69, 70].

1.7.6 Secretory Carcinoma

Secretory carcinoma is a newly recognized subtype with similar morphology to their mammary gland counterpart. This new entity has been extracted from acinic cell carcinoma following the recognition of a morphologically similar subset of secretory carcinoma in a review of acinic cell carcinomas of the mammary gland [71, 72]. As in mammary and acinic cell carcinomas, they are low to intermediate in grade and typically managed similarly to acinic cell carcinoma. A subset of this entity, as in mammary tumors, manifests (12, 15) resulting in gene fusion transcript of the ETV6 and the NTRK3 genes [73–75]. Although this fusion has not been reported in other salivary gland carcinomas, it has been detected in multiple tumor entities of diverse cell origins including carcinoma, lymphoma, thyroid, and rare lung tumors. The incorporation of this fusion in the diagnosis and differential diagnosis of primary and metastatic salivary tumors must supersede the morphologic diagnosis. The diagnostic and biological significance of this fusion is currently uncertain and must await large studies with long-term follow-up. The clinical course and management is similar to acinic cell carcinoma [76].

1.7.7 Adenocarcinoma: Not Otherwise Specified (NOS)

Adenocarcinoma, NOS, is defined as a salivary gland malignancy with ductal and glandular features that cannot be categorized as epithelial salivary carcinomas. This entity includes adenocarcinoma, NOS, cribriform adenocarcinoma, and mucinous, papillary, and intestinal carcinoma subtypes. The majority of tumors are of parotid origin, but minor and major salivary glands can be the source. In general, they can be considered intermediate in grade and behavior. Surgical excision remains to be the primary treatment [77–80].

1.7.8 Basal Cell Adenocarcinoma (BCAC)

BCAC, a distinctive low-grade malignancy of salivary glands, is characterized by uniform basaloid cell composition forming ductal, acinar, and tubular structures. Their pathologic classification into benign and malignant forms is based on the presence of lack of infiltrative extension into host tissue. BCAC may present as de novo or as carcinoma arising from basal cell salivary adenoma especially the membranous form [81–83]. Some of these tumors share striking resemblance to dermal adnexal tumors, and both types of tumors may occur in the same patient. Tumors should be differentiated from metastatic basal cell carcinoma of the skin, and sialoblastoma in infants. Complete excision with clear margins is generally curative. Recurrence may occur if close margins or satellite nodules are reported. Neck dissection is rarely recommended. Not uncommonly, carcinoma may arise from preexisting adenoma and may manifest high-grade features. Patients with these tumors should be managed similar to a high-grade salivary malignancy.

1.7.9 Clear Cell Carcinoma (CCC)

CCC is a rare entity typically composed of clear epithelial cells with and without fibrosis. Among tumors that may exhibit significant clear cell features are mucoepidermoid, oncocytic, and myoepithelial carcinomas. Grossly, tumors are generally less well-circumscribed, soft, and tan with and without visible sclerosis. The most common site for these tumors is the oral cavity. Females are thought to be more affected than males, but the rarity of these tumors precludes confirmation. Complete excision of this low–/intermediate-grade tumor is curative. Rarely nodal metastasis and recurrence may occur [84–87].

1.7.10 Myoepithelial Carcinoma

Myoepithelial carcinoma, similar to myoepithelioma, is composed entirely of malignant myoepithelial cells of hybrid epithelial and smooth muscle characteristics. Pre-surgical classification into benign and myoepithelial-rich PA may not be possible by FNA screening. Grossly, tumors are generally ill-defined, gray to tan in color, and firm in consistency. Histopathologically, they may display spindle, epithelioid, plasmacytoid, and/or mixed cell composition with infiltrative and ill-defined boundaries. The differentiation from the benign tumor is largely based on the infiltrative nature and extension into surrounding soft tissue. Myoepithelial carcinoma presents either in a pure form or as the malignant component of long-standing pleomorphic adenomas. These tumors are generally low grade and managed by complete surgical excision. Infiltrative spindle cell forms can be prone to recurrence [88–91].

1.7.11 Epithelial-Myoepithelial Carcinoma (EMC)

EMC is a low-grade salivary malignancy composed of dual cell types; outer clear myoepithelial and inner epithelial cells in ductal and nesting formation. EMC is uncommon with an estimated incidence of 5% of salivary malignancies. The most common sites of these tumor types are the parotid and the submandibular glands. The majority is of low-intermediate grade and is generally cured by complete surgical excision. Because of their dual cell formation, they may cause differential diagnostic difficulties with adenoid cystic, myoepithelial, and clear cell carcinomas. High-grade transformation has been reported and should be managed as high-grade malignancy [92–94].

1.7.12 Carcinosarcoma

Carcinosarcoma is a rare salivary malignancy composed of two distinct high-grade epithelial carcinoma and heterologous mesenchymal derived components. The epithelial form in commonly high-grade adenocarcinoma and the mesenchyme form is osteo-chrondro rhabdo and/or angiosarcoma subtypes. Tumors are large and grossly variable with solid, hemorrhagic, and osteo-chondromatous features with extension into surrounding host tissue. Generally, they are de novo in presentation but may rarely originate from pleomorphic adenoma and both instances are managed in a multidisciplinary setting. These tumors should be considered high-grade malignancy and if not surgically eradicated can be managed by either sarcoma or carcinoma medical oncology [95–98].

1.7.13 Poorly Differentiated and Undifferentiated Carcinomas

Primary poorly differentiated carcinoma may exhibit either small (slightly larger than lymphocytes) or large cell formation typically in cohesive sheets and nests. These tumors may manifest neuroendocrine differentiation and can be diagnosed as poorly differentiated carcinoma with neuroendocrine features or small- and large-cell neuroendocrine carcinoma. The latter tumors, particularly, should be differentiated from metastatic or unknown primary Merkel cell carcinoma. Tumors typically run aggressive clinically and frequently show lymph node metastasis. Management remains to be initial surgery with postoperative XRT and/or chemotherapy [99–101].

1.7.14 Undifferentiated (Lymphoepithelial) Carcinoma

Morphologically these tumors mimic nasopharyngeal carcinoma and are rare in Caucasian populations. Tumor is characteristically composed of malignant epithelial cells forming synthetial nests with intra- and peritumoral lymphoid infiltrate of undifferentiated tumor cells. Primary intraparotid tumor may arise de novo or from lymphoepithelial lesions. Tumor may or may not be positive for EBV. The tumor may present with lymph node metastasis. Surgical treatment is the primary approach with postoperative radiation and/or chemotherapy [102–105].

1.7.15 Primary Squamous Carcinoma

Primary squamous carcinoma of the salivary gland is exceedingly rare, and the diagnosis mostly only is made after the exclusion of dermal squamous malignancy even if remote. Primary squamous carcinoma can rarely occur in patients with long-standing sialolithiasis and chronic inflammation and squamous metaplasia of the main duct that primary squamous diagnosis can develop. The differential diagnosis from tumors with squamous features includes MEC and salivary duct carcinomas. Proximity to the main duct with evidence of squamous metaplasia and/or dysplasia is necessary to confirm the primary origin. Typically they are well to moderately differentiated and their surgical excision is curative [106–108].

1.7.16 Sialoblastoma

This is a tumor of infancy and has, until recently, been considered of uncertain malignant potential. In the fourth WHO edition of H&N tumor classification, it was considered low-grade malignant neoplasm of infancy. Histologically, tumors manifest basal cell proliferation with remarkable resemblance to salivary gland anlage.

This entity shares common cellular features with basaloid salivary tumors and adenoid cystic carcinoma. Their presentation at birth or shortly afterward is critical to proper classification. Complete surgical excision is curative in most cases. Recurrence and nodal metastasis have been reported in approximately 25%. Rare instance of concurrent presentation with hepatoblastoma and congenital nevi has been reported [109–112].

References

1. Batsakis JG, Luna MA, El-Naggar AK. Histopathologic grading of salivary gland neoplasms: II. Acinic cell carcinomas. Ann Otol Rhinol Laryngol. 1990;99(11):929–33.
2. Ianez RF, et al. Human salivary gland morphogenesis: myoepithelial cell maturation assessed by immunohistochemical markers. Histopathology. 2010;57(3):410–7.
3. Bilgin CC, et al. Multiscale feature analysis of salivary gland branching morphogenesis. PLoS One. 2012;7(3):e32906.
4. Knox SM, et al. Parasympathetic innervation maintains epithelial progenitor cells during salivary organogenesis. Science. 2010;329(5999):1645–7.
5. Batsakis JG, et al. Histogenesis of salivary gland neoplasms: a postulate with prognostic implications. J Laryngol Otol. 1989;103(10):939–44.
6. Klijanienko J, Vielh P. Fine-needle sampling of salivary gland lesions. IV. Review of 50 cases of mucoepidermoid carcinoma with histologic correlation. Diagn Cytopathol. 1997;17(2):92–8.
7. Klijanienko J, Vielh P. Fine-needle sampling of salivary gland lesions. III. Cytologic and histologic correlation of 75 cases of adenoid cystic carcinoma: review and experience at the Institut Curie with emphasis on cytologic pitfalls. Diagn Cytopathol. 1997;17(1):36–41.
8. Sivars L, et al. Human papillomavirus and p53 expression in cancer of unknown primary in the head and neck region in relation to clinical outcome. Cancer Med. 2014;3(2):376–84.
9. Strojan P, et al. Contemporary management of lymph node metastases from an unknown primary to the neck: II. a review of therapeutic options. Head Neck. 2013;35(2):286–93.
10. Klijanienko J, Vielh P. Salivary carcinomas with papillae: cytology and histology analysis of polymorphous low-grade adenocarcinoma and papillary cystadenocarcinoma. Diagn Cytopathol. 1998;19(4):244–9.
11. Kawahara A, et al. Salivary duct carcinoma cytologically diagnosed distinctly from salivary gland carcinomas with squamous differentiation. Diagn Cytopathol. 2008;36(7):485–93.
12. Spiro RH. Salivary neoplasms: overview of a 35-year experience with 2,807 patients. Head Neck Surg. 1986;8(3):177–84.
13. Skalova A, et al. Pleomorphic adenoma of the salivary glands with intravascular tumor deposits: a diagnostic pitfall. Am J Surg Pathol. 2012;36(11):1674–82.
14. Knight J, Ratnasingham K. Metastasising pleomorphic adenoma: Systematic review. Int J Surg. 2015;19:137–45.
15. Manucha V, Ioffe OB. Metastasizing pleomorphic adenoma of the salivary gland. Arch Pathol Lab Med. 2008;132(9):1445–7.
16. Dardick I, et al. Immunohistochemical and ultrastructural correlates of muscle-actin expression in pleomorphic adenomas and myoepitheliomas based on comparison of formalin and methanol fixation. Virchows Arch A Pathol Anat Histopathol. 1992;421(2):95–104.
17. Simpson RH, Jones H, Beasley P. Benign myoepithelioma of the salivary glands: a true entity? Histopathology. 1995;27(1):1–9.
18. Turgut S, et al. Myoepithelioma of the parotid gland: a report of two cases. Ear Nose Throat J. 2001;80(3):155–8.

19. Hyman BA, et al. Membranous basal cell adenoma of the parotid gland. Malignant transformation in a patient with multiple dermal cylindromas. Arch Pathol Lab Med. 1988;112(2):209–11.
20. Scott AR, Faquin WC, Deschler DG. Parotid mass in a woman with multiple cutaneous cylindromas. Head Neck. 2010;32(5):684–7.
21. Yu GY, Ubmuller J, Donath K. Membranous basal cell adenoma of the salivary gland: a clinicopathologic study of 12 cases. Acta Otolaryngol. 1998;118(4):588–93.
22. Deutsch E, et al. Synchronous bilateral oncocytoma of the parotid glands. A case report. ORL J Otorhinolaryngol Relat Spec. 1984;46(2):66–8.
23. Sorensen M, et al. Multifocal adenomatous oncocytic hyperplasia of the parotid gland (unusual clear cell variant in two female siblings.). Pathol Res Pract. 1986;181(2):254–9.
24. Hyde J, et al. Bilateral multinodular oncocytomas of the parotid arising in a background of bilateral oncocytic nodular hyperplasia. Ear Nose Throat J. 2008;87(1):51–4.
25. Ellies M, Laskawi R, Arglebe C. Extraglandular Warthin's tumours: clinical evaluation and long-term follow-up. Br J Oral Maxillofac Surg. 1998;36(1):52–3.
26. Lam KH, et al. Multifocal nature of adenolymphoma of the parotid. Br J Surg. 1994;81(11):1612–4.
27. Gnepp DR, Schroeder W, Heffner D. Synchronous tumors arising in a single major salivary gland. Cancer. 1989;63(6):1219–24.
28. Bastaki JM, et al. Secretory myoepithelial carcinoma: a histologic and molecular survey and a proposed nomenclature for mucin producing signet ring tumors. Head Neck Pathol. 2014;8(3):250–60.
29. Tasaki T, et al. Sclerosing mucoepidermoid carcinoma with eosinophilia of the salivary gland: case report and review of the literature. Pathol Int. 2013;63(2):125–31.
30. Brandwein MS, et al. Mucoepidermoid carcinoma: a clinicopathologic study of 80 patients with special reference to histological grading. Am J Surg Pathol. 2001;25(7):835–45.
31. McHugh CH, et al. Prognostic factors in mucoepidermoid carcinoma of the salivary glands. Cancer. 2012;118(16):3928–36.
32. Pires FR, et al. Prognostic factors in head and neck mucoepidermoid carcinoma. Arch Otolaryngol Head Neck Surg. 2004;130(2):174–80.
33. Nakayama T, et al. Clinicopathological significance of the CRTC3-MAML2 fusion transcript in mucoepidermoid carcinoma. Mod Pathol. 2009;22(12):1575–81.
34. Jee KJ, et al. Genomic profiles and CRTC1-MAML2 fusion distinguish different subtypes of mucoepidermoid carcinoma. Mod Pathol. 2013;26(2):213–22.
35. Shinawi T, et al. KIBRA gene methylation is associated with unfavorable biological prognostic parameters in chronic lymphocytic leukemia. Epigenetics. 2012;7(3):211–5.
36. Ellington CL, et al. Adenoid cystic carcinoma of the head and neck: Incidence and survival trends based on 1973-2007 Surveillance, Epidemiology, and End Results data. Cancer. 2012;118(18):4444–51.
37. Dal Maso M, Lippi L. Adenoid cystic carcinoma of the head and neck: a clinical study of 37 cases. Laryngoscope. 1985;95(2):177–81.
38. Spiro RH, Huvos AG, Strong EW. Adenoid cystic carcinoma of salivary origin. A clinicopathologic study of 242 cases. Am J Surg. 1974;128(4):512–20.
39. Nagao T. "Dedifferentiation" and high-grade transformation in salivary gland carcinomas. Head Neck Pathol. 2013;7(Suppl 1):S37–47.
40. Brayer KJ, et al. Recurrent fusions in MYB and MYBL1 define a common, transcription factor-driven oncogenic pathway in salivary gland adenoid cystic carcinoma. Cancer Discov. 2016;6(2):176–87.
41. Persson M, et al. Recurrent fusion of MYB and NFIB transcription factor genes in carcinomas of the breast and head and neck. Proc Natl Acad Sci U S A. 2009;106(44):18740–4.
42. Nordkvist A, et al. Non-random chromosome rearrangements in adenoid cystic carcinoma of the salivary glands. Genes Chromosomes Cancer. 1994;10(2):115–21.
43. van Weert S, et al. Histopathological grading of adenoid cystic carcinoma of the head and neck: analysis of currently used grading systems and proposal for a simplified grading scheme. Oral Oncol. 2015;51(1):71–6.

44. Szanto PA, et al. Histologic grading of adenoid cystic carcinoma of the salivary glands. Cancer. 1984;54(6):1062–9.
45. Rettig EM, et al. MYB rearrangement and clinicopathologic characteristics in head and neck adenoid cystic carcinoma. Laryngoscope. 2015;125(9):E292–9.
46. Jayaprakash V, et al. Survival rates and prognostic factors for infiltrating salivary duct carcinoma: analysis of 228 cases from the surveillance, epidemiology, and end results database. Head Neck. 2014;36(5):694–701.
47. LiVolsi VA, Perzin KH. Malignant mixed tumors arising in salivary glands. I. Carcinomas arising in benign mixed tumors: a clinicopathologic study. Cancer. 1977;39(5):2209–30.
48. Katabi N, et al. Consistent PLAG1 and HMGA2 abnormalities distinguish carcinoma ex-pleomorphic adenoma from its de novo counterparts. Hum Pathol. 2015;46(1):26–33.
49. Weiler C, et al. Carcinoma ex pleomorphic adenoma with special reference to the prognostic significance of histological progression: a clinicopathological investigation of 41 cases. Histopathology. 2011;59(4):741–50.
50. Griffith CC, et al. Salivary duct carcinoma and the concept of early carcinoma ex pleomorphic adenoma. Histopathology. 2014;65(6):854–60.
51. Di Palma S, et al. Non-invasive (intracapsular) carcinoma ex pleomorphic adenoma: recognition of focal carcinoma by HER-2/neu and MIB1 immunohistochemistry. Histopathology. 2005;46(2):144–52.
52. Jaehne M, et al. Clinical and immunohistologic typing of salivary duct carcinoma: a report of 50 cases. Cancer. 2005;103(12):2526–33.
53. Locati LD, et al. Clinical activity of androgen deprivation therapy in patients with metastatic/relapsed androgen receptor-positive salivary gland cancers. Head Neck. 2016;38(5):724–31.
54. Masubuchi T, et al. Clinicopathological significance of androgen receptor, HER2, Ki-67 and EGFR expressions in salivary duct carcinoma. Int J Clin Oncol. 2015;20(1):35–44.
55. Di Palma S, et al. Salivary duct carcinomas can be classified into luminal androgen receptor-positive, HER2 and basal-like phenotypes. Histopathology. 2012;61(4):629–43.
56. Kapadia SB, Barnes L. Expression of androgen receptor, gross cystic disease fluid protein, and CD44 in salivary duct carcinoma. Mod Pathol. 1998;11(11):1033–8.
57. Williams L, et al. Salivary duct carcinoma: the predominance of apocrine morphology, prevalence of histologic variants, and androgen receptor expression. Am J Surg Pathol. 2015;39(5):705–13.
58. Mitani Y, et al. Alterations associated with androgen receptor gene activation in salivary duct carcinoma of both sexes: potential therapeutic ramifications. Clin Cancer Res. 2014;20(24):6570–81.
59. Saintigny P, et al. Frequent PTEN loss and differential HER2/PI3K signaling pathway alterations in salivary duct carcinoma: implications for targeted therapy. Cancer. 2018;124(18):3693–705.
60. Kimple AJ, et al. Polymorphous low-grade adenocarcinoma: a case series and determination of recurrence. Laryngoscope. 2014;124(12):2714–9.
61. Castle JT, et al. Polymorphous low grade adenocarcinoma: a clinicopathologic study of 164 cases. Cancer. 1999;86(2):207–19.
62. Patel TD, et al. Polymorphous low-grade adenocarcinoma of the head and neck: a population-based study of 460 cases. Laryngoscope. 2015;125(7):1644–9.
63. Michal M, et al. Cribriform adenocarcinoma of the tongue: a hitherto unrecognized type of adenocarcinoma characteristically occurring in the tongue. Histopathology. 1999;35(6):495–501.
64. Simpson RH, et al. Polymorphous low-grade adenocarcinoma of the salivary glands with transformation to high-grade carcinoma. Histopathology. 2002;41(3):250–9.
65. Klijanienko J, Vielh P. Cytologic characteristics and histomorphologic correlations of 21 salivary duct carcinomas. Diagn Cytopathol. 1998;19(5):333–7.
66. Patel NR, et al. Demographic trends and disease-specific survival in salivary acinic cell carcinoma: an analysis of 1129 cases. Laryngoscope. 2014;124(1):172–8.

67. Chiosea SI, et al. The profile of acinic cell carcinoma after recognition of mammary analog secretory carcinoma. Am J Surg Pathol. 2012;36(3):343–50.
68. Spiro RH, Huvos AG, Strong EW. Acinic cell carcinoma of salivary origin. A clinicopathologic study of 67 cases. Cancer. 1978;41(3):924–35.
69. Skalova A, et al. Acinic cell carcinoma with high-grade transformation: a report of 9 cases with immunohistochemical study and analysis of TP53 and HER-2/neu genes. Am J Surg Pathol. 2009;33(8):1137–45.
70. Thompson LD, et al. Clinicopathologic and immunophenotypic characterization of 25 cases of acinic cell carcinoma with high-grade transformation. Head Neck Pathol. 2016;10(2):152–60.
71. Reis-Filho JS, et al. Is acinic cell carcinoma a variant of secretory carcinoma? A FISH study using ETV6'split apart' probes. Histopathology. 2008;52(7):840–6.
72. Skalova A, et al. Mammary analogue secretory carcinoma of salivary glands, containing the ETV6-NTRK3 fusion gene: a hitherto undescribed salivary gland tumor entity. Am J Surg Pathol. 2010;34(5):599–608.
73. Ito Y, et al. Mammary analogue secretory carcinoma of salivary glands: a clinicopathologic and molecular study including 2 cases harboring ETV6-X fusion. Am J Surg Pathol. 2015;39(5):602–10.
74. Sethi R, et al. Mammary analogue secretory carcinoma: update on a new diagnosis of salivary gland malignancy. Laryngoscope. 2014;124(1):188–95.
75. Skalova A, et al. Mammary analogue secretory carcinoma of salivary glands with high-grade transformation: report of 3 cases with the ETV6-NTRK3 gene fusion and analysis of TP53, beta-catenin, EGFR, and CCND1 genes. Am J Surg Pathol. 2014;38(1):23–33.
76. Majewska H, et al. Mammary analogue secretory carcinoma of salivary glands: a new entity associated with ETV6 gene rearrangement. Virchows Arch. 2015;466(3):245–54.
77. Wahlberg P, et al. Carcinoma of the parotid and submandibular glands--a study of survival in 2465 patients. Oral Oncol. 2002;38(7):706–13.
78. Whittaker JS, Turner EP. Papillary tumours of the minor salivary glands. J Clin Pathol. 1976;29(9):795–805.
79. Gillenwater AM, et al. Primary intestinal-like adenocarcinoma of major salivary glands: 2 instances of previously undocumented phenotype. Head Neck. 2013;35(8):E234–6.
80. Slova D, et al. Colonic-type adenocarcinoma of the base of the tongue: a case report of a rare neoplasm. Head Neck Pathol. 2012;6(2):250–4.
81. Ellis GL, Wiscovitch JG. Basal cell adenocarcinomas of the major salivary glands. Oral Surg Oral Med Oral Pathol. 1990;69(4):461–9.
82. Choi HR, et al. Molecular analysis of chromosome 16q regions in dermal analogue tumors of salivary glands: a genetic link to dermal cylindroma? Am J Surg Pathol. 2002;26(6):778–83.
83. Rito M, et al. Frequent and differential mutations of the CYLD gene in basal cell salivary neoplasms: linkage to tumor development and progression. Mod Pathol. 2018;31(7):1064–72.
84. Milchgrub S, et al. Hyalinizing clear cell carcinoma of salivary gland. Am J Surg Pathol. 1994;18(1):74–82.
85. Solar AA, Schmidt BL, Jordan RC. Hyalinizing clear cell carcinoma: case series and comprehensive review of the literature. Cancer. 2009;115(1):75–83.
86. Tanguay J, Weinreb I. What the EWSR1-ATF1 fusion has taught us about hyalinizing clear cell carcinoma. Head Neck Pathol. 2013;7(1):28–34.
87. Shah AA, et al. EWSR1 genetic rearrangements in salivary gland tumors: a specific and very common feature of hyalinizing clear cell carcinoma. Am J Surg Pathol. 2013;37(4):571–8.
88. Batsakis JG, Luna MA, el-Naggar A. Histopathologic grading of salivary gland neoplasms: III. Adenoid cystic carcinomas. Ann Otol Rhinol Laryngol. 1990;99(12):1007–9.
89. Gnepp DR. Mucinous myoepithelioma, a recently described new myoepithelioma variant. Head Neck Pathol. 2013;7(Suppl 1):S85–9.
90. Skalova A, et al. Clear cell myoepithelial carcinoma of salivary glands showing EWSR1 rearrangement: molecular analysis of 94 salivary gland carcinomas with prominent clear cell component. Am J Surg Pathol. 2015;39(3):338–48.

91. Kong M, et al. Prognostic factors in myoepithelial carcinoma of salivary glands: a clinicopathologic study of 48 cases. Am J Surg Pathol. 2015;39(7):931–8.
92. Seethala RR, Barnes EL, Hunt JL. Epithelial-myoepithelial carcinoma: a review of the clinicopathologic spectrum and immunophenotypic characteristics in 61 tumors of the salivary glands and upper aerodigestive tract. Am J Surg Pathol. 2007;31(1):44–57.
93. Seethala RR. Oncocytic and apocrine epithelial myoepithelial carcinoma: novel variants of a challenging tumor. Head Neck Pathol. 2013;7(Suppl 1):S77–84.
94. Roy P, et al. Epithelial-myoepithelial carcinoma with high grade transformation. Am J Surg Pathol. 2010;34(9):1258–65.
95. Stephen J, et al. True malignant mixed tumors (carcinosarcoma) of salivary glands. Oral Surg Oral Med Oral Pathol. 1986;61(6):597–602.
96. Kwon MY, Gu M. True malignant mixed tumor (carcinosarcoma) of parotid gland with unusual mesenchymal component: a case report and review of the literature. Arch Pathol Lab Med. 2001;125(6):812–5.
97. Love GL, Sarma DP. Spindle cell mucoepidermoid carcinoma of submandibular gland. J Surg Oncol. 1986;31(1):66–8.
98. Manuel S, et al. Carcinosarcoma of the parotid gland with epithelial-myoepithelial carcinoma and pleomorphic sarcoma components. Br J Oral Maxillofac Surg. 2002;40(6):480–3.
99. Kawaratani H, et al. Large cell neuroendocrine carcinoma presenting with neck swelling in the submandibular gland: a case report. J Med Case Rep. 2013;7(1):81.
100. Walters DM, et al. Small cell carcinoma of the submandibular gland: a rare small round blue cell tumor. Am J Otolaryngol. 2007;28(2):118–21.
101. Pang B, et al. Desmoplastic small round cell tumor of major salivary glands: report of 1 case and a review of the literature. Appl Immunohistochem Mol Morphol. 2011;19(1):70–5.
102. Kuo T, Hsueh C. Lymphoepithelioma-like salivary gland carcinoma in Taiwan: a clinicopathological study of nine cases demonstrating a strong association with Epstein-Barr virus. Histopathology. 1997;31(1):75–82.
103. Auclair PL, Goode RK, Ellis GL. Mucoepidermoid carcinoma of intraoral salivary glands. Evaluation and application of grading criteria in 143 cases. Cancer. 1992;69(8):2021–30.
104. Wang CP, et al. Lymphoepithelial carcinoma versus large cell undifferentiated carcinoma of the major salivary glands. Cancer. 2004;101(9):2020–7.
105. Li F, et al. A clinical analysis of 37 cases with lymphoepithelial carcinoma of the major salivary gland treated by surgical resection and postoperative radiotherapy: a single institution study. Med Oncol. 2014;31(5):957.
106. Gaughan RK, Olsen KD, Lewis JE. Primary squamous cell carcinoma of the parotid gland. Arch Otolaryngol Head Neck Surg. 1992;118(8):798–801.
107. Marks MW, et al. Squamous cell carcinoma of the parotid gland. Plast Reconstr Surg. 1987;79(4):550–4.
108. Wang W, Li Y, Tang Y. Keratocystoma of the parotid gland: a case report and review of previous publications. Br J Oral Maxillofac Surg. 2015;53(7):655–7.
109. Ortiz-Hidalgo C, et al. Sialoblastoma: report of a congenital case with dysembryogenic alterations of the adjacent parotid gland. Histopathology. 2001;38(1):79–80.
110. Canalis RF, et al. Congenital basal cell adenoma of the submandibular gland. Arch Otolaryngol. 1980;106(5):284–6.
111. Vawter GF, Tefft M. Congenital tumors of the parotid gland. Arch Pathol. 1966;82(3):242–5.
112. Taylor GP. Congenital epithelial tumor of the parotid-sialoblastoma. Pediatr Pathol. 1988;8(4):447–52.

Molecular Characterization of Salivary Gland Carcinomas

2

André Fehr, Jörn Bullerdiek, Thorsten Jaekel, and Thomas Löning

Abbreviations

a.k.a.	Also known as
ACC	Acinic cell carcinoma
AdCC	Adenoid cystic carcinoma
AR	Androgen receptor
CAMSG	Cribriform adenocarcinoma of minor salivary glands
CREB	cAMP response element-binding protein
CXPA	Carcinoma ex pleomorphic adenoma
FGF-IGF-PI3K	Fibroblast growth factor-insulin-like growth factor-phosphatidylinositol 3-kinase pathway
FISH	Fluorescence in situ hybridization
HCCC	Hyalinizing clear-cell carcinoma
IDC	Low-grade intraductal carcinoma
MAPK	Mitogen-activated protein kinase
MASC	Mammary analogue secretory carcinoma
MEC	Mucoepidermoid carcinoma

A. Fehr (✉)
Sahlgrenska Cancer Center, University of Gothenburg, Gothenburg, Sweden
e-mail: andre.fehr@gu.se

J. Bullerdiek
Institut für Medizinische Genetik, Universitätsmedizin Rostock, Rostock, Germany
e-mail: joern.bullerdiek@med.uni-rostock.de

T. Jaekel
Pathologie Bremen, Bremen, Germany
e-mail: Jaekel@pathologie-bremen.de

T. Löning
Gerhard-Seifert-Referenzzentrum, Hamburg, Germany
e-mail: loening@hansepathnet.de

© Springer Nature Switzerland AG 2019
L. Licitra, L. D. Locati (eds.), *Salivary Gland Cancer*,
https://doi.org/10.1007/978-3-030-02958-6_2

NOS	Not otherwise specified
PA	Pleomorphic adenoma
PAC	Polymorphous adenocarcinoma
PI3K	Phosphatidylinositol 3-kinase
RT-PCR	Reverse transcription polymerase chain reaction
SC	Secretory breast carcinoma
SDC	Salivary duct carcinoma
SGC	Salivary gland carcinomas

2.1 Introduction

The advent and widespread use of new genetic methods (e.g., next-generation sequencing or array technologies) has paved the way for promising advancements in our understanding of molecular tumor biology. This is also true for salivary gland carcinomas (SGC) which comprise a widely heterogeneous group of cancers [1]. Diagnosis is challenging, due to the diversity of histologic subtypes and the overlapping morphological patterns among many of these lesions. The phenotypic heterogeneity is reflected by the variety of aberrant genetic and molecular pathways contributing to the development and progression of each tumor. There are unique molecular alterations for some SGCs (Table 2.1), which will be the focus of this chapter, pointing out molecular markers that could become relevant in clinical practice. This chapter highlights markers that can be used for typization of tumors and sporadically reported and research-based markers that can be found elsewhere in the literature.

Table 2.1 Overview of recurrent alterations in salivary gland carcinomas

Diagnosis	Alteration	Gene fusion	Comments	References
MEC	t(11;19)(q21~22;p13) t(11;15)(q21;q26)	*CRTC1-MAML2* *CRTC3-MAML2*	Usual good prognosis; occurs mainly in low- and intermediate-grade MECs	[2–4] [5, 6]
	Loss of *CDKN2A*		Indicator for worse prognosis	[7]
	Hotspot mutation in *HRAS*		Occurs in ~20% of MECs	[8]
	t(6;15)(p21;q12)	*EWSR1-POU5F1*	Occur in high-grade MEC-like tumors	[9]
	Mutation of *TP53*		Occurs in intermediate- and high-grade MECs	[10]
	In-frame deletion in *POU6F2*		187Q > –	
AdCC	t(6;9)(q22~23;p23~24) t(8;9) t(8;14)	*MYB-NFIB* *MYBL1-NFIB* *MYBL1-RAD51B*		[11–13]

Table 2.1 (continued)

Diagnosis	Alteration	Gene fusion	Comments	References
MASC	t(12;15)(p13;q25)	*ETV6-NTRK3*	Same fusion as in SC of the breast	[14]
	t(12;?)	*ETV6-X* (unknown fusion partner)	Potential more aggressive than MASC with *ETV6-NTRK3* fusion	[15, 16]
HCCC	t(12;22)(q13;q12)	*EWSR1-ATF1*	Occur in high frequency in HCCC and CCOC, indicates a biologic link between these entities	[17, 18]
CXPA	t(8q12)	*CTNNB1-PLAG1* *FGFR1-PLAG1* *TCEA1-PLAG1* *CHCHD7-PLAG1* *LIFR-PLAG1*	Same fusions as described for PAs	[19–22]
	t(12q14–15)	*HMGA2-WIF1* *HMGA2-FHIT* *HMGA2-NFIB*		
	Amplification 12q13–15		Amplification of *HMGA2* and/or *MDM2*	
	Mutation of *TP53* Mutation or amplification of *ERBB2* (HER2)			
SDC	Mutations of *TP53*, *HRAS*, *PIK3CA*, or *BRAF* Loss or mutation of *PTEN* Amplification of *ERBB2* Gain of *EGFR* Gain and/or overexpression of *AR* (androgen receptor)			[21, 23]
PAC	Hotspot mutation in *PRKD1*		p.Glu710Asp	[24]
CAMSG	t(1;14) t(14;X)	*ARID1A-PRKD1* *DDX3X-PRKD1*		[25]

AdCC adenoid cystic carcinoma, *CAMSG* cribriform adenocarcinoma of minor salivary glands, *CXPA* carcinoma ex pleomorphic adenoma, *HCCC* hyalinizing clear-cell carcinoma, *MASC* mammary analogue secretory carcinoma, *MEC* mucoepidermoid carcinoma, *PA* pleomorphic adenoma, *PAC* polymorphous adenocarcinoma, *SC* secretory carcinoma of the breast, *SDC* salivary duct carcinoma

2.2 Mucoepidermoid Carcinoma

Mucoepidermoid carcinoma (MEC) is the most common salivary gland malignancy. MECs are composed of mucinous, intermediate (clear-cell), and squamoid tumor cells forming cystic and solid patterns [1]. Rarely they can also occur in other anatomic locations such as the skin, lung, maxillary sinus, and upper respiratory tract

[26–29]. MEC is traditionally graded in low-, intermediate-, and high-grade tumors. Low-grade MECs have an excellent prognosis after surgical excision with a 10-year survival rate of over 90%. In contrast, high-grade MECs have a poor prognosis. Despite intense treatment strategies, the 10-year survival rate is about 25% [1, 30]. Previous cytogenetic studies have identified a t(11;19)(q21~22;p13) translocation as a recurrent and tumor-type-specific rearrangement in MECs of the salivary glands [2]. Recent studies have shown that this rearrangement results in a fusion of *CRTC1* (a.k.a. *MECT1*, *TORC1*, and *WAMTP1*) exon 1 with exon 2–5 of *MAML2* [5], whereas a small subset of MEC shows a t(11;15)(q21;q26) translocation cytogenetically reflecting a *CRTC3-MAML2* fusion [31].

MAML2 belongs to a family of Mastermind-like nuclear proteins that act as transcriptional coactivators for Notch receptors. CRTC1 and CRTC3 are part of a family of highly conserved CREB coactivators [5, 32]. The *CRTC1-MAML2* fusion encodes a chimeric protein consisting of the CREB-binding domain of CRTC1 linked to the transactivation domain of MAML2. In particular, the fusion protein activates transcription of cAMP/CREB target genes [33, 34]. Previous studies have shown that sustained expression of the fusion is essential for tumor cell growth in salivary gland cancers that carrying the t(11;19) translocation [3]. Tumors with *CRTC1/CRTC3-MAML2* gene fusion tend to be low- or intermediate-grade. High-grade MEC are rarely fusion positive. Moreover, some clinical studies have demonstrated that patients with *CRTC1/CRTC3-MAML2*-positive MECs have increased survival and a better prognosis [4, 6, 35–37], although there is still an ongoing debate on this query [38]. In addition, detection of the *CRTC1-MAML2* fusion might be useful for diagnostic purposes since it is very characteristic of MEC, irrespective of anatomical location. Nevertheless, an identical fusion has also been identified in look-alikes of the so-called metaplastic Warthin tumor and in clear-cell hidradenomas of the skin [32, 39–41], thus broadening the spectrum of neoplasms associated with this gene fusion.

Recently, genomic studies have shown that fusion-positive MECs can be subdivided in low- and intermediate-grade tumors by copy number alterations [4, 6]. Tumors with no or only a few copy number alterations have a good prognosis, while tumors with numerous copy number alterations, including loss of the tumor suppressor *CDKN2A*, tend to be high-grade tumors and have a poor prognosis [7, 35, 36, 42]. It is noteworthy that there is a subgroup of tumors that may be classified morphologically as high-grade MEC but are negative for the fusion [6, 31, 35, 36]. Moreover, it has been speculated that at least some of the cases classified as high-grade tumors that do not carry the translocation might in fact not represent MEC but rather a more aggressive squamous carcinoma or a SDC [35, 36]. Irrespective of the *MAML2* fusion status, gene copy number alterations of either *HER2* or *EGFR* are associated with high- and extremely rarely low- and intermediate-grade MEC [10]. *HER2* or *EGFR* gene abnormality might play an important role in the development of high-grade MEC and also in the progression from *MAML2* fusion-positive low-/intermediate- to high-grade in a subset of MEC [10]. Whole-exome sequencing and gene copy number analyses performed on 18 MEC have shown that *TP53* is the most common mutated gene in MEC (28%). Interestingly, the mutations were only found in intermediate- and high-grade MECs, and the mutated tumors had more mutations overall than tumors without *TP53* mutations ($p = 0.006$). The second most frequent mutated gene *POU6F2* was found in three low-grade MECs encoding the same in-frame deletion (187Q>-) [43]. The *POU6F2* gene encodes a member of the POU protein family; the family members are transcriptional regulators, many of which are known to control cell-type-specific differentiation pathways [44]. Loss of heterozygosity in regions containing *POU6F2* or overexpression of *POU6F2* has been reported in Wilms tumor [9, 45]. The authors proposed that beside the *CRTC1/CRTC3-MAML2* gene fusions as the main oncogenic driver, somatic *TP53* mutation may act as an alternate mechanism of tumorigenesis, and *POU6F2* mutations may act as drivers of oncogenesis in low-grade MEC [43].

In addition to *CRTC1/CRTC3-MAML2* fusions, rare cases with t(6;22)(p21;q12) translocation and *EWSR1-POU5F1* gene fusion have been reported [8]. Although these findings have been validated, analyses of larger tumor series are required to evaluate the diagnostic or biological significance of these findings. Last but not least, hotspot mutations in *HRAS* have been found in approximately 20% of MECs. The presence of *HRAS* mutations strongly correlates with high-grade tumor [46].

2.3 Adenoid Cystic Carcinoma

Adenoid cystic carcinoma (AdCC) is one of the most common cancers of the salivary glands. It is composed of epithelial and myoepithelial neoplastic cells that form various patterns, including tubular, cribriform, and solid [1]. Although AdCC of the salivary gland is a slow-growing tumor, long-term prognosis is poor due to frequent local recurrences, distant metastases, and tendency for perineural invasion [1, 47].

Genomic studies of AdCC have shown that losses of 1p and 6q are associated with high-grade tumors and poor prognosis, whereas loss of 14q is exclusively seen in low-grade tumors [11, 48]. Key genomic alteration in AdCC is a recurrent t(6;9)(q22~23;p23~24) chromosomal translocation that results in a fusion of the transcription factor genes *MYB* and *NFIB* (Fig. 2.1) [49]. The *MYB* oncogene acts as a regulator of stem cells. The gene is highly expressed in immature, proliferating cells and is downregulated during differentiation [50]. *NFIB* encodes a transcription factor that controls cell proliferation and cell viability [19]. The MYB-NFIB fusions, which consist of the DNA binding and transactivation domains of MYB fused to different parts of the three-end of NFIB, interrupt the C-terminal part of MYB, leading to loss of negative regulatory sequence elements and, subsequently, to overexpression of the fusion protein [49]. In addition to gene fusion, *MYB* may be activated by copy number gain or juxtaposition of enhancer elements from other genes, including *NFIB*, *RAD51B*, or *TGFBR3*, to the *MYB* locus [48, 51, 52]. The latter events result in overexpression of a normal MYB protein, whereas the fusion events usually result in expression of truncated MYB proteins.

Recent molecular analyses, including whole-exome sequencing of AdCCs, have revealed a wide mutational diversity and low somatic mutation rate, with gene mutations influencing a wide variety of pathways, such as mutations

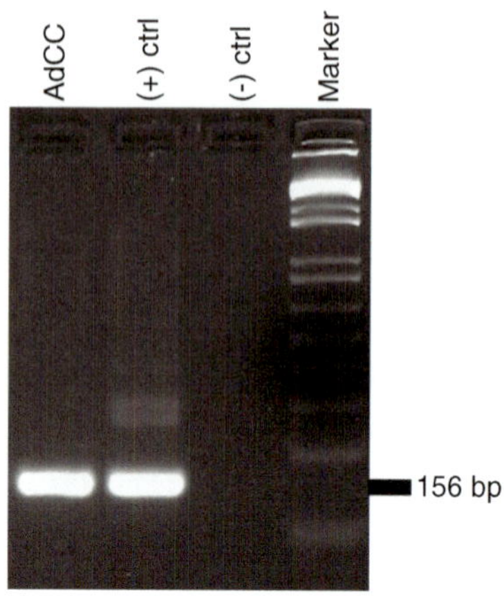

Fig. 2.1 AdCC carrying the *MYB-NFIB* gene fusion, detected by RT-PCR. (+) positive, (−) negative, ctrl control

affecting the FGF-IGF-PI3K pathway in 30% of samples as well as in the NOTCH1 pathway in 13% of the cases [12, 53]. Interestingly, *KIT* and *EGFR*, which are frequently overexpressed in AdCC, are rarely mutated or amplified. The translocation t(6;9) is the only highly recurrent genetic alteration in these tumors suggesting that the product of the *MYB-NFIB* fusion gene is a key driver mutation in the development of AdCC. In a subset of AdCC, t(8;9) and t(8;14) translocations are detected, fusing the *MYBL1* gene to *NFIB* and *RAD51B*, respectively [13, 54].

In summary, *MYB/MYBL1* activation due to gene fusion or other mechanisms occurs in the vast majority (60–80%) of AdCC and is a novel diagnostic biomarker for this tumor entity [13, 14, 55]. Also, its clinical application as new molecular target for therapy in AdCC patients is promising though functional studies are necessary.

2.4 Mammary Analogue Secretory Carcinoma

Certain types of SGCs have striking histological similarities with mammary tumors and indeed share overlap in molecular features. Mammary analogue secretory carcinoma (a.k.a. secretory carcinoma or MASC) is a newly described salivary gland carcinoma that is defined by its histologic, immunophenotypic, and genetic similarities to secretory breast carcinoma (SC) (Fig. 2.2a) [56, 57]. Key genomic alteration in both SC of the breast and MASC is the *ETV6-NTRK3* chimeric tyrosine kinase generated by a balanced chromosomal translocation t(12;15)(p13;q25) [56, 58]. The chromosomal alteration can be detected by *ETV6*-fluorescence in situ hybridization or by RT-PCR for the *ETV6-NTRK3* fusion transcript (Fig. 2.2b). The *ETV6-NTRK3* fusion can be found in the vast majority of MASC [56]. MASC typically has an indolent clinical course, although sporadic cases with high-grade transformation have been reported [59]. Further studies are needed to clarify whether the clinical behavior of MASC matches the tumor's low-grade histologic appearance. Before their initial description, these salivary gland tumors were generally diagnosed as ACC or adenocarcinoma, NOS.

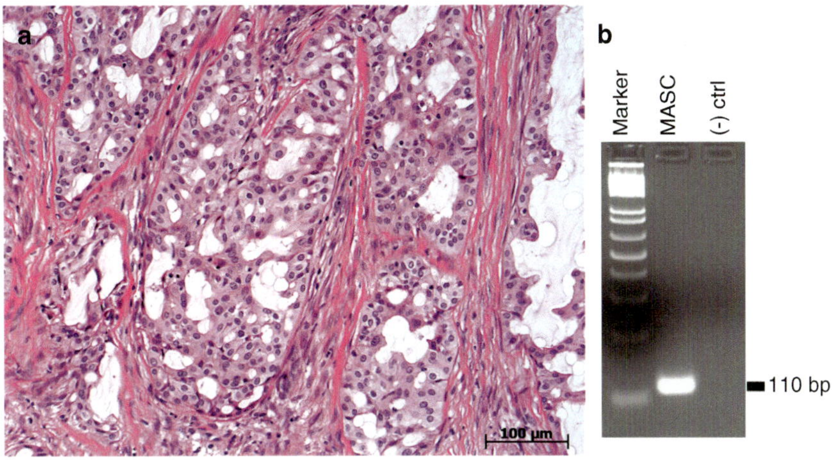

Fig. 2.2 (**a**) Typical MASC with partly confluent tumor complexes containing abundant (foamy) secretory material. The eosinophilic tumor cells are cuboidal in shape and contain moderately atypical nuclei. (**b**) MASC-specific *ETV6-NTRK3* gene fusion detected by RT-PCR. (–) negative, ctrl control

Expression of the *ETV6-NTRK3* gene fusion leads to constitutive activation of the Ras-MAPK and the PI3K-AKT pathways [15, 56, 58]. Recent studies have shown that a subset of fusion-negative MASCs have variant fusions involving *ETV6* and an unknown fusion partner, designated as *ETV6-X* fusions, and tumors with these fusions may behave more aggressively than *ETV6-NTRK3*-positive cases [16, 60]. The presence of the *ETV6-NTRK3* fusion gene has not been demonstrated in any other salivary gland tumor so far. Interestingly, the same t(12;15) translocation with the same fusion gene was also described in congenital mesoblastic nephroma [61], congenital fibrosarcoma [62], and some cases of myelogenous leukemia [63], indicating that this chimeric tyrosine kinase has transforming activity in multiple cell lineages. Studies that have identified MASCs retrospectively have demonstrated that they had previously most often been classified as ACC, MEC, or adenocarcinoma/cystadenocarcinoma, NOS [56, 64–68]. Taking into account the different tumor biology of these neoplasias, it is mandatory to exploit all immunohistochemical and molecular tools prior to the final diagnosis.

2.5 Hyalinizing Clear-Cell Carcinoma

Hyalinizing clear-cell carcinoma (a.k.a. clear-cell adenocarcinoma, clear-cell carcinoma, or HCCC) is a unique low-grade tumor with rare metastases and a very good prognosis. The tumor has a typical clear-cell morphology and pattern of hyalinization often with focal mucinous differentiation [1, 17, 69].

Recurrent t(12;22)(q13;q12) translocation consistent with *EWSR1-ATF1* gene fusion in HCCC has been described [70]. Rearrangements of *EWSR1* not only have been found in about 85% of HCCC [17, 18, 70] but also in a high percentage of clear-cell odontogenic carcinomas (CCOC), suggesting a biologic link between these two malignancies [71]. In contrast, the fusion has not been detected in any of the morphological mimics: epithelial-myoepithelial carcinoma, myoepithelial carcinoma, or MEC, demonstrating its usefulness as a diagnostic biomarker for HCCC [70]. The translocation appears to be very specific to HCCC. Interestingly, high-grade transformation of HCCC with *EWSR1* rearrangement has been reported recently [72].

2.6 Carcinoma Ex Pleomorphic Adenoma

Carcinoma ex pleomorphic adenoma (CXPA) is defined as a carcinoma arising from a primary or recurrent benign pleomorphic adenoma (PA). It amounts to approximately 10–15% of all SGCs. The malignant component is frequently an adenocarcinoma, NOS, or SDC or may be any other histological subtype of SGC, such as MEC or AdCC (Fig. 2.3) [1]. CXPA is often a high-grade malignancy and especially when associated with deep (extracapsular) invasion has to be regarded as neoplasia with high risk of progression. High-grade adenocarcinoma, NOS, and

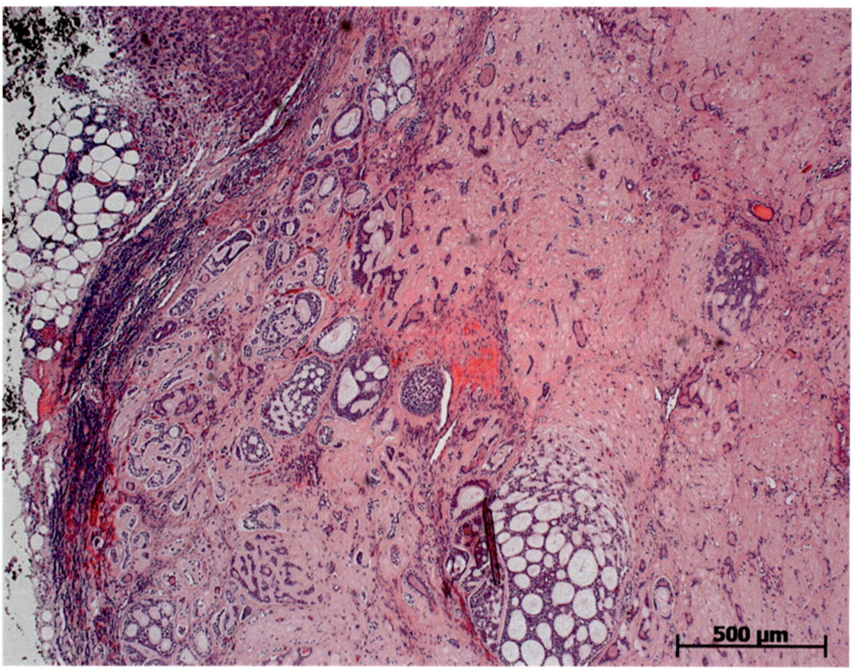

Fig. 2.3 H and E staining of CXPA. Tumor is partly encapsulated and shows residues of PA (right) with abortive ductal formation and dissociated myoepithelial cells in a sclerosing background. At the bottom of the figure and in the lower left part, several typical (pseudo-) cribriform manifestations of an AdCC. In addition, the upper left part shows invasion into the surrounding fatty tissues, the tumor component later classified as SDC (positive for AR and p53, data not shown)

SDC are the most common histologic subtypes, counting for approximately 80% of the carcinomatous components [1, 20]. However, some cases of CXPA are low-grade tumors, following a more indolent course [20]. The understanding of molecular mechanism causal for the transformation process of a benign PA into a CXPA is still very limited. Because of the tremendous diversity in histologic appearance, recent molecular studies have attempted to identify the genetic abnormalities that define this tumor. CXPA can express PA-specific gene fusions involving the transcription factor genes *PLAG1* (e.g., *CTNNB1-PLAG1*) and *HMGA2* (e.g., *HMGA2-WIF1*) [51, 73–76]. Subsets of CXPA also show amplification of *MDM2* and *HMGA2* in 12q13–15, mutations of *TP53* and/or amplification of *ERBB2* (HER2) as markers of malignant transformation [23, 73, 75, 77]. Most CXPA with *ERBB2* amplification are SDCs developing within PAs; these patients may benefit from treatment with trastuzumab [21].

2.7 Salivary Duct Carcinoma and Low-Grade Intraductal Carcinoma

Salivary duct carcinoma (a.k.a. high-grade ductal carcinoma or SDC) is one of the most aggressive malignancies of the salivary gland representing about 10% of all SGCs. Local recurrences as well as regional lymph node involvement and distant metastases are common. It can occur de novo or as the malignant component of CXPA and shows many genetic and histologic similarities to invasive ductal carcinoma of the breast [1, 78, 79]. Recent molecular analyses, including whole-exome sequencing, have revealed a wide mutational diversity and a high mutational burden (1.7 mutations/megabase) for SDC [80]. Frequently detected genetic alterations were mutations in *TP53* (55%), *HRAS* (23%), and *PIK3CA* (23%) and amplification of *ERBB2* (35%). The majority (74%) of tumors had alterations in either MAP-kinase genes (*BRAF/HRAS/NF1*) or *ERBB2* [80]. These results are in line with previous studies, which reported that the most common alterations in SDC are mutations in *TP53* (>50%), *PIK3CA* (~30%), *HRAS* (~30%), *BRAF* (7%), and *EGFR* gain (~80%), and loss, or mutation of *PTEN* (~40%) [81]. Additionally, more than 70% of SDCs have copy number gain and/or overexpression of the androgen receptor (*AR*) [79, 80, 82, 83]. Knockdown of AR expression in SDC cells in vitro markedly inhibits growth, suggesting that SDC patients with AR-positive tumors may benefit from androgen deprivation therapy [83]. Dalin and coworkers have emphasized the fact that the majority (61%) of SDCs have genetic alterations for which published clinical evidence supporting specific targeted therapies exists [80]. Taken together, the molecular data of SDC suggest that for this disease tumor sequencing on a routine basis is likely to be of clinical value.

There is also a very uncommon low-grade variant of SDC, with a favorable prognosis after complete excision. After a long discussion, the term low-grade SDC for these entities was replaced by low-grade intraductal carcinoma (a.k.a. low-grade cribriform cystadenocarcinoma, ductal carcinoma in situ, low-grade salivary duct carcinoma, or IDC), to clarify that these tumors are biologically different from ordinary SDC [1, 84, 85]. These lesions are indolent but can be graded as low-, intermediate-, or high-grade tumors depending on the degree of the cytologic abnormalities present. Reported tumors have been described as typically small, unencapsulated, and cystic [85, 86]. In contrast to SDC, no amplification of *ERBB2* was found in low-grade IDCs [87]. Interestingly, approximately 13% of IDCs show focal transformations into a high-grade morphology [85, 86, 88]. However, the clinical impact of this transition is not clear, since the number of high-grade IDCs is very small and the median follow-up is only 27 months [84]. Nevertheless, there is indication that high-grade IDC have good prognosis [88].

2.8 Acinic Cell Carcinoma

Acinic cell carcinoma (ACC) is a low-grade, slow-growing tumor [1]. Histopathologically, variable architectural patterns have been described: solid, microcystic, papillary-cystic, and follicular [89]. Classifying ACC according to these subtypes can be challenging, as different patterns may occur in a single lesion [90]. Since the emergence of MASCs as a distinct tumor entity, the defining characteristics of ACC have come under question. New evidence suggests that it may be a far more aggressive tumor than originally reported [91]. As mentioned above, tumors previously classified as ACC were often retrospectively identified as MASC.

The knowledge of the associated molecular background is still very limited. Only in a minority of ACC, an abnormal karyotypic profile has been found, and the only common change observed was trisomy 8 in three cases [92]. No gene fusions or recurrent mutations have been identified so far. Studies on growth factor receptors using tissue microarrays with 168 ACCs have shown epidermal growth factor receptor (EGFR, HER1) immunoreactivity in 30 ACC (18%) [93] and overexpression of epidermal growth factor receptor 2 (ERBB2, HER2) in 1 single case out of 170 ACC (0.6%) [94]. However, in situ hybridization suggests overexpression of *ERBB2* on mRNA level in ACC [24]. Recently, it was shown that mice with constitutive activation of the Wnt and mTOR signaling pathways develop tumors that have remarkable morphologic similarity to human ACCs [25]. Treatment of tumor-bearing mice with the mTOR inhibitor rapamycin resulted in complete regression of the tumors. Immunohistochemical analysis of human ACC samples showed that mTOR signaling is also activated in human ACCs, indicating that mTOR inhibitors such as rapamycin or temsirolimus might be useful for treatment of patients with ACC [25, 95].

2.9 Polymorphous Adenocarcinoma and Cribriform Adenocarcinoma

Polymorphous adenocarcinoma (a.k.a. polymorphous low-grade adenocarcinoma, PLGA, or PAC) is a usually indolent low-grade salivary gland malignancy characterized by uniform cytology and histologic diversity [1]. Histopathologically, PAC is a challenging diagnosis. The two main differential diagnoses are AdCC and PA. The tumor occurs mainly at intraoral sites and sporadically in the major glands [1].

Cribriform adenocarcinoma of minor salivary glands (CAMSG) is a low-grade carcinoma, mainly found in the tongue and oropharynx, that shares morphologic, clinical, and molecular features with PAC [1, 22].

A variety of molecular and genetic findings have been reported in PAC lately. The majority of PACs (~75%) harbor somatic rearrangements of *PRKD1*, *PRKD2*, and *PRKD3* or somatic mutations of *PRKD1* encoding p.Glu710Asp, distinguishing them from other salivary malignancies [96, 97]. Thus, *PRKD1* mutations could be tested as a biomarker to distinguish PAC from its mimics. Interestingly, CAMSG has also alterations of *PRKD* family genes. *PRKD1* and *PRKD3* rearrangements were found in ~80% of CAMSG. In some cases recurrent *ARID1A-PRKD1* and *DDX3X-PRKD1* gene fusions were detected [97, 98]. These findings indicate a shared molecular pathogenesis for PAC and CAMSG. These facts raise the question whether PAC and CAMSG represent separate entities or variants of one spectrum [1, 97].

2.10 Conclusions

The discovery of specific and recurring translocations, point mutations, and amplifications in some types of SGC has given pathologists new and highly specific diagnostic tools and in some cases prognostic and possibly treatment-relevant markers. While diagnosis, i.e., confirmation of tumor-type and its related prognostic impact, may be supported in all tumors listed above, the detection of the MEC-related fusion gene and other molecular markers may provide segregation of tumors with low and high risk of progression. Also, the detection of fusion gene characteristic for certain SGC (particularly AdCC) may facilitate a tailored therapeutic approach in a multimodal setting, analogous to what is aimed for in the EORTC study 1206 for patients with SDC (see Chap. 13).

References

1. El-Naggar AK, Chan JKC, Grandis JR, Takata T, Slootweg PJ, editors. Pathology and genetics of head and neck tumours. World Health Organization Classification of Tumours. 4th ed. Lyon: IARC Press; 2017.
2. Nordkvist A, Gustafsson H, Juberg-Ode M, Stenman G. Recurrent rearrangements of 11q14-22 in mucoepidermoid carcinoma. Cancer Genet Cytogenet. 1994;74(2):77–83.
3. Komiya T, Park Y, Modi S, Coxon AB, Oh H, Kaye FJ. Sustained expression of Mect1-Maml2 is essential for tumor cell growth in salivary gland cancers carrying the t(11;19) translocation. Oncogene. 2006;25(45):6128–32.
4. Behboudi A, Enlund F, Winnes M, Andren Y, Nordkvist A, Leivo I, et al. Molecular classification of mucoepidermoid carcinomas-prognostic significance of the MECT1-MAML2 fusion oncogene. Genes Chromosomes Cancer. 2006;45(5):470–81.
5. Tonon G, Modi S, Wu L, Kubo A, Coxon AB, Komiya T, et al. t(11;19)(q21;p13) translocation in mucoepidermoid carcinoma creates a novel fusion product that disrupts a Notch signaling pathway. Nat Genet. 2003;33(2):208–13.
6. Fehr A, Meyer A, Heidorn K, Röser K, Löning T, Bullerdiek J. A link between the expression of the stem cell marker HMGA2, grading, and the fusion CRTC1-MAML2 in mucoepidermoid carcinoma. Genes Chromosomes Cancer. 2009;48(9):777–85.

7. Verdorfer I, Fehr A, Bullerdiek J, Scholz N, Brunner A, Krugmann J, et al. Chromosomal imbalances, 11q21 rearrangement and MECT1-MAML2 fusion transcript in mucoepidermoid carcinomas of the salivary gland. Oncol Rep. 2009;22(2):305–11.
8. Möller E, Stenman G, Mandahl N, Hamberg H, Molne L, van den Oord JJ, et al. POU5F1, encoding a key regulator of stem cell pluripotency, is fused to EWSR1 in hidradenoma of the skin and mucoepidermoid carcinoma of the salivary glands. J Pathol. 2008;215(1): 78–86.
9. Di Renzo F, Doneda L, Menegola E, Sardella M, De Vecchi G, Collini P, et al. The murine Pou6f2 gene is temporally and spatially regulated during kidney embryogenesis and its human homolog is overexpressed in a subset of Wilms tumors. J Pediatr Hematol Oncol. 2006;28(12):791–7.
10. Nakano T, Yamamoto H, Hashimoto K, Tamiya S, Shiratsuchi H, Nakashima T, et al. HER2 and EGFR gene copy number alterations are predominant in high-grade salivary mucoepidermoid carcinoma irrespective of MAML2 fusion status. Histopathology. 2013;63(3):378–92.
11. Rao PH, Roberts D, Zhao Y-J, Bell D, Harris CP, Weber RS, et al. Deletion of 1p32-p36 is the most frequent genetic change and poor prognostic marker in adenoid cystic carcinoma of the salivary glands. Clin Cancer Res. 2008;14(16):5181–7.
12. Stephens PJ, Davies HR, Mitani Y, Van Loo P, Shlien A, Tarpey PS, et al. Whole exome sequencing of adenoid cystic carcinoma. J Clin Invest. 2013;123(7):2965–8.
13. Mitani Y, Liu B, Rao PH, Borra VJ, Zafereo M, Weber RS, et al. Novel MYBL1 gene rearrangements with recurrent MYBL1-NFIB fusions in salivary adenoid cystic carcinomas lacking t(6;9) translocations. Clin Cancer Res. 2015;22(3):725–33.
14. Stenman G, Persson F, Andersson MK. Diagnostic and therapeutic implications of new molecular biomarkers in salivary gland cancers. Oral Oncol. 2014;50(8):683–90.
15. Lannon CL, Sorensen PH. ETV6-NTRK3: a chimeric protein tyrosine kinase with transformation activity in multiple cell lineages. Semin Cancer Biol. 2005;15(3):215–23.
16. Ito Y, Ishibashi K, Masaki A, Fujii K, Fujiyoshi Y, Hattori H, et al. Mammary analogue secretory carcinoma of salivary glands: a clinicopathologic and molecular study including 2 cases harboring ETV6-X fusion. Am J Surg Pathol. 2015;39(5):602–10.
17. Weinreb I. Hyalinizing clear cell carcinoma of salivary gland: a review and update. Head Neck Pathol. 2013;7(Suppl 1):S20–9.
18. Shah AA, LeGallo RD, van Zante A, Frierson HF Jr, Mills SE, Berean KW, et al. EWSR1 genetic rearrangements in salivary gland tumors: a specific and very common feature of hyalinizing clear cell carcinoma. Am J Surg Pathol. 2013;37(4):571–8.
19. Dooley AL, Winslow MM, Chiang DY, Banerji S, Stransky N, Dayton TL, et al. Nuclear factor I/B is an oncogene in small cell lung cancer. Genes Dev. 2011;25(14):1470–5.
20. Lewis JE, Olsen KD, Sebo TJ. Carcinoma ex pleomorphic adenoma: pathologic analysis of 73 cases. Hum Pathol. 2001;32(6):596–604.
21. Sharon E, Kelly R, Szabo E. Sustained response of carcinoma ex pleomorphic adenoma treated with trastuzumab and capecitabine. Head Neck Oncol. 2010;2(1):12.
22. Skalova A, Sima R, Kaspirkova-Nemcova J, Simpson RH, Elmberger G, Leivo I, et al. Cribriform adenocarcinoma of minor salivary gland origin principally affecting the tongue: characterization of new entity. Am J Surg Pathol. 2011;35(8):1168–76.
23. Ihrler S, Weiler C, Hirschmann A, Sendelhofert A, Lang S, Guntinas-Lichius O, et al. Intraductal carcinoma is the precursor of carcinoma ex pleomorphic adenoma and is often associated with dysfunctional p53. Histopathology. 2007;51(3):362–71.
24. Jordan R, Dardick I, Lui E, Birek C. Demonstration of c-erbB-2 oncogene overexpression in salivary gland neoplasms by in situ hybridization. J Oral Pathol Med. 1994;23(5):226–31.
25. Diegel CR, Cho KR, El-Naggar AK, Williams BO, Lindvall C. Mammalian target of rapamycin-dependent acinar cell neoplasia after inactivation of Apc and Pten in the mouse salivary gland: implications for human acinic cell carcinoma. Cancer Res. 2010;70(22):9143–52.
26. Chan RC, Chan JY. Head and neck mucoepidermoid carcinoma: a curious association with second primary malignancy. Otolaryngol Head Neck Surg. 2014;151(5):797–801.

27. Wolfish EB, Nelson BL, Thompson LD. Sinonasal tract mucoepidermoid carcinoma: a clinicopathologic and immunophenotypic study of 19 cases combined with a comprehensive review of the literature. Head Neck Pathol. 2012;6(2):191–207.
28. Fonseca FP, de Andrade BA, Lopes MA, Pontes HA, Vargas PA, de Almeida OP. P63 expression in papillary cystadenoma and mucoepidermoid carcinoma of minor salivary glands. Oral Surg Oral Med Oral Pathol Oral Radiol. 2013;115(1):79–86.
29. Lennerz JK, Perry A, Mills JC, Huettner PC, Pfeifer JD. Mucoepidermoid carcinoma of the cervix: another tumor with the t(11;19)-associated CRTC1-MAML2 gene fusion. Am J Surg Pathol. 2009;33(6):835–43.
30. Pires FR, de Almeida OP, de Araujo VC, Kowalski LP. Prognostic factors in head and neck mucoepidermoid carcinoma. Arch Otolaryngol Head Neck Surg. 2004;130(2):174–80.
31. Fehr A, Röser K, Heidorn K, Hallas C, Löning T, Bullerdiek J. A new type of MAML2 fusion in mucoepidermoid carcinoma. Genes Chromosomes Cancer. 2008;47(3):203–6.
32. Enlund F, Behboudi A, Andren Y, Oberg C, Lendahl U, Mark J, et al. Altered Notch signaling resulting from expression of a WAMTP1-MAML2 gene fusion in mucoepidermoid carcinomas and benign Warthin's tumors. Exp Cell Res. 2004;292(1):21–8.
33. Coxon A, Rozenblum E, Park YS, Joshi N, Tsurutani J, Dennis PA, et al. Mect1-Maml2 fusion oncogene linked to the aberrant activation of cyclic AMP/CREB regulated genes. Cancer Res. 2005;65(16):7137–44.
34. Wu L, Liu J, Gao P, Nakamura M, Cao Y, Shen H, et al. Transforming activity of MECT1-MAML2 fusion oncoprotein is mediated by constitutive CREB activation. EMBO J. 2005;24(13):2391–402.
35. Seethala RR, Dacic S, Cieply K, Kelly LM, Nikiforova MN. A reappraisal of the MECT1/MAML2 translocation in salivary mucoepidermoid carcinomas. Am J Surg Pathol. 2010;34(8):1106–21.
36. Jee KJ, Persson M, Heikinheimo K, Passador-Santos F, Aro K, Knuutila S, et al. Genomic profiles and CRTC1-MAML2 fusion distinguish different subtypes of mucoepidermoid carcinoma. Mod Pathol. 2013;26(2):213–22.
37. Nakayama T, Miyabe S, Okabe M, Sakuma H, Ijichi K, Hasegawa Y, et al. Clinicopathological significance of the CRTC3-MAML2 fusion transcript in mucoepidermoid carcinoma. Mod Pathol. 2009;22(12):1575–81.
38. Seethala RR, Chiosea SI. MAML2 status in mucoepidermoid carcinoma can no longer be considered a prognostic marker. Am J Surg Pathol. 2016;40(8):1151–3.
39. Behboudi A, Winnes M, Gorunova L, van den Oord JJ, Mertens F, Enlund F, et al. Clear cell hidradenoma of the skin-a third tumor type with a t(11;19)-associated TORC1-MAML2 gene fusion. Genes Chromosomes Cancer. 2005;43(2):202–5.
40. Tirado Y, Williams MD, Hanna EY, Kaye FJ, Batsakis JG, El-Naggar AK. CRTC1/MAML2 fusion transcript in high grade mucoepidermoid carcinomas of salivary and thyroid glands and Warthin's tumors: implications for histogenesis and biologic behavior. Genes Chromosomes Cancer. 2007;46(7):708–15.
41. Fehr A, Röser K, Belge G, Löning T, Bullerdiek J. A closer look at Warthin tumors and the t(11;19). Cancer Genet Cytogenet. 2008;180(2):135–9.
42. Anzick SL, Chen WD, Park Y, Meltzer P, Bell D, El-Naggar AK, et al. Unfavorable prognosis of CRTC1-MAML2 positive mucoepidermoid tumors with CDKN2A deletions. Genes Chromosomes Cancer. 2009;49(1):59–69.
43. Kang H, Tan M, Bishop JA, Jones S, Sausen M, Ha PK, Agrawal N, et al. Whole-exome sequencing of salivary gland mucoepidermoid carcinoma. Clin Cancer Res. 2017;23(1):283–8.
44. Besch R, Berking C. POU transcription factors in melanocytes and melanoma. Eur J Cell Biol. 2014;93(1–2):55–60.
45. Perotti D, De Vecchi G, Testi MA, Lualdi E, Modena P, Mondini P, et al. Germline mutations of the POU6F2 gene in Wilms tumors with loss of heterozygosity on chromosome 7p14. Hum Mutat. 2004;24(5):400–7.
46. Yoo J, Robinson RA. H-ras gene mutations in salivary gland mucoepidermoid carcinomas. Cancer. 2000;88(3):518–23.

47. Laurie SA, Ho AL, Fury MG, Sherman E, Pfister DG. Systemic therapy in the management of metastatic or locally recurrent adenoid cystic carcinoma of the salivary glands: a systematic review. Lancet Oncol. 2011;12(8):815–24.
48. Persson M, Andren Y, Moskaluk CA, Frierson HF Jr, Cooke SL, Futreal PA, et al. Clinically significant copy number alterations and complex rearrangements of MYB and NFIB in head and neck adenoid cystic carcinoma. Genes Chromosomes Cancer. 2012;51(8):805–17.
49. Persson M, Andren Y, Mark J, Horlings HM, Persson F, Stenman G. Recurrent fusion of MYB and NFIB transcription factor genes in carcinomas of the breast and head and neck. Proc Natl Acad Sci U S A. 2009;106(44):18740–4.
50. Ramsay RG, Gonda TJ. MYB function in normal and cancer cells. Nat Rev Cancer. 2008;8(7):523–34.
51. von Holstein SL, Fehr A, Persson M, Nickelsen M, Therkildsen MH, Prause JU, et al. Lacrimal gland pleomorphic adenoma and carcinoma ex pleomorphic adenoma: genomic profiles, gene fusions, and clinical characteristics. Ophthalmology. 2014;121(5):1125–33.
52. Drier Y, Cotton MJ, Williamson KE, Gillespie SM, Ryan RJ, Kluk MJ, et al. An oncogenic MYB feedback loop drives alternate cell fates in adenoid cystic carcinoma. Nat Genet. 2016;48(3):265–72.
53. Ho AS, Kannan K, Roy DM, Morris LG, Ganly I, Katabi N, et al. The mutational landscape of adenoid cystic carcinoma. Nat Genet. 2013;45(7):791–8.
54. Brayer KJ, Frerich CA, Kang H, Ness SA. Recurrent fusions in MYB and MYBL1 define a common, transcription factor-driven oncogenic pathway in salivary gland adenoid cystic carcinoma. Cancer Discov. 2016;6(2):176–87.
55. Brill LB 2nd, Kanner WA, Fehr A, Andrén Y, Moskaluk CA, Löning T, et al. Analysis of MYB expression and MYB-NFIB gene fusions in adenoid cystic carcinoma and other salivary neoplasms. Mod Pathol. 2011;24(9):1169–76.
56. Skálová A, Vanecek T, Sima R, Laco J, Weinreb I, Perez-Ordonez B, et al. Mammary analogue secretory carcinoma of salivary glands, containing the ETV6-NTRK3 fusion gene: a hitherto undescribed salivary gland tumor entity. Am J Surg Pathol. 2010;34(5):599–608.
57. Fehr A, Löning T, Stenman G. Mammary analogue secretory carcinoma of the salivary glands with ETV6-NTRK3 gene fusion. Am J Surg Pathol. 2011;35(10):1600–2.
58. Tognon C, Knezevich SR, Huntsman D, Roskelley CD, Melnyk N, Mathers JA, et al. Expression of the ETV6-NTRK3 gene fusion as a primary event in human secretory breast carcinoma. Cancer Cell. 2002;2(5):367–76.
59. Skalova A, Vanecek T, Majewska H, Laco J, Grossmann P, Simpson RH, et al. Mammary analogue secretory carcinoma of salivary glands with high-grade transformation: report of 3 cases with the ETV6-NTRK3 gene fusion and analysis of TP53, beta-catenin, EGFR, and CCND1 genes. Am J Surg Pathol. 2014;38(1):23–33.
60. Skalova A, Vanecek T, Simpson RH, Laco J, Majewska H, Baneckova M, et al. Mammary analogue secretory carcinoma of salivary glands: molecular analysis of 25 ETV6 gene rearranged tumors with lack of detection of classical ETV6-NTRK3 fusion transcript by standard RT-PCR: report of 4 cases harboring ETV6-X gene fusion. Am J Surg Pathol. 2016;40(1):3–13.
61. Rubin BP, Chen CJ, Morgan TW, Xiao S, Grier HE, Kozakewich HP, et al. Congenital mesoblastic nephroma t(12;15) is associated with ETV6-NTRK3 gene fusion: cytogenetic and molecular relationship to congenital (infantile) fibrosarcoma. Am J Pathol. 1998;153(5):1451–8.
62. Knezevich SR, McFadden DE, Tao W, Lim JF, Sorensen PH. A novel ETV6-NTRK3 gene fusion in congenital fibrosarcoma. Nat Genet. 1998;18(2):184–7.
63. Kralik JM, Kranewitter W, Boesmueller H, Marschon R, Tschurtschenthaler G, Rumpold H, et al. Characterization of a newly identified ETV6-NTRK3 fusion transcript in acute myeloid leukemia. Diagn Pathol. 2011;6:19.
64. Griffith C, Seethala R, Chiosea SI. Mammary analogue secretory carcinoma: a new twist to the diagnostic dilemma of zymogen granule poor acinic cell carcinoma. Virchows Arch. 2011;459(1):117–8.
65. Connor A, Perez-Ordonez B, Shago M, Skalova A, Weinreb I. Mammary analog secretory carcinoma of salivary gland origin with the ETV6 gene rearrangement by FISH: expanded

morphologic and immunohistochemical spectrum of a recently described entity. Am J Surg Pathol. 2012;36(1):27–34.
66. Chiosea SI, Griffith C, Assaad A, Seethala RR. Clinicopathological characterization of mammary analogue secretory carcinoma of salivary glands. Histopathology. 2012;61(3):387–94.
67. Pinto A, Nose V, Rojas C, Fan YS, Gomez-Fernandez C. Searching for mammary analogue secretory carcinoma of salivary gland among its mimics. Mod Pathol. 2014;27(1):30–7.
68. Bishop JA, Yonescu R, Batista D, Eisele DW, Westra WH. Most nonparotid "acinic cell carcinomas" represent mammary analog secretory carcinomas. Am J Surg Pathol. 2013;37(7):1053–7.
69. Solar AA, Schmidt BL, Jordan RC. Hyalinizing clear cell carcinoma: case series and comprehensive review of the literature. Cancer. 2009;115(1):75–83.
70. Antonescu CR, Katabi N, Zhang L, Sung YS, Seethala RR, Jordan RC, et al. EWSR1-ATF1 fusion is a novel and consistent finding in hyalinizing clear-cell carcinoma of salivary gland. Genes Chromosomes Cancer. 2011;50(7):559–7.
71. Bilodeau EA, Weinreb I, Antonescu CR, Zhang L, Dacic S, Muller S, et al. Clear cell odontogenic carcinomas show EWSR1 rearrangements: a novel finding and a biological link to salivary clear cell carcinomas. Am J Surg Pathol. 2013;37(7):1001–5.
72. Jin R, Craddock KJ, Irish JC, Perez-Ordonez B, Weinreb I. Recurrent hyalinizing clear cell carcinoma of the base of tongue with high-grade transformation and EWSR1 gene rearrangement by FISH. Head Neck Pathol. 2012;6(3):389–94.
73. Persson F, Andrén Y, Winnes M, Wedell B, Nordkvist A, Gudnadottir G, et al. High-resolution genomic profiling of adenomas and carcinomas of the salivary glands reveals amplification, rearrangement, and fusion of HMGA2. Genes Chromosomes Cancer. 2009;48(1):69–82.
74. Queimado L, Lopes CS, Reis AM. WIF1, an inhibitor of the Wnt pathway, is rearranged in salivary gland tumors. Genes Chromosomes Cancer. 2007;46(3):215–25.
75. Roijer E, Nordkvist A, Strom AK, Ryd W, Behrendt M, Bullerdiek J, et al. Translocation, deletion/amplification, and expression of HMGIC and MDM2 in a carcinoma ex pleomorphic adenoma. Am J Pathol. 2002;160(2):433–40.
76. Stenman G. Fusion oncogenes in salivary gland tumors: molecular and clinical consequences. Head Neck Pathol. 2013;7(Suppl 1):S12–9.
77. Nordkvist A, Roijer E, Bang G, Gustafsson H, Behrendt M, Ryd W, et al. Expression and mutation patterns of p53 in benign and malignant salivary gland tumors. Int J Oncol. 2000;16(3):477–83.
78. Jaehne M, Roeser K, Jaekel T, Schepers JD, Albert N, Loning T. Clinical and immunohistologic typing of salivary duct carcinoma: a report of 50 cases. Cancer. 2005;103(12):2526–33.
79. Jaspers HC, Verbist BM, Schoffelen R, Mattijssen V, Slootweg PJ, van der Graaf WT, et al. Androgen receptor-positive salivary duct carcinoma: a disease entity with promising new treatment options. J Clin Oncol. 2011;29(16):e473–6.
80. Dalin MG, Desrichard A, Katabi N, Makarov V, Walsh LA, Lee KW, et al. Comprehensive molecular characterization of salivary duct carcinoma reveals actionable targets and similarity to apocrine breast cancer. Clin Cancer Res. 2016;22(18):4623–33.
81. Andersson MK, Stenman G. The landscape of gene fusions and somatic mutations in salivary gland neoplasms - implications for diagnosis and therapy. Oral Oncol. 2016;57:63–9.
82. Simpson RH. Salivary duct carcinoma: new developments--morphological variants including pure in situ high grade lesions; proposed molecular classification. Head Neck Pathol. 2013;7(Suppl 1):S48–58.
83. Mitani Y, Rao PH, Maity SN, Lee YC, Ferrarotto R, Post JC, et al. Alterations associated with androgen receptor gene activation in salivary duct carcinoma of both sexes: potential therapeutic ramifications. Clin Cancer Res. 2014;20(24):6570–81.
84. Kuo YJ, Weinreb I, Perez-Ordonez B. Low-grade salivary duct carcinoma or low-grade intraductal carcinoma? Review of the literature. Head Neck Pathol. 2013;7(Suppl 1):S59–67.
85. Delgado R, Klimstra D, Albores-Saavedra J. Low grade salivary duct carcinoma. A distinctive variant with a low grade histology and a predominant intraductal growth pattern. Cancer. 1996;78(5):958–67.

86. Brandwein-Gensler M, Hille J, Wang BY, Urken M, Gordon R, Wang LJ, et al. Low-grade salivary duct carcinoma: description of 16 cases. Am J Surg Pathol. 2004;28(8):1040–4.
87. Stevens TM, Kovalovsky AO, Velosa C, Shi Q, Dai Q, Owen RP, et al. Mammary analog secretory carcinoma, low-grade salivary duct carcinoma, and mimickers: a comparative study. Mod Pathol. 2015;28(8):1084–100.
88. Weinreb I, Tabanda-Lichauco R, Van der Kwast T, Perez-Ordonez B. Low-grade intraductal carcinoma of salivary gland: report of 3 cases with marked apocrine differentiation. Am J Surg Pathol. 2006;30(8):1014–21.
89. Abrams AM, Cornyn J, Scofield HH, Hansen LS. Acinic cell adenocarcinoma of the major salivary glands. A clinicopathologic study of 77 cases. Cancer. 1965;18:1145–62.
90. Ellis GL, Auclair PL. Tumors of the salivary glands, AFIP atlas of tumor pathology. 4th ed. Washington, D.C.: American Registry of Pathology; 2008.
91. Chiosea SI, Griffith C, Assaad A, Seethala RR. The profile of acinic cell carcinoma after recognition of mammary analog secretory carcinoma. Am J Surg Pathol. 2012;36(3):343–50.
92. Mitelmann F, Johansson B, Mertens F, editors. Mitelman database of chromosome aberrations and gene fusions in cancer; 2016. Available from: http://cgap.nci.nih.gov/Chromosomes/Mitelman.
93. Clauditz TS, Gontarewicz A, Lebok P, Tsourlakis MC, Grob TJ, Munscher A, et al. Epidermal growth factor receptor (EGFR) in salivary gland carcinomas: potentials as therapeutic target. Oral Oncol. 2012;48(10):991–6.
94. Clauditz TS, Reiff M, Gravert L, Gnoss A, Tsourlakis MC, Munscher A, et al. Human epidermal growth factor receptor 2 (HER2) in salivary gland carcinomas. Pathology. 2011;43(5):459–64.
95. Ettl T, Schwarz-Furlan S, Haubner F, Muller S, Zenk J, Gosau M, et al. The PI3K/AKT/mTOR signalling pathway is active in salivary gland cancer and implies different functions and prognoses depending on cell localisation. Oral Oncol. 2012;48(9):822–30.
96. Weinreb I, Piscuoglio S, Martelotto LG, Waggott D, Ng CK, Perez-Ordonez B, et al. Hotspot activating PRKD1 somatic mutations in polymorphous low-grade adenocarcinomas of the salivary glands. Nat Genet. 2014;46(11):1166–9.
97. Weinreb I, Zhang L, Tirunagari LM, Sung YS, Chen CL, Perez-Ordonez B, et al. Novel PRKD gene rearrangements and variant fusions in cribriform adenocarcinoma of salivary gland origin. Genes Chromosomes Cancer. 2014;53(10):845–56.
98. Majewska H, Skalova A, Weinreb I, Stodulski D, Hyrcza M, Stankiewicz C, et al. Giant cribriform adenocarcinoma of the tongue showing PRKD3 rearrangement. Pol J Pathol. 2016;67(1):84–90.

3 The Role of Imaging in Staging and Follow-Up of Salivary Gland Tumors

Silvana Sdao, Enrico Civelli, Alessandra Alessi, and Giuseppina Calareso

Abbreviations

ACC	Adenoid cystic carcinoma
ADC	Apparent diffusion coefficient
CNB	Core needle biopsy
CT	Computed tomography
DCE-MRI	Dynamic contrast-enhanced Magnetic Resonance Imaging
DWI	Diffusion-weighted imaging
FDG PET-CT	Positron emission tomography-computed tomography with fluorine-18-deoxy-D-glucose
FNAC	Fine needle aspiration cytology
FS	Fat saturation
GE	Gradient echo
MET	11C-methionine
MRI	Magnetic resonance imaging
NOS	Not otherwise specified
SGTs	Salivary gland tumor
SUV	Standardized uptake value
T1W	T1-weighted
T2W	T2-weighted
T-peak	Time-to-peak enhancement
US	Ultrasound
WR	Washout ratio

S. Sdao (✉) · E. Civelli · G. Calareso
Department of Radiology, Fondazione IRCCS Istituto Nazionale dei Tumori, Milan, Italy
e-mail: silvana.sdao@istitutotumori.mi.it; Enrico.Civelli@istitutotumori.mi.it; giuseppina.calareso@istitutotumori.mi.it

A. Alessi
Nuclear Medicine Department, Fondazione IRCCS Istituto Nazionale dei Tumori, Milan, Italy
e-mail: Alessandra.Alessi@istitutotumori.mi.it

© Springer Nature Switzerland AG 2019
L. Licitra, L. D. Locati (eds.), *Salivary Gland Cancer*,
https://doi.org/10.1007/978-3-030-02958-6_3

3.1 Introduction

The role of imaging in salivary gland tumors (SGTs) is primarily to detect the lesion, possibly classifying it as benign or malignant. Imaging helps to stage malignant tumor according to the TNM classification, in order to plan therapy (including surgical, radiation, and oncological treatment) [1, 2].

Imaging provides information about tumor location (regarding anatomical relationship with nervous and vascular structures), local extension, perineural spread, nodal and distant metastases.

For superficial tumors, especially within the parotid and the submandibular glands, ultrasound (US) is the modality of choice for initial workup and may be combined with fine needle aspiration cytology (FNAC) or core needle biopsy (CNB) to obtain tissue diagnosis [2]. If US does not allow for the evaluation of the whole lesion (because of deep location) or there are signs that suggests extra-glandular extension, advanced techniques such as magnetic resonance imaging (MRI) or computed tomography (CT) should be carried out [1, 2]. For SGTs arising from the upper aerodigestive tract, endoscopy and CT examination are essentials for diagnosis [3, 4].

3.2 Ultrasound

Ultrasound (US) is the first step in the diagnostic algorithm of patients presenting with a palpable salivary gland mass. It can be used to distinguish solid from cystic lesion, perform nodal staging and, in addition to Doppler technique, assess vascular structures and tumor vascularity [5]. US is also an optimal guide to perform invasive diagnostic procedure such as FNAC or CNB.

The examination is usually carried out with high-frequency transducers, such as 5–12-MHz wideband linear transducers [6]. All the parenchyma and all the lesion should be scanned in at least two orthogonal planes. The whole neck should also be evaluated to assess the lymph node status [6].

The normal echogenicity of salivary glands is usually homogeneous and varies from bright and strongly hyperechoic to lightly hyperechoic in comparison to adjacent muscles, depending on the amount of fat within the gland.

Regarding the parotid gland, facial nerves and its branches conventionally represent anatomical markers to distinguish superficial from deep portion; since these nerves' structures are not well visible at US examination, the retromandibular vein (which generally lies above the nerve) is used as landmark. Of note, deeper areas of glandular parenchyma may be hidden in the acoustic shadow behind the mandibular ramus. Lymph nodes may be normally found in glandular parenchyma, usually in the upper and lower poles [7]. The normal appearance of intraglandular nodes is that of oval-shaped, slightly hypoechoic structures with hyperechoic hilum and short axis up to 5–6 mm [7].

3.2.1 Benign Neoplasm

The most common benign neoplasm of salivary gland is pleomorphic adenoma, which typically presents at US as a hypoechoic, well-circumscribed and lobulated lesion with posterior acoustic enhancement, sometimes with calcifications (Fig. 3.1) [6, 8]. The use of power Doppler usually shows poor or absent vascularization within the lesion.

The second most common benign neoplasm is Warthin's tumor. The US appearance of this tumor is that of a hypoechoic, oval-shaped lesion with well-defined margins, commonly containing multiple, small and spongelike anechoic areas (Fig. 3.2) [6, 8]. This appearance may vary according to the size. In fact, tumors larger than 4–5 cm tend to show high cystic content compared to smaller lesions, with some cases presenting totally cystic content. Despite the difference being sometimes subtle, Warthin's tumor is usually hyper-vascularized at power Doppler compared to pleomorphic adenoma [9].

It has been reported that lobulated shape is frequently encountered in pleomorphic adenomas, while cystic areas may be commonly found in Warthin's tumor; nevertheless, these features are not pathognomonic of these neoplasms, as they can be found in many other lesions. For example, cystic areas may be frequently found also in malignant tumors, such as mucoepidermoid or acinic cell carcinoma, as well as in abscessed or necrotic metastatic node [10]. As a consequence, attention should be paid to these features as certain degree of overlap may exist.

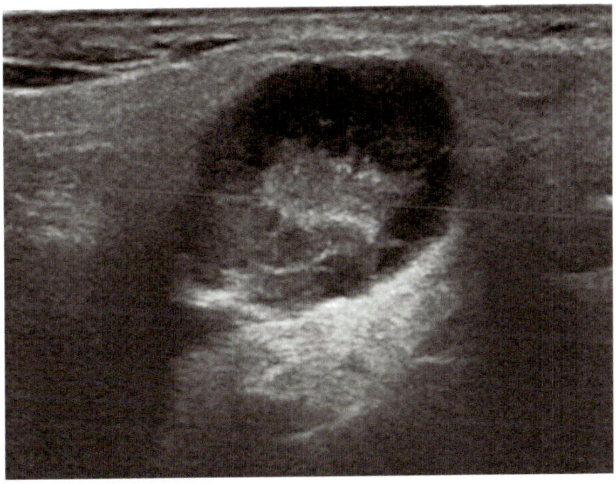

Fig. 3.1 US imaging of pleomorphic adenoma of the parotid gland. The lesion is inhomogeneous, predominantly hypoechoic with well-defined borders and posterior acoustic enhancement

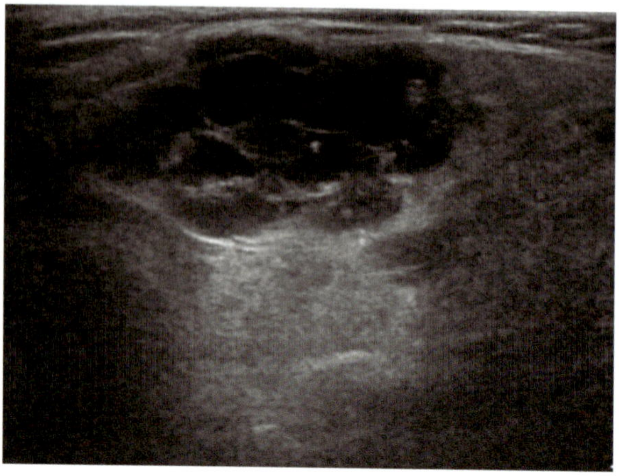

Fig. 3.2 US imaging of Warthin's tumor of the parotid gland. The lesion is hypoechoic with multiple, spongelike anechoic areas. The lesion shows lobulated margins and posterior acoustic enhancement (similar to pleomorphic adenoma)

3.2.2 Malignant Neoplasms

Imaging features of malignant tumor mostly depend on the degree of malignancy. *Well-differentiated* malignant SGTs generally present with US features that are similar to that of benign tumors. *Poorly differentiated* malignant SGTs presents in many cases with irregular shape, ill-defined margins and hypoechoic, inhomogeneous, structure [6]. The internal echo-structure of malignant tumors at US may be different: predominantly solid, cystic, mainly cystic with a mural solid nodule. As vascularization is not pathognomonic, Doppler techniques are not usually helpful in differentiating between benign and malignant SGTs [6, 11]. Perilesional adenopathies are additional findings that may suggest malignancy.

Metastases from other tumors to salivary glands are very rare. The most common primary tumors metastasizing to salivary glands are head and neck neoplasm, melanoma, squamous carcinoma of the skin, breast and lung cancer [12]. At US they usually are well-defined, hypoechoic, oval-shaped lesions [6].

The sensitivity of US is reported to range from 62% to 84%, the specificity from 88% to 96% while the accuracy from 57% to 96% [1, 13]. US-guided FNAC may provide further information regarding the nature of a lesion [14]; however, considering that negative predictive value of FNAC is reported to be low (66%), attention should be paid to negative results [1]. In case of US-guided FNAC failure, a reliable diagnosis can be obtained by US-guided CNB which reach a sensitivity of 93% and an accuracy of 98% [15]. Complications, such as hematomas or temporary facial weakness, are uncommon; rare cases of tumor seeding following both FNAC and CNB are reported in literature [1, 15, 16].

The use of US is limited to superficial structures and the accuracy depends on specialist expertise [2]. Furthermore, minor salivary gland lesions, deep tissue/bone involvement and perineural spread are not evaluable with conventional US technique.

3.3 Magnetic Resonance Imaging

Magnetic resonance imaging (MRI) is the modality of choice for staging SGTs due to its optimal soft tissue contrast [1]. High-resolution turbo-spin-echo T1-weighted (T1W) and T2-weighted (T2W) sequences, in addition to post-contrast images with fat saturation (FS), are the essentials for the assessment of salivary gland neoplasms [1, 17].

Post-contrast 3D gradient echo (GE) sequences have been recently introduced and are usually combined with FS techniques. These sequences allow for multiplanar reconstructions thus offering anatomic details of great importance. Multiplanar images are reconstructed from isotropic, axial, acquisitions with slice thickness up to 0.8 mm.

In adult population most of the tumors arising from the parotid gland can be efficiently visualized on non-contrast T1W images, because of their relatively low signal compared to the hyperintense background of the gland, which is due to physiological fatty involution [17]. For this reason, T1W sequences provide excellent information regarding tumor margins, tumor deep extention and pattern of infiltration. In addition, post-contrast T1W images with FS technique are useful to best address bone invasion, meningeal infiltration or perineural spread [18]. In fact, when using T1W fat-saturated sequences the bone marrow, the cortex and the skull base will have suppressed signal compared to the hyperintense, enhancing, tumorallowing for the detection of bony and meningeal invasion as well as tumor spread along the facial and trigeminal nerves (up the stylomastoid foramen, the foramen ovale and the foramen rotundum) [18].

As for US imaging, the MRI appearance of benign and *low-grade* malignant SGTs may show overlapping features, especially with regard to well-defined margins and to the homogeneity of signal intensity. On the other side, *high-grade* neoplasms often present with more aggressive features such as irregular borders, invasion into adjacent compartments (parapharyngeal space, muscles or bone), low signal on T2W images, heterogeneous enhancement, cystic changes or central necrosis (Fig. 3.3 a, b) [1, 2]. Among these characteristics, signal intensity on T2W images has been reported to be helpful in predicting whether a salivary gland neoplasm is benign or malignant [18]; usually a mass with low to intermediate signal intensity on T2W images is associated with malignancy while hyperintense masses on T2W images might be considered benign. An exception is represented by malignant tumor that shows cystic/necrotic changes, which may be a confounding factor with benign ones.

MRI sensitivity and the specificity in predicting malignancy were reported to be 70% and 73%, respectively [17]. However, conventional MRI in the differential diagnosis of SGTs has some limitations [1, 2].

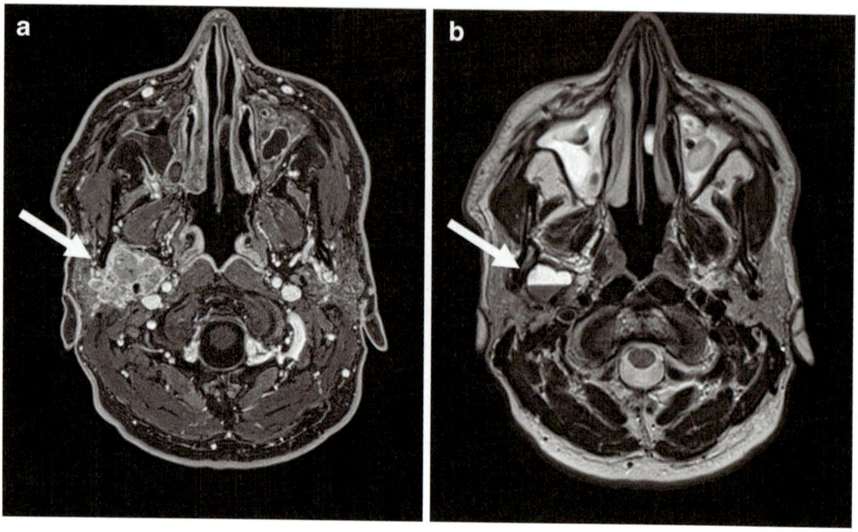

Fig. 3.3 MRI examination of high-grade neoplasm located in the deep lobe of the parotid gland. On post-contrast T1W-FS sequence (**a**) the lesion shows inhomogeneous enhancement and irregular borders; on T2W sequence (**b**) the same lesion shows cystic component with fluid-fluid level within

3.4 Additional MR Imaging Techniques

Diffusion-weighted imaging (DWI) is an MRI technique which provides information about tissues *cellular density* in relation to freedom of motion of their water molecules. In highly cellular tissues and dense fluids water motion is restricted, while in pure fluids water motion is not.

Simplifying, a tissue or tumor characterized by high cellular density shows high signal on DWI sequence. The signal on DWI sequence can be quantitatively expressed by means of apparent diffusion coefficient (ADC), value that is automatically calculated and shown separately in a specific map (Fig. 3.4 a–d)

Regarding SGTs, an overlap in terms of ADC values has been reported between a large part of low-/high-grade malignant neoplasm and benign lesion [19, 20]. This overlapping could be in part explained by the fact that some high-grade malignant neoplasms show cystic or necrotic component (with no water motion restriction), while some benign tumors (such as Warthin's tumor) have high cellularity (and subsequently significant water motion restriction). Therefore, it is not possible to differentiate between malignant and benign SGTs based on DWI imaging alone [19].

Dynamic contrast-enhanced MRI (DCE-MRI) is another additional MRI technique that evaluates the different degrees of tumor contrast enhancement over time. This technique is mostly based on two parameters: the time-to-peak enhancement (T-peak) and the washout ratio (WR). According to these parameters, four different

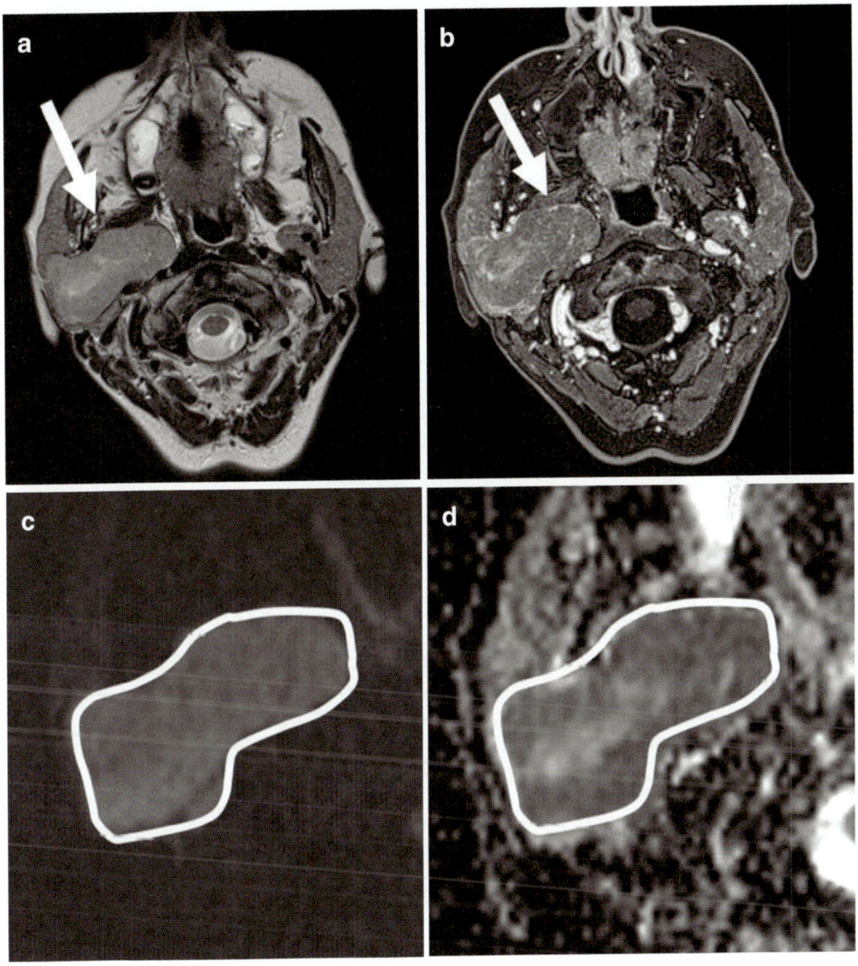

Fig. 3.4 MRI examination of a huge lesion within the parotid gland that shows intermediate signal on T2W image (**a**) and inhomogeneous enhancement on post-contrast fat-saturated T1W image (**b**). The tumor shows high cellularity (and restricted diffusion) which correspond to high signal on DWI sequence (**c**) and low ADC value on the specific map (**d**)

curves of enhancement pattern have been developed (A, B, C, D: persistent enhancement, washout, plateau and no enhancement, respectively) [21]. Most malignant SGTs show a type C curve (typically associated with a T-peak < 120 s and a WR < 30%) but, also in this case, overlap with benign lesion exists.

Currently, the use of DWI or DCE-MR alone to differentiate between benign and malignant SGTs is not advised. Conversely, the combined use of DWI and DCE-MR imaging features is more advisable and shows promise to increase diagnostic accuracy for discriminating between different tumor types [22].

3.5 Computed Tomography

Computed tomography (CT) is the preferred modality in patients with MR contraindication (claustrophobia, cardiac pacemakers, metallic devices) or when further information about bone structures is required. A satisfactory CT examination should always provide images with thin slices (up to 1mm) and multiplanar reconstruction with bone and soft tissue algorithms [1].

It is well known that soft tissue contrast of CT images is lower compared to MRI; in fact, perineural spread could be suspected only in the case of skull base foramina asymmetry, due to cortical erosion consequent to neural thickening. The use of iodinated contrast medium is mandatory to increase soft tissue resolution and depict pathology with better accuracy (attention should always be paid in patients with suspected nephropathy or previous allergic reactions). On the other hand, CT scans are more widely available and easier to perform, compared to MRI, due to shorter time of acquisition [18].

3.6 Perineural Spread

The incidence of perineural spread is reported to occur in up to 50% of high-grade malignant SGT, being particularly common for adenoid cystic carcinoma (ACC) [2]. The assessment of neural involvement is of utmost importance for tumor staging and treatment. As previously stated, both CT and MRI can detect perineural spread; however MRI is definitively superior. MRI allows to suspect perineural

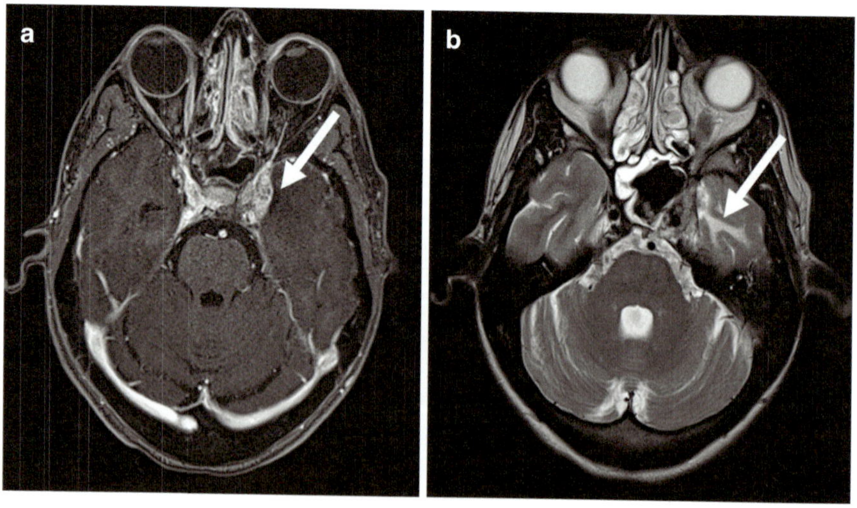

Fig. 3.5 Gadolinium-enhanced T1-weighted magnetic resonance imaging (**a**) demonstrating enhancing thickening along the mandibular branch (V3) of the trigeminal nerve, conditioning lateral bulging of cavernous sinus dural membranes (arrow). On T2W image (**b**), brain edema is present due to mass effect of the cavernous sinus bulging

spread both on pre-contrast T1W images (due to the replacement of fat in neural foramina) and on post-contrast T1W images with FS, as diffuse or nodular enhanced thickening of the cranial nerves (Fig. 3.5 a, b) [1, 18].The first and most commonly involved nerves in SGTs are the facial and trigeminal nerves due to the close anatomical relationship with the major salivary glands. The auriculotemporal nerve represents an important connection between facial and trigeminal nerves [1]. In more advanced disease, other cranial nerves may be involved.

MRI sensitivity for perineural spread has been reported to be up to 95% [1, 23]. False-positive findings due to inflammatory changes reduce MRI specificity (85%). Microscopic neoplastic infiltration may cause inaccuracy in diagnosing neural involvement and may explain the presence of skip lesions [1].

3.7 Follow-Up of Salivary Gland Tumors

Clinical examination in patients who underwent surgery and radiotherapy is difficult in relation to anatomical changes related to surgery and radiation-induced tissue fibrosis. For this reason, in some cases, deeper recurrences or perineural spread may be overlooked [1].

It has been reported that up to 70% of recurrence of high-grade SGTs manifest within 3 years of treatment [1, 24] and that up to 50% of patients affected by SGTs show distant metastasis during follow-up, most of which [1, 25] arising from high-grade ACC, adenocarcinoma NOS (not otherwise specified) and carcinoma ex pleomorphic adenoma. In most of cases, metastases involve the lungs while less than 15% affect the bones, liver, brain and other sites [3].

Imaging, during follow up of SGTs, has the role to detect early recurrence; this role is crucial for those relapse that can be still treated and is essential to improve the prognosis of these patients which is generally poor [24, 25].

As reported above, US is an easy and fast modality to assess superficial masses characterizing them as solid or cystic but has the well-known limitation of poor assessment of deeper tissues. After irradiation, salivary glands may become hypoechoic and inhomogeneous at US. Of note, the salivary glands may enlarge immediately after radiotherapy and later become smaller because of subsequent atrophy. As a consequence, during follow-up, US is primarily used for guiding FNAC or CNB to discriminate recurrence from post-treatment changes.

MRI is the most sensitive techniques to perform follow-up in patients with SGTs. The use of paramagnetic contrast medium is mandatory to increase soft tissue resolution and to detect perineural spread, as already mentioned. Baseline examination is usually performed 3 months after the end of treatments [1]. Attention should be paid to post-irradiation changes such as edema, which correspond on high signal on T2W images. DWI may be helpful in monitoring treatment and diagnosing recurrence only in SGTs with high cellular density at the baseline, such as for squamous cell carcinoma [26].

CT is an easy and fast modality to follow-up SGTs and is of utmost importance for imaging distant metastases (Fig. 3.6) [27].

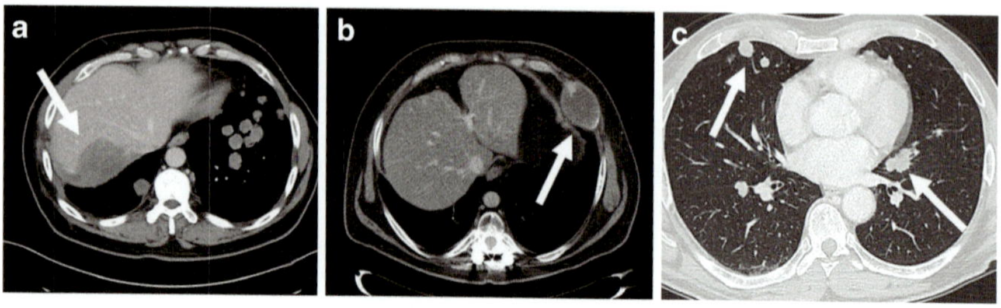

Fig. 3.6 CT examination during follow-up of a patient affected by submandibular adenoid cystic carcinoma shows distant metastasis within the liver (**a**), left thoracic wall (**b**), and lungs (**c**)

3.8 Positron Emission Tomography-CT with Fluorine-18-Deoxy-D-Glucose (FDG PET-CT)

SGTs are an uncommon clinical indication for FDG PET-CT that is the most widely used functional imaging modality based on the assessment of tumor glucose metabolism. An increase of FDG uptake, expressed by standardized uptake value (SUV), is associated with cell vitality and proliferative activity [28]. FDG PET-CT is not a useful imaging method for distinguishing between benign and malignant SGTs. In fact, benign tumors such as Warthin's tumors and pleomorphic adenomas usually show increased FDG uptake without significant difference in SUV compared to malignant SGTs [29, 30]. Furthermore, *low-grade* malignant tumors (clear cell carcinoma, etc.) are often biologically hard to differentiate from benign lesions. Considering the metabolic features of these tumors, FDG PET-CT is not routinely recommended for the diagnosis and initial staging, especially in histotypes with low glucose avidity. FDG PET-CT might be useful in the detection of cervical lymph nodes and distant metastases in patient with *high-grade* SGTs, modifying the therapeutic management in up to 15–25% of patient and sometimes avoiding unnecessary surgery [1, 31, 32]. On the contrary, literature data doesn't show consensus about the role of FDG PET-CT on surveillance/follow up of malignant SGTs. Particular attention should be made for ACC which is a biologically and clinically distinct subtype of SGTs with lower FDG uptake, slow development but strong tendency for local invasion and poor prognosis. In ACC patients the use of alternative radiopharmaceutical like 11C-methionine (MET) might be considered. MET is an essential amino acid that plays a role in cancer cell metabolism [33]; its uptake is often increased in tumors with low glucose uptake. The main limitation of this tracer is the short half-life which implies the presence of on-site cyclotron and dedicated radiochemistry laboratories for the production and clinical utilization. The use of hybrid PET/MRI images might offer a higher sensitivity and specificity to assess the presence of malignancy on initial staging, providing high-quality complimentary morphological and multi-parametric functional information in one setting [34]. However, at present, sufficient data are still lacking.

References

1. Freling N, Crippa F, Maroldi R. Staging and follow-up of high-grade malignant salivary gland tumours: the role of traditional versus functional imaging approaches - a review. Oral Oncol. 2016;60:157–66. https://doi.org/10.1016/j.oraloncology.2016.04.016. Epub 2016 May 25.
2. Lee YY, Wong KT, King AD, Ahuja AT. Imaging of salivary gland tumours. Eur J Radiol. 2008;66(3):419–36. https://doi.org/10.1016/j.ejrad.2008.01.027. Epub 2008 Mar 11.
3. Wyszyńska-Pawelec G, Gontarz M, Zapała J, Szuta M. Minor salivary gland tumours of upper aerodigestive tract: a clinicopathological study. Gastroenterol Res Pract. 2012;2012:780453. https://doi.org/10.1155/2012/780453. Epub 2012 May 21.
4. Guzzo M, Locati LD, Prott FJ, Gatta G, McGurk M, Licitra L. Major and minor salivary gland tumors. Crit Rev Oncol Hematol. 2010;74(2):134–48. https://doi.org/10.1016/j.critrevonc.2009.10.004. Epub 2009 Nov 24.
5. Thoeny HC. Imaging of salivary gland tumours. Cancer Imaging. 2007;7:52–62.
6. Bialek EJ, Jakubowski W, Zajkowski P, Szopinski KT, Osmolski A. US of the major salivary glands: anatomy and spatial relationships, pathologic conditions, and pitfalls. Radiographics. 2006;26(3):745–63.
7. Ying M, Ahuja A. Sonography of neck lymph nodes. Part I: normal lymph nodes. Clin Radiol. 2003;58(5):351–8.
8. Shimizu M, Ussmüller J, Hartwein J, Donath K, Kinukawa N. Statistical study for sonographic differential diagnosis of tumorous lesions in the parotid gland. Oral Surg Oral Med Oral Pathol Oral Radiol Endod. 1999;88(2):226–33.
9. Kim J, Kim EK, Park CS, Choi YS, Kim YH, Choi EC. Characteristic sonographic findings of Warthin's tumor in the parotid gland. J Clin Ultrasound. 2004;32(2):78–81.
10. Zajkowski P, Jakubowski W, Białek EJ, Wysocki M, Osmólski A, Serafin-Król M. Pleomorphic adenoma and adenolymphoma in ultrasonography. Eur J Ultrasound. 2000;12(1):23–9.
11. Schick S, Steiner E, Gahleitner A, Böhm P, Helbich T, Ba-Ssalamah A, Mostbeck G. Differentiation of benign and malignant tumors of the parotid gland: value of pulsed Doppler and color Doppler sonography. Eur Radiol. 1998;8(8):1462–7.
12. Dequanter D, Lothaire P, Andry G. Secondary malignant tumors of the parotid. Ann Otolaryngol Chir Cervicofac. 2005;122(1):18–20.
13. Bozzato A, Zenk J, Greess H, Hornung J, Gottwald F, Rabe C, Iro H. Potential of ultrasound diagnosis for parotid tumors: analysis of qualitative and quantitative parameters. Otolaryngol Head Neck Surg. 2007;137(4):642–6.
14. Wong DS, Li GK. The role of fine-needle aspiration cytology in the management of parotid tumors: a critical clinical appraisal. Head Neck. 2000;22(5):469–73.
15. Novoa E, Gürtler N, Arnoux A, Kraft M. Role of ultrasound-guided core-needle biopsy in the assessment of head and neck lesions: a meta-analysis and systematic review of the literature. Head Neck. 2012;34(10):1497–503. https://doi.org/10.1002/hed.21821. Epub 2011 Aug 24.
16. Wan YL, Chan SC, Chen YL, Cheung YC, Lui KW, Wong HF, Hsueh C, See LC. Ultrasonography-guided core-needle biopsy of parotid gland masses. AJNR Am J Neuroradiol. 2004;25(9):1608–12.
17. Christe A, Waldherr C, Hallett R, Zbaeren P, Thoeny H. MR imaging of parotid tumors: typical lesion characteristics in MR imaging improve discrimination between benign and malignant disease. AJNR Am J Neuroradiol. 2011;32(7):1202–7. https://doi.org/10.3174/ajnr.A2520. Epub 2011 Jun 30.
18. Yousem DM, Kraut MA, Chalian AA. Major salivary gland imaging. Radiology. 2000;216(1):19–29.
19. Habermann CR, Arndt C, Graessner J, Diestel L, Petersen KU, Reitmeier F, Ussmueller JO, Adam G, Jaehne M. Diffusion-weighted echo-planar MR imaging of primary parotid gland tumors: is a prediction of different histologic subtypes possible? AJNR Am J Neuroradiol. 2009;30(3):591–6. https://doi.org/10.3174/ajnr.A1412. Epub 2009 Jan 8.

20. Thoeny HC, De Keyzer F, Boesch C, Hermans R. Diffusion-weighted imaging of the parotid gland: influence of the choice of b-values on the apparent diffusion coefficient value. J Magn Reson Imaging. 2004;20(5):786–90.
21. Yabuuchi H, Fukuya T, Tajima T, Hachitanda Y, Tomita K, Koga M. Salivary gland tumors: diagnostic value of gadolinium-enhanced dynamic MR imaging with histopathologic correlation. Radiology. 2003;226(2):345–54.
22. Assili S, Fathi Kazerooni A, Aghaghazvini L, Saligheh Rad HR, Pirayesh Islamian J. Dynamic contrast magnetic resonance imaging (DCE-MRI) and diffusion weighted MR imaging (DWI) for differentiation between benign and malignant salivary gland tumors. J Biomed Phys Eng. 2015;5(4):157–68. eCollection 2015 Dec.
23. Shimamoto H, Chindasombatjaroen J, Kakimoto N, Kishino M, Murakami S, Furukawa S. Perineural spread of adenoid cystic carcinoma in the oral and maxillofacial regions: evaluation with contrast-enhanced CT and MRI. Dentomaxillofac Radiol. 2012;41(2):143–51. https://doi.org/10.1259/dmfr/21825064.
24. Gillespie MB, Albergotti WG, Eisele DW. Recurrent salivary gland cancer. Curr Treat Options in Oncol. 2012;13(1):58–70. https://doi.org/10.1007/s11864-011-0174-0.
25. Terhaard CH, Lubsen H, Van der Tweel I, Hilgers FJ, Eijkenboom WM, Marres HA, Tjho-Heslinga RE, de Jong JM, Roodenburg JL, Dutch Head and Neck Oncology Cooperative Group. Salivary gland carcinoma: independent prognostic factors for locoregional control, distant metastases, and overall survival: results of the Dutch head and neck oncology cooperative group. Head Neck. 2004;26(8):681–92; discussion 692-3.
26. Thoeny HC, De Keyzer F, King AD. Diffusion-weighted MR imaging in the head and neck. Radiology. 2012;263(1):19–32. https://doi.org/10.1148/radiol.11101821.
27. Sood S, McGurk M, Vaz F. Management of salivary gland tumours: United Kingdom national multidisciplinary guidelines. J Laryngol Otol. 2016;130(Suppl 2):S142–9. https://doi.org/10.1017/S0022215116000566.
28. Minn H, Clavo AC, Grénman R, Wahl RL. In vitro comparison of cell proliferation kinetics and uptake of tritiated fluorodeoxyglucose and L-methionine in squamous-cell carcinoma of the head and neck. J Nucl Med. 1995;36(2):252–8.
29. Park SB, Choi JY, Lee EJ, Yoo J, Cheon M, Cho SK, Choe YS, Lee KH, Kim BT. Diagnostic criteria on (18)F-FDG PET/CT for differentiating benign from malignant focal hypermetabolic lesions of parotid gland. Nucl Med Mol Imaging. 2012;46(2):95–101.
30. Toriihara A, Nakamura S, Kubota K, Makino T, Okochi K, Shibuya H. Can dual-time-point 18F-FDG PET/CT differentiate malignant salivary gland tumors from benign tumors? AJR Am J Roentgenol. 2013;201(3):639–44.
31. Jeong HS, Chung MK, Son YI, Choi JY, Kim HJ, Ko YH, Baek CH. Role of 18F-FDG PET/CT in management of high-grade salivary gland malignancies. J Nucl Med. 2007;48(8):1237–44.
32. Razfar A, Heron DE, Branstetter BF 4th, Seethala RR, Ferris RL. Positron emission tomography-computed tomography adds to the management of salivary gland malignancies. Laryngoscope. 2010;120(4):734–8.
33. Toubaru S, Yoshikawa K, Ohashi S, Tanimoto K, Hasegawa A, Kawaguchi K, Saga T, Kamada T. Accuracy of methionine-PET in predicting the efficacy of heavy particle therapy on primary adenoid cystic carcinomas of the head and neck. Radiat Oncol. 2013;8:143.
34. Rasmussen JH, Nørgaard M, Hansen AE, Vogelius IR, Aznar MC, Johannesen HH, Costa J, Engberg AM, Kjær A, Specht L, Fischer BM. Feasibility of multiparametric imaging with PET/MR in head and neck squamous cell carcinoma. J Nucl Med. 2017;58(1):69–74.

4 Surgery for Malignant Parotid Gland Tumours

Vincent Vander Poorten

4.1 Introduction

Malignancy involving the parotid can arise primarily from the parotid tissue (primary parotid cancer), primarily in the lymph nodes in the realm of lymphoma, or can be due to a non-parotid cancer that metastasizes to or directly invades the parotid. Cancers metastasizing to the parotid lymph nodes are mainly skin cancer of the forehead, eyelid and temple area, but cancers anywhere in the body can do so. Cancers directly invading the parotid are mainly skin cancer, external acoustic meatus cancer and oropharyngeal cancer with very deep extension [1]. Successful treatment depends on a maximally informative preoperative workup that allows for careful individualized planning of surgery and the often needed postoperative radiotherapy [2].

4.2 Surgery for Primary Parotid Cancer

Eighty to ninety percent of parotid tissue is located laterally to the course of the facial nerve. In parallel, 80–90% of epithelial neoplasms arise laterally to the course of the facial nerve [3]. The remainder of the tumours is located below the level of the facial nerve, in the deep lobe. In less than 1%, a tumour arises from the accessory parotid tissue along Stensen's duct.

One in four parotid tumours is cancer, and their histopathological appearance is extremely diverse (Table 4.1). Their malignant nature is frequently unclear before surgery but is suggested in many other instances by clinical signs, rapid growth,

V. Vander Poorten (✉)
Otorhinolaryngology, Head and Neck Surgery, University Hospitals Leuven, Leuven, Belgium

Head and Neck Oncology, Department of Oncology, KU Leuven, Leuven, Belgium
e-mail: vincent.vanderpoorten@uzleuven.be

© Springer Nature Switzerland AG 2019
L. Licitra, L. D. Locati (eds.), *Salivary Gland Cancer*,
https://doi.org/10.1007/978-3-030-02958-6_4

Table 4.1 The WHO[a] 2017 histologic classification of malignant salivary gland tumours [4]

Type WHO	Abbreviation
1. Mucoepidermoid carcinoma	MEC
2. Adenoid cystic carcinoma	AdCC
3. Acinic cell carcinoma	AcCC
4. Polymorphous adenocarcinoma	
5. Clear cell carcinoma	
6. Basal cell adenocarcinoma	
7. Intraductal carcinoma	
8. Adenocarcinoma, NOS	ACNOS
9. Salivary duct carcinoma	SDC
10. Myoepithelial carcinoma	
11. Epithelial-myoepithelial carcinoma	
12. Carcinoma ex pleomorphic adenoma	
13. Secretory carcinoma	
14. Sebaceous adenocarcinoma	
15. Carcinosarcoma	
16. Undifferentiated carcinoma	
17. Large cell neuroendocrine carcinoma	
18. Small cell neuroendocrine carcinoma	
19. Lymphoepithelial carcinoma	
20. Squamous cell carcinoma	
21. Oncocytic carcinoma	
22. Sialoblastoma (uncertain malignant potential)	

[a]*WHO* World Health Organization
Modified from the WHO publication to include only the malignancies [4]

enlarged neck lymph nodes (29%), deep fixation or skin invasion (9%) (Fig. 4.1), pain (44%) and CN VII dysfunction (19%), a finding independent of the tumour diameter [5–10]. Clinical TNM staging summarizes this clinical information on the size of the primary, the nodal extension, the function of the facial nerve and the invasion of surrounding structures [11, 12] (Table 4.2).

Surgical excision of parotid cancer with—on indication—a course of postoperative radiotherapy is the treatment modality providing the best chance of cure [1, 2, 12–14]. The extent of surgery of the primary tumour is determined by the size of the lesion, the relationship to the facial nerve and eventual extraparotid tissue invasion. A thorough preoperative workup aims at anticipating these tumour characteristics. In this way the extent of surgery and eventual reconstruction can be planned, and a realistic estimate of expected prognosis can already be made in the preoperative situation [8]. Table 4.3 displays expected treatment results of multidisciplinary treatment of patients with parotid cancer in terms of disease-specific survival.

4.2.1 Workup: Diagnostic Radiology

For small, slowly growing mobile tumours, imaging will not frequently alter the approach. Imaging is mandatory, however, when confronted with a large tumour (>4 cm), impaired tumour mobility, facial nerve dysfunction or, in the case of palpable cervical lymph nodes [12], ultrasound is well suited for evaluation of

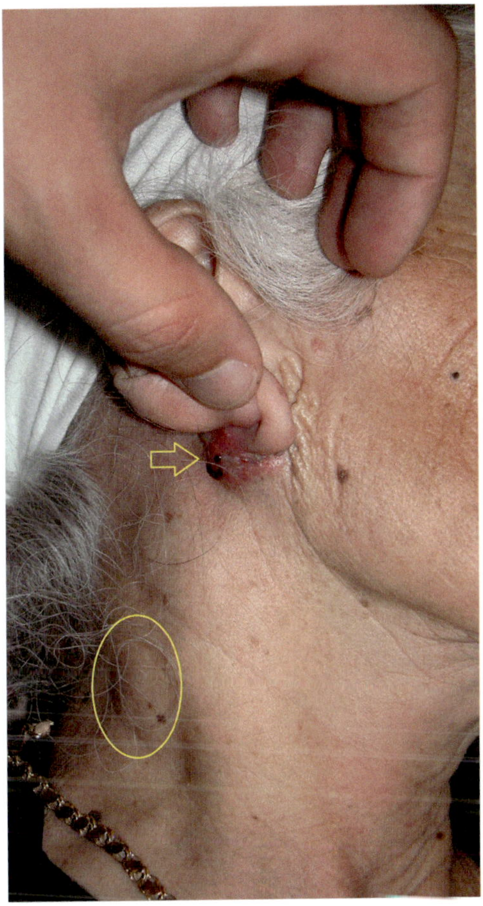

Fig. 4.1 Parotid cancer with skin invasion. Source: Prognosis in Head and Neck Cancer, Robert J Baatenburg de Jong, editor. V. Vander Poorten: Prognosis in patients with parotid carcinoma; Chap. 21, p. 356. Reprinted by permission of Taylor and Francis

relatively small and superficially localized neoplasms and may optimize results of fine needle aspiration cytology (FNAC). A magnetic resonance imaging study (MRI) is superior to a computerized tomography (CT) in evaluating parotid tumours and is especially useful in visualizing the retromandibular parotid and parapharyngeal space, the area of the stylomastoid foramen and eventual facial nerve invasion and perineural extension (Fig. 4.2). Also for recurrent tumours, the exact assessment of tumour extent needs MR imaging. Additionally, conventional MRI also has specific signs suggesting malignancy [26], and a specific pattern on diffusion-weighted MRI (DW-MRI) may result in an even improved identification of potential malignancy [27]. CT scanning may be required in instances where bone invasion is suspected (mastoid, mandible, infratemporal fossa) [1]. In suspected malignancy, based on clinical, radiological or FNAC elements, positron emission tomography (PET) with or without CT can be considered to exclude distant metastases, before embarking on locoregional therapy. A recognized pitfall of PET-CT is the high false-positive and false-negative rate in differentiating benign from malignant salivary disease [28].

Table 4.2 UICC eighth edition TNM classification and stage regrouping for major salivary gland malignancies [11]

T—primary tumour			
Tx	Primary tumour cannot be assessed		
T0	No evidence of primary tumour		
T1	Tumour 2 cm or less, without extraparenchymal extension[a]		
T2	Tumour >2 to 4 cm, without extraparenchymal extension		
T3	Tumour >4 to 6 cm, and/or extraparenchymal extension		
T4a	Tumour invades the skin, mandible, ear canal and/or seventh nerve involvement		
T4b	Tumour invades the base of skull, and/or pterygoid plates and/or encases carotid artery		
N—regional lymph nodes			
NX	Regional lymph nodes cannot be assessed		
N0	No regional lymph node metastasis		
N1	Metastasis in a single ipsilateral node, 3 cm or less in greatest dimension, without extranodal extension		
N2a	Single ipsilateral node >3 to 6 cm, without extranodal extension		
N2b	Multiple ipsilateral nodes <6 cm, without extranodal extension		
N2c	Bilateral or contralateral nodes <6 cm, without extranodal extension		
N3a	Metastasis in a lymph node >6 cm without extranodal extension		
N3b	Metastasis in 1 or more lymph nodes with extranodal extension		
M—distant metastasis			
M0	No distant metastasis		
M1	Distant metastasis		
Stage grouping			
Stage 0	Tis	N0	M0
Stage I	T1	N0	M0
Stage II	T2	N0	M0
Stage III	T3	N0	M0
	T1, T2, T3	N1	M0
Stage IVa	T4a	N0, N1	M0
	T1, T2, T3, T4a	N2	M0
Stage IVb	T4b	Any N	M0
	Any T	N3	M0
Stage IVc	Any T	Any N	M1

[a]Extraparenchymal extension is clinical or macroscopic invasion of soft tissues or nerve, other than those listed under T4a and T4b

4.2.2 Workup: Pretreatment Pathology

In specific situations we will attempt to obtain tissue before embarking on treatment, when we expect this information to alter management. Aims then are (1) to confirm salivary tissue origin, (2) to discriminate between benign and malignant lesions and (3) to obtain, if possible, information on histopathologic typing (Table 4.1). For this purpose, we dispose of (ultrasound-guided) fine needle aspiration cytology (UgFNAC), US-guided thru-cut biopsy and open biopsy.

Using FNAC, an experienced cytologist can quite accurately (accuracy 79%) differentiate between malignant and benign tumours [29–31]. Cytologic features of a lymphocyte-predominant lesion should raise the suspicion of lymphoma, and a thru-cut or open biopsy may ensue. In case of salivary tissue found on FNAC, correct tumour typing is difficult, but maximizing pretreatment probability of the

Table 4.3 Disease-specific survival (DSS) following treatment of patients with parotid carcinoma [12]

Authors	Year of publication	DSS 5 years (%)	DSS 10 years (%)
Frankenthaler et al. [5]	1991	75	70
Kane et al. [15]	1991	69	68
Pedersen et al. [16]	1992		52
Poulsen et al. [17]	1992	71	65
Renehan [18]	1999	78	65
Spiro [13]	1986	55	47
Spiro and Wang [19]	1993	77	65
Spiro et al. [14]	1989	63	47
Therkildsen et al. [20]	1998	76	72
Leverstein et al. [21]	1998	75	67
Vander Poorten et al. [7]	1999	59	54
Harbo et al. [22]	2002	57	51
Vander Poorten et al. [9]	2003	62	
Godballe et al. [23]	2003	52	
Mendenhall et al. [24]	2005		57
Lima et al. [25]	2005	72	69
Vander Poorten et al. [8]	2009	69	58

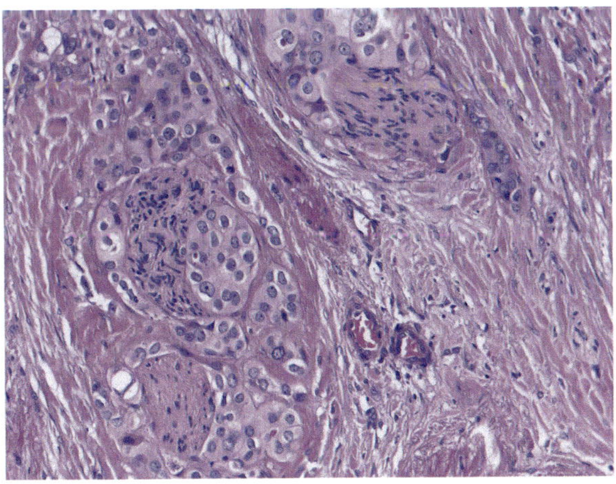

Fig. 4.2 Massive perineural spread of undifferentiated parotid carcinoma. Source: Prognosis in Head and Neck Cancer, Robert J Baatenburg de Jong, editor. V. Vander Poorten: Prognosis in patients with parotid carcinoma; Chap. 21, p. 364. Reprinted by permission of Taylor and Francis

benign or malignant nature remains a feasible goal. This then allows for appropriate counselling of the patient and guides timing and prioritization of treatment and planning of the extent of resection and possible reconstruction. Ultrasound guidance of FNAC increases its accuracy and simultaneously helps in evaluating the neck [32]. Direct on-site evaluation of the cellular quality of the aspirate by the pathologist is a means of further increasing accuracy, implying immediate repetition of the FNAC when the aspirate is deemed unsatisfactory [33]. The obtainable daily practice accuracy of FNAC is reflected in the findings of a series of 1355 aspirates by the Institut Curie group in Paris, who found an 80.5% correct identification of malignancy (true positive), 11.9% false negatives, 4.6% suspicious lesions and 3%

of uninterpretable samples [30]. The 12% false negativity implies that removal of the tumour for further histopathology analysis remains required, also when the FNAC suggests benign disease [12]. The difficulty in increasing accuracy of FNAC lies in the fact that the different salivary gland tumour types have overlapping histological features and that individual cells, obtained by FNAC, are not embedded in their tissue architecture.

Controversy surrounds the use of thru-cut biopsies for parotid lesions. While some studies report safety and higher accuracy than FNAC [34, 35], the author has seen several cases of damage to facial nerve branches in patients subjected to parotid thru-cut biopsies. Open biopsy is rarely indicated but can be considered in (1) skin invading tumours where an incisional biopsy is in the area where the skin will have to be resected anyway in an eventual subsequent extended parotidectomy and in (2) advanced tumours that, at presentation, are already beyond surgical cure, so the biopsy may be the only tissue sample obtained. Increasingly, molecular biological studies can be carried out, also on the incisional biopsy material [36].

4.2.3 Extent of Surgery for the Primary Tumour

The different types of parotidectomies that are classically described all have identification of the facial nerve—and preservation if possible—as common principle and are listed below:

1. Partial superficial parotidectomy implies resection of the tumour with a cuff of normal tissue where possible.
2. Superficial or lateral parotidectomy implies removal of all tissue lateral to the facial nerve.
3. Total parotidectomy implies removal of all tissue lateral and medial to the facial nerve.
4. Radical parotidectomy implies all tissue, including the nerve.
5. Extended parotidectomy implies a radical parotidectomy with adjacent invaded structures such as the skin, bone of mastoid or mandible, temporomandibular joint, masticatory muscles and infratemporal fossa.

Recently the European salivary gland society (ESGS) published a proposal for a rational and logical description of parotidectomies, performed for both benign and malignant diseases in the parotid gland, numbering the levels of the parotid in reference to a plane formed by an imaginary line connecting the bifurcation of the facial nerve trunk into its two major branches (temporofacial and cervicofacial) with Stensen's duct [37]. The parotidectomy performed is described by an enumeration of the levels resected in combination with additional non-parotid structures that are sacrificed. These are represented by capital letters placed in between brackets after the resected levels (CN VII, facial nerve trunk and/or all the main branches; CN VII t-z-b-m-c, when only facial nerve branches have been resected; ECA, external carotid artery; GAN, greater auricular nerve; LTB, lateral temporal resection; MB, mastoid bone; MM, masseter muscle; S, skin) (Table 4.4).

Table 4.4 ESGS parotidectomy classification applied to common surgical situations [37]

Parotidectomy I	Partial superficial parotidectomy
Parotidectomy II	Partial superficial parotidectomy
Parotidectomy I–II	Superficial parotidectomy
Parotidectomy I–II–III	Superficial parotidectomy extended to the inferior deep lobe
Parotidectomy III–IV	Deep lobe parotidectomy
Parotidectomy I–IV	Total parotidectomy with facial nerve preservation
Parotidectomy V	Accessory lobe removal
Parotidectomy I–IV (VII)	Total parotidectomy with facial nerve resection
Parotidectomy I–IV (VII, S, MM)	Extended total parotidectomy with facial nerve resection plus skin and masseter muscle resection
ECD I	Extracapsular dissection with tumour in level I
ECD II	Extracapsular dissection with tumour in level II
ECD V	Extracapsular dissection with tumour in level V

Table 4.3 shows a number of situations described by this system.

4.2.3.1 Less-Than-Total Parotidectomy (Nos. 1 and 2)

There is quite some debate about the extent of surgery needed to remove a preoperatively known parotid cancer, and in our recent paper, we pointed out that the controversy mainly regards stage I and II tumours [2].

Because the majority of parotid cancers (80–90%) are located in the superficial or lateral parotid lobe, with a normally functioning facial nerve, several authors agree that performing the standard superficial or lateral parotidectomy would appear to be adequate in the majority of small tumour cases without regional metastasis [12, 38], and in the same line, many authors, retrospectively reviewing their institutional patient series, find that a less-than-total parotidectomy had been employed in a subset of their treated patients. This is frequently the case in patients where the diagnosis of malignancy is made in retrospect, following a limited parotidectomy that is judged to have adequately removed the tumour. In these instances, a decision to go back, to perform a completion parotidectomy, is not taken. Already in 1975 Ronald Spiro reported that 58% of malignant tumours in his series of the MSKCC had been adequately removed by less-than-total parotidectomy.

In our own nationwide review of patients with parotid cancer in the Netherlands, 27% of patients were treated with a superficial parotidectomy [9], and in our study including Belgian and German patients, this was the case in 21% of patients. It is unclear how these patients would have done with more radical primary surgery [8].

4.2.3.2 Total Conservative Parotidectomy (No. 3) (Fig. 4.3)

Proponents of more radical surgery especially stress the presence of intraparotid lymph nodes. These are to be considered the first echelon nodes for metastatic cells on their way to the neck nodes and thus at the highest risk of being involved with lymph node metastasis [3, 39–41]. Indeed, Armstrong et al. showed that the parotid lymph nodes are involved in 53% of elective neck dissections [42]. Similarly, Klussman et al., in their series of patients that all had undergone total parotidectomy and elective neck dissection, found that 65% of pN+ necks had metastatic disease in the parotid lymph nodes [43].

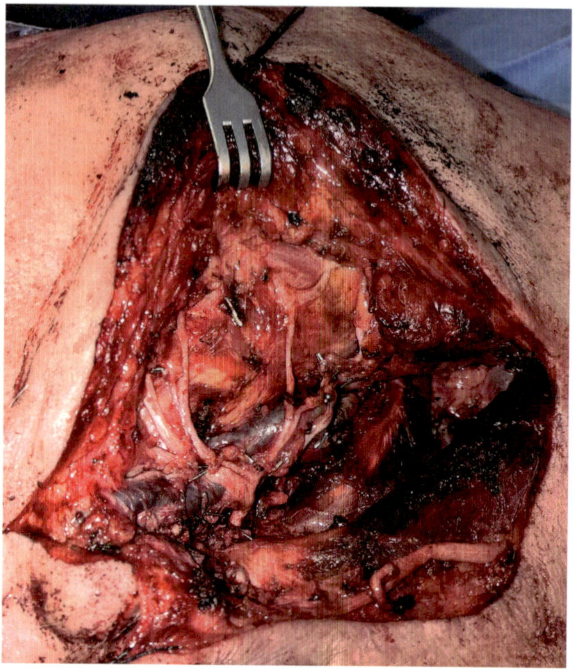

Fig. 4.3 Total conservative parotidectomy. The facial nerve, preoperatively functioning, is preserved intact, but all salivary tissue has been removed

This reasoning entails performing a deep lobe parotidectomy in patients with metastatic skin cancer to a superficial intraparotid node (see further below), primary parotid cancer that has metastasized to the neck nodes or to a superficial parotid node and high-grade primary parotid cancer [3].

There is far less discussion on the need for total parotidectomy tumours located in the parapharyngeal or deep lobe or even in the more advanced tumours located in the superficial lobe (tumours >4 cm or with facial nerve dysfunction, i.e. UICC stages III and IV disease). Especially in these high-stage, high-grade parotid carcinomas, the intraparotid lymph nodes may harbour metastatic disease that would be overlooked or not resected should a lesser procedure be performed [43–45].

Until a prospective randomized evaluation proves the oncological benefit of removing the deep lobe to address occult metastatic disease, to date very little local recurrence has been observed in primary parotid tumours that are well localized in the superficial lobe and that are adequately removed. It is very likely that the use of postoperative radiotherapy will also aid with the control of possible microscopic lymph node deposits located in the deep lobe [46–48]. On the other hand, regarding metastatic skin cancer, several reports point at the importance of resecting the deep lobe. A large Australian series of patients with metastatic cancer to the parotid underwent superficial parotidectomy and neck dissection without removal of the deep lobe. Even with postoperative radiation therapy, a recurrence rate of 20% was observed, of which two out of three recurrences occurred in the area of the deep parotid lobe [49] (see *Metastatic Cancer to the Parotid*). Authors of the Mayo Clinic, resecting the deep lobe parotid in these patients, found a metastatic rate of 22% in the deep lobe parotid nodes [50].

4.2.3.3 Nerve Sacrifying Total Parotidectomy (No. 4 and Higher) (Fig. 4.4)

As a general rule, facial nerve branches are only to be resected when preoperatively paralysed, preoperatively invaded or circumferentially surrounded by tumour. Most preoperative normally functioning nerve branches can be dissected macroscopically free from the tumour [1, 2, 12, 51]. Nerve sacrifice in these instances will induce disproportionate morbidity at the expense of minor gain in tumour control [51–53]. A good suggestion is to perform electromyography in preoperatively suspected malignant tumours. This is more sensitive than clinical examination and can help in counselling the patient on the possible need for nerve resection and reconstruction [54]. In the situation where the tumour has to be dissected off the nerve, it is important not to leave macroscopic tumour behind. The consensus regarding the safety of using postoperative radiotherapy to control disease left behind on a spared nerve branch only regards microscopical disease, not macroscopical disease [2, 14, 18, 21, 32, 51, 52].

When one or more branches of the facial nerve are not functioning preoperatively, or the nerve is preoperatively found encased in tumour, we add a more or less extended nerve resection to a total parotidectomy [1, 2, 12]. When doing a facial trunk or branch resection, it is recommended to do frozen section of the cut margins to avoid leaving tumour skip metastases. Especially AdCC is notorious for this feature [55]. A mastoidectomy or lateral temporal bone resection may be needed to obtain free margins (Fig. 4.4).

Following resection, immediate cable grafting guarantees the best function. After trimming of the nerve endings, tension-free anastomosis of the epineurium is

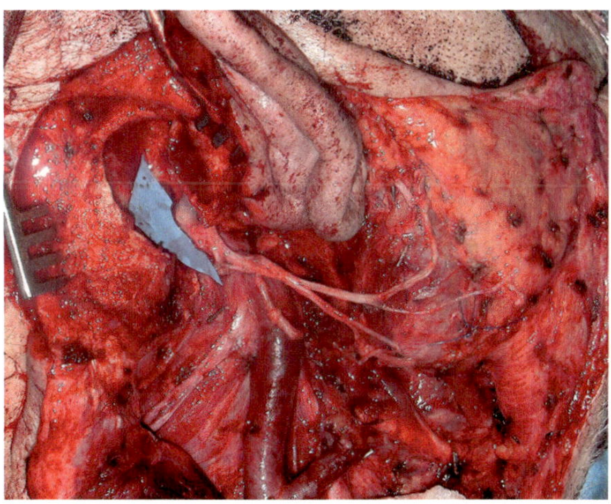

Fig. 4.4 Extended radical parotidectomy with GAN as cable graft, proximal anastomosis in the mastoid

a prerequisite for successful reinnervation [54, 56]. To this purpose, the greater auricular nerve is the first choice. It is in the operative field, has an ideal arborization, a good proximal diameter of the main trunk for coaptation to the cut main trunk of the facial nerve and also the distal branches nicely adapt to the diameter of the peripheral branches [2, 12, 56–58]. Both the GAN and the facial nerve share a monofascicular character, which is also an advantage [56]. For longer defects the same donor nerve can be backtraced to include cervical sensory branches [12, 56]. A key issue in facial nerve cable grafting is to overcome the numerical and size discrepancies. Stennert described the key principles to obtain (1) size augmentation by unifying two smaller branches to increase the diameter of the nerve graft and (2) size reduction (distal splitting of nerves and suturing the peripheral epineurium) [56]. The sural nerve is less ideal, as it is polifascicular, has almost no arborization and requires opening of a second surgical field [56, 59, 60].

Two years following cable grafting, one can expect the final result: a light to obvious paresis with synkinesis but possible eye closure (House Brackmann grades II and III) [54, 61]. EMG signs of reinnervation appear after 4.5 months, followed by the first movements from 6 months on [57–59]. Radiotherapy does not impair these results, but a preoperative nerve dysfunction (and, increasingly so, the longer this exists) and age over 60 do affect the final result in a negative way [54]. The radiotherapy effect has been studied by Brown et al. These authors find a House-Brackmann grade III or IV in 69% of irradiated patients versus in 78% of nonirradiated patients, a difference which is non-significant ($p = 0.54$) [57]. This finding was recently confirmed by a Spanish study, where the authors compared six cable-grafted patients without RT to seven cable-grafted patients undergoing radiotherapy. Again, at a median follow-up of about 3 years, there was no difference in facial movements [62]. On the other hand, highly complex reconstructions such as microneurovascular free muscle flaps do suffer from postoperative radiotherapy, and as such these are rarely used in this patient population which consists of a majority of elderly patients [63].

Immediate facial nerve reconstruction outperforms delayed reconstruction: the longer the lag time between resection and reconstruction, and the longer the defect length, the less favourable the reinnervation outcome will be. In delayed reconstruction, decreasing muscle fibres and motor endplates, degenerating Schwann cells and increasing fibrosis will result in a longer duration and less successful bridging of the defect by the regenerating axons [56].

In patients where surgery implies a mastoidectomy and proximal facial nerve resection that results in too short nerve stump in the middle ear, cable grafting becomes technically impossible. Here, a hypoglossal-distal facial nerve anastomosis can result in a quick reinnervation of the facial musculature, over a period of 3–4 months. Initially this procedure was mainly performed as an end-to-end XII–VII anastomosis, but subsequently, it was found that adequate results can also be obtained using a GAN interposition graft in a hypoglossal-facial-jump-anastomosis (HFJA). This implies incising the XII nerve only over half its circumference—thus preserving half of the hypoglossal motor input to the tongue—and then suturing a GAN interposition graft in this defect, allowing ingrowth of hypoglossal axons within the GAN perineurium into the distal facial nerve stump. This significantly reduces tongue musculature dysfunction [64]. For very extensive facial nerve resections, there are some other options to consider. The hypoglossal nerve can be mobilized up to the separate branches that run into the floor of mouth and tongue muscles, and after mobilizing the main trunk of the XIIth nerve, as well as the descending ansa hypoglossi branch, all these branches then can be anastomosed without tension to the distal facial nerve. Alternatively, a combination of facio-facial interposition grafts for the orbicularis oculi with a HFJA anastomosis for the orbicularis oris can give excellent results too [2, 56, 65].

During the period of 1–2 years that is needed for the above-mentioned nerve grafts to take effect, the crucial facial motor functions of eye closure and oral competence have to be guaranteed by static measures. These are routinely applied in patients undergoing cable grafting or hypoglossal nerve-based anastomoses in order to bridge the recovery period. These static measures can of course also be the only measures taken in elderly patients, where cable grafting is not performed because of an estimated limited effect [2, 66].

Taking care of a paralysed orbicularis oculi muscle aims at countering the unopposed action of the superior levator palpebrae muscle. To this end, a gold or platinum weight implant of 1–1.2 g on the upper tarsal plate, combined with a lateral canthopexy/canthoplasty, is very effective [67]. Secondarily, a brow lift can additionally compensate for brow ptosis. Further, a lateral tarsorrhaphy can help, in patients where a canthopexy or canthoplasty is insufficient in promoting eye closure [2].

Different measures to tackle the effect of the paralysis of the lower facial musculature aim at restoring the oral commissure, the nasolabial fold and the nasal ala. Reinforcing the ala nasi aims at reducing inspiratory collapse and at improving nasal flow [68]. A first possibility is the dynamic temporalis muscle transfer. In this technique, three divergent strips of fascia are sutured in between the temporalis tendon at its release point from the coronoid process on one hand and the three key midfacial structures on the other (upper lip—modulus—lower lip). Alternatively, a semi-dynamic solution consists of deep temporalis fascial slings left attached to the temporalis muscle. A third, less frequently used option is a static suspension of fascial slings to the zygomatic periosteum [2, 63]. The typical lower lip elevation and inversion following lower lip depressor paralysis can be addressed by transferring the anterior belly of the digastric muscle to the angle of the mouth. In this technique, the tendon that joins the anterior to the posterior belly of the digastric is inserted superiorly to the orbicularis oris muscle, through a lower lip vermillion incision at the angle of the mouth. When the anterior belly muscle, which is still attached to its mandibular insertion, then contracts, it provides for a new depressor function [69].

Common to these static measures is the frequent need for secondary corrections, due to the untoward and continuing effect of gravity on the initial reconstructive efforts. Inserting a cartilage graft onto the inferior orbital rim, anteriorly of the inferior tarsal plate, may counter lower eyelid ectropion; a further wedge excision may be needed to reduce eventual continuing lower lip elongation [63].

4.2.3.4 Extended Parotidectomies: Reconstructive Issues Regarding the Skin and Soft Tissue (Fig. 4.5)

Complete resection of extensive tumours may require, besides a removal of the facial nerve as described above under "Sect. 4.2.3.3", also a resection of the skin, mandibular or temporal bone or adjacent deep soft tissues such as the masticatory muscles [2, 12, 70]. Additional procedures required to do so may be—alone or in combination—an ascending ramus mandibulectomy, an infratemporal fossa dissection and a lateral temporal bone resection [1]. Logic dictates that it is best to reconstruct the resulting composite defect in the same session, in order to restore form and function and thus quality of life. This approach also facilitates a timely postoperative radiotherapy, which is always indicated in tumours that require such an extensive resection [63, 71]. Delayed reconstruction in post-RT contracted and fibrotic tissues implies a significantly increased risk of wound breakdown and failure of the reconstructive efforts [63]. In order to reach the best functional and aesthetic result in the long run, the surgical team generally will combine cable grafting of the resected facial nerve with static measures with a selection of procedures for defect filling and restoring the skin, as enumerated here below [72].

Primary closure or a cervicofacial rotation flap is satisfactory for limited skin defects, while larger defects may need a cervicodeltopectoral flap [2]. These flaps are raised while creating access for a neck dissection. After the resection, the skin with a good texture and colour match can be rotated into the area where the skin was resected, while the donor site can be primarily closed [63, 73, 74]. For large defects (up to 7 by 13 cm) in patients that are unfit for free flaps, one option is a "keystone island flap" based on occipital and posterior auricular perforators [75], and another option is the "supraclavicular artery island flap", a pedicled flap, that

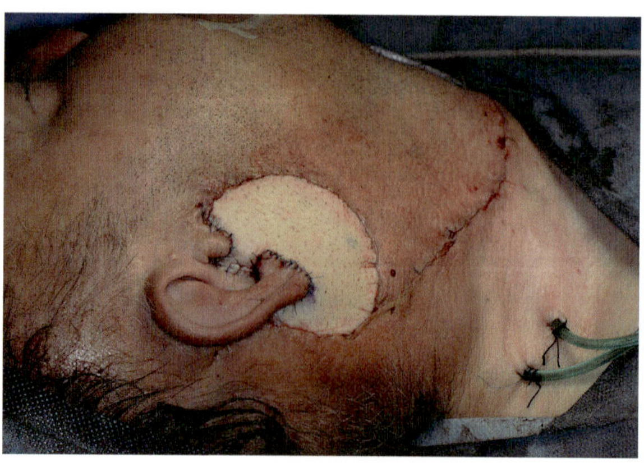

Fig. 4.5 Reconstruction with anterolateral thigh flap. After comprehensive neck dissection and extended radical parotidectomy with skin resection, external acoustic meatus, lateral temporal bone resection, reconstruction by GAN facial nerve cable grafting, static reconstruction including gold weight in the upper eyelid and temporalis fascial sling to the angle of the mouth and covering the defect with replacement of resected skin in view of postoperative radiotherapy. Patient at this moment 4y NED

can bring in a substantial amount of skin and subcutaneous soft tissue without having to perform a microvascular anastomosis [76]. After deepithelialization, this flap can also be used as a "filler" flap when there is substantial soft tissue loss without a skin defect [77].

It is common for tumours necessitating skin resections to also require removal of deep and supporting tissues. It may be needed to resect the masseter muscle which results in a denuded mandible, to clear the parapharyngeal space and/or infratemporal fossa tissues or to perform a lateral temporal bone resection [63] (Fig. 4.5). Reconstruction then requires free or pedicled composite flaps. Pedicled flaps that reliably provide significant skin and soft tissue volume are the pedicled latissimus dorsi flap [78] and the pectoralis major myocutaneous flap [79]. These still have an important role to play in difficult situations: the medically compromised patient, in salvaging failed free flap reconstructions, or in combination with free flap reconstructions. In general, however, microvascular free flaps are preferred, and especially the anterolateral thigh (ALT) perforator flap is frequently chosen. It is a flap with a relatively constant anatomy, which facilitates its harvesting, and with a comfortable vascular axis combining a long length (8–16 cm) and a large calibre (2–2.5 mm) [80, 81]. Flap volume can be adapted to the needs of the defect. When a thin cutaneous flap is needed, one can go for a suprafascial dissection, and if more volume is needed, the surgeon can include vastus lateralis or rectus femoris muscle in a musculocutaneous ALT flap. If mainly volume is needed, the combination of a deepithelialized ALT flap with a cervicofacial rotation flap can give a very nice aesthetic result [63]. Identifying and preserving the nerve to the vastus lateralis and the fascia lata can be considered for facial reanimation [72, 80]. Because the donor site is separate from the resection field, a two-team approach is possible and speeds up the total procedure time. Primary closure for skin defects less than 9 cm wide results in low donor site morbidity. In considering the volume that needs restoring, the surgeon has to take expected flap shrinkage over time into account. The post-RT volume loss of ALT flaps in parotidectomy reconstruction was recently very elegantly quantified as limited to 8%, a number to keep in mind when preparing this flap [82]. For restoring the skin and soft tissue, less-used alternative free flaps are the scapular and parascapular flaps [83] and the rectus abdominis free flap (the latter especially for very large defects) [84].

A parotid cancer that requires mandibular resection will typically result in a lateral mandibular defect with or without the condyle. Bony reconstruction generally only works well when the condyle and the temporomandibular joint can be preserved and then an osteocutaneous fibula flap can restore bone and limited skin defects. If needed the surgeon can provide additional soft tissue by including the soleus muscle [85]. Extensive defects that cannot be adequately addressed by a single flap may require using two free flaps [86, 87]. On the other hand, one should keep in mind that it may be indicated for medically unfit patients to minimize the surgical complexity and address the bony defect with only a soft tissue reconstruction (ALT, latissimus dorsi, or rectus abdominis). One then provides acceptable speech, mastication and frontal facial symmetry in rest but accepts malocclusion and deviation to the resected side on mouth opening [63].

4.2.4 Surgery for Cancer Metastatic to the Parotid

As already stated above under “Sect. 4.2.3.2”, the parotid gland is a lymphatic basin for melanoma and non-melanoma skin cancer (cutaneous squamous cell carcinoma, SCC; metastatic basal cell carcinoma; Merkel cell carcinoma) located on the conjunctiva, eyelid, cheek, forehead, temple, scalp, auricle and middle ear [88, 89], but also oropharyngeal cancer can drain to these lymph nodes.

The most frequent cancer metastasizing to the parotid is cutaneous SCC, with parotid metastasis (including the external jugular node) accounting for 75% of nodal metastases. Level II nodes are affected in two out of five patients with N+ disease [88]. This disease is increasingly encountered, and one important factor is the steadily increasing number of patients undergoing solid organ transplantation, needing immunosuppression.

Regarding the surgical approach, there is the same discussion that surrounds the need to perform a total parotidectomy in all of these patients. There is agreement on the prognostic value of finding metastatic lymph nodes in the deep lobe of the parotid in these instances [50], which heralds poor outcome (disease recurrence, distant metastasis and death from disease) for metastatic skin cancer to the parotid. A clear link was also described between not addressing these nodes and the observation of local recurrences in that area in one in five patients [49]. Parotid bed recurrences have even been reported in up to 44% [90–92]. Whereas performance of a deep lobe parotidectomy for parotid metastasis of non-melanoma skin cancer implied an excellent locoregional control in the series of the Mayo Clinic, overall oncological outcome and survival remained relatively low. Only one in three patients was free of distant metastasis at 5 years. The authors conclude that, in patients with a high risk of metastatic involvement of the deep parotid lymph nodes, such as those that have a skin malignancy that has clinically metastasized to the parotid, there is evidence that deep lobe parotid removal improves local parotid bed control [3, 50].

Important to note is that, once there is a surgical indication for a parotidectomy because of a parotid metastasis of cutaneous SCC, the neck also has to be addressed, even if clinically N0. This can be done surgically, and then selective neck dissection should address levels I–III for facial primaries, levels II–III for SCC of the anterior scalp and external ear and levels II–V for SCC of the posterior scalp and neck [93]. If pN0, the postoperative radiotherapy can be limited to the parotid bed. Alternatively both the parotid bed and the neck can be irradiated [94].

For parotid metastasis of melanoma, many authors perform a superficial parotidectomy [88], but in the series of the Mayo Clinic, the authors also performed a deep lobe parotidectomy, which implied an excellent local control. Again, overall oncological outcome and survival remained low: patients with parotid metastatic melanoma were either dead of disease or alive with distant metastasis at the end of follow-up (1/3 of patients) [3, 50]. Indeed, once there is obvious melanoma metastatic disease in the parotid, it is advisable to screen for distant metastatic disease using PET-CT scan and brain MRI [88].

4.2.5 Treatment of the Neck

4.2.5.1 The cN+ Neck

Clinically and/or radiologically apparent regional metastasis (cN+ disease) at presentation is reported in 14–29% of patients [8, 9, 42, 45] and involves most frequently levels II, III and IV [42] and requires a (modified) radical neck dissection, removing levels I to V, with radicality towards the non-lymphatic structures (nerve XI, jugular vein or sternocleidomastoid muscle) depending on proximity of the lymph node metastasis [95]. This old knowledge has recently been confirmed again in recent studies from the Memorial Sloan Kettering Cancer Center, where the rates of pN+ involvement in level I were 51.6%, in level II 77%, in level III 73%, in level IV 53% and finally 40% in level V [96], as well as from Korea, where rates of pN+ involvement in level I were 42.9%, in level II 90%, in level III 40%, in level IV 57.1% and still 42.9% in level V [97]. Besides the well-accepted prognostic value of clinical neck disease as such [7–9, 98], recent reports have focused on the independent negative prognostic significance of an increasing ratio of the number positive nodes over the total number of lymph nodes removed, the so-called lymph node density [99, 100].

As stated above, a significant proportion (53–65%) of patients with pN+ disease on neck dissection will also have metastatic deposits in the intraparotid lymph nodes [42, 43], and in this way it is logical and consequent that, when a neck dissection is needed for removal of cN+ disease, a deep lobe parotidectomy is performed too.

In pN+ patients, radiotherapy applied to the parotid and the ipsilateral neck doubles locoregional control and improves survival [71, 95, 101–103].

4.2.5.2 The cN0 Neck

The reported rates of pN+ disease in patients that are defined as cN0, based on clinical and high-quality radiological examination, vary widely. They range between 12% and 49%, and this derives from the high number of salivary gland cancer histotypes and grades within histotypes, each with a different tendency to regional metastasis [42, 43, 45, 102, 104–106].

In these patients with a cN0 neck at presentation, we usually solve this problem by looking at the presence of the risk factors for occult neck disease and deciding to treat the neck when the probability, based on the combined presence of different risk factors, exceeds the threshold of 15–20%. These risk factors predicting micrometastases are clinical factors such as age in the sixth decade, pain and seventh nerve function and local size and extension as reflected in T-classification, as well as histological factors such as histotype and grade, extraglandular extension and lymphatic invasion [42, 104, 105, 107, 108].

Histologies that have classically been associated with a high prevalence of cN0pN+ disease are high-grade mucoepidermoid carcinoma, salivary duct carcinoma, undifferentiated carcinoma, adenocarcinoma NOS and squamous cell carcinoma [42, 45, 109, 110]. Although until recently generally thought to have a low tendency to regional metastasis, parotid AdCC seems to have a high-grade subgroup

(AdCC-HGT) that implies a pN+ rate of up to 57% [111]. Generally considered as having a low rate of pN+ disease are acinic cell carcinoma (AcCC) and low-grade mucoepidermoid carcinoma, although series routinely doing an elective neck dissection on all patients also find higher than expected rates here [43, 45], and also in AcCC nowadays a high-grade subtype is defined that implies a higher risk [112, 113]. That said, also low-grade cancers and early-stage cancers can present with cN0pN+ disease [96, 104, 114].

When it is then decided to treat the neck, the first possible option is by elective neck surgery. Some groups propose a routine elective neck dissection for every patient with parotid carcinoma [45, 106]. Zbären et al. base this recommendation on their observation of a 22% occult rate in operated patients, who then show an improved 5-year locoregional control as compared to patients where the neck was merely observed. These findings have to be appreciated in the context that none of the patients in this series did receive radiotherapy [106, 115]. Stennert reports even a 45% occult rate in a series of patients who all underwent neck dissection [45]. A Brazilian series reported an occult metastasis rate of 37% that was predicted by T-classification, severe desmoplasia and histology (adenocarcinoma, undifferentiated carcinoma, high-grade MEC, SDC and SCC, together resulting in a 68% occult rate) [105].

The second option that has also been shown effective is elective radiotherapy [46, 47, 71, 102, 107, 108] in high-risk patients that end up in this category depending on definitive histopathology of the resected primary. This strategy is appealing because the indications for elective neck treatment concur with the indications for postoperative radiotherapy to the primary and also because many of the factors that imply high risk only become clear following pathological examination of the resected primary (exact histotype, exact grade, extraparenchymal extension, lymphovascular invasion). Indeed, pre- and perioperative typing of salivary carcinomas frequently proves very difficult (accuracy 51–62%) [95, 107, 116, 117]. Furthermore, radiotherapy may still be indicated a cN0 neck turns out to be pN+ [46–48, 71]. The answer as to which approach to the cN0 neck is the best one, elective neck surgery with—on indication—postoperative radiotherapy or immediate elective radiotherapy, can only reliably obtained by conducting a prospective randomized trial, which will be difficult to organize.

Alternative approaches that have been postulated to fine-tune the choice between the two modalities are (1) using preoperative USgFNAC of the neck and (2) using of perioperative frozen section [32, 118]. In our own policy, we perform—in preoperatively known malignancies with a cN0 neck—a standard selective level II dissection before doing the parotidectomy. By the time the parotidectomy is performed, frozen section analysis of the level II nodes is available. If frozen section reveals macrometastases, we consider the neck as cN+ and perform a modified neck dissection [7, 12]. Other authors have described "levels I and II node sampling" in high-risk patients [119].

The levels to address with either surgery or radiotherapy became clear by analysing elective neck dissection specimens. A pivotal study dates already from 1992 [42] and concludes that the neck levels to address are levels II, III and IV. Recent studies confirmed that in cN0 necks, disease is rather rarely found in levels I and V indeed [96, 108].

In our recent paper, we therefore made up an overview of three possible scenarios that can be encountered in the clinical reality in dealing with the cN0 neck in salivary gland cancer [2]:

First Scenario
Low risk of occult nodal disease (T1–T2, low-grade tumour, young patient): a wait-and-see policy can be defended [96], a level II dissection at the beginning of the procedure with frozen section can be performed [12] with extension to a comprehensive neck dissection in the rare occasion that disease is present or an elective neck dissection may be carried out [43, 45, 106, 114].

Second Scenario
Risk factors for occult disease discovered only at definitive histology (high grade and/or high stage): elective irradiation of the neck [47, 107].

Third Scenario
High risk of occult nodal disease preoperatively certain:

1. Elective neck dissection (II–IV or Ib–IV) and postoperative radiotherapy to the neck based on the histopathological findings in the resected primary and the END specimen [102].
2. Elective irradiation of the neck, especially if adjuvant radiotherapy for the primary tumour is already likely [5, 46, 47, 107].
3. Super-selective dissection of level II with extension to a comprehensive neck dissection when disease is present [12, 120]. One should consider also resecting level I and level V in some specific anatomical situations, like for a primary located more anteriorly where metastases to level I are more likely and like for a large tumour located in the parotid tail where there is increased risk of spread to level. If no disease is present, radiotherapy to the neck can be decided upon based on the definitive pathology report of the resected primary. Other authors dissect levels I–II [119] or levels I–III [121] neck dissection with frozen sections and conversion to comprehensive neck dissection in presence of occult nodal disease, but the rationale to dissect level I is doubtful given the low incidence of disease in level I as seen in the pivotal study of Armstrong et al. [42]. Furthermore, in this study, the few patients with a positive node in level I all had also positive level II nodes that would also have been detected if limiting the dissection for frozen section to level II. Recent studies confirmed a low rate of cN0pN+ in level I [96, 108].

4.2.6 Conclusion

Parotid carcinoma is a particularly demanding tumour for both patient and the multidisciplinary team trying to offer the best treatment. Every step in the management is complicated: the clinical assessment, the radiological evaluation, the histopathology, the ablative surgery and the realm of reconstructive options, the radiotherapy and the eventual chemotherapy, as well as the management of arising complications. Undoubtedly care for patients with this rare disease is best, when centralized in specialized tertiary referral centres.

References

1. Cracchiolo JR, Shaha AR. Parotidectomy for parotid cancer. Otolaryngol Clin N Am. 2016;49:415–24.
2. Lombardi D, McGurk M, Vander Poorten V, Guzzo M, Accorona R, Rampinelli V, Nicolai P. Surgical treatment of salivary malignant tumors. Oral Oncol. 2017;65:102–13.
3. Olsen KD, Moore EJ. Deep lobe parotidectomy: clinical rationale in the management of primary and metastatic cancer. Eur Arch Otorhinolaryngol. 2014;271:1181–5.
4. WHO classification of tumours of salivary glands. In: El-Naggar AK, John KC, Grandis JR, Takata T, Slootweg PJ, editors. WHO classification of head and neck tumours. Lyon: IARC; 2017. p. 160–84.
5. Frankenthaler RA, Luna MA, Lee SS, Ang KK, Byers RM, Guillamondegui OM, Wolf P, Goepfert H. Prognostic variables in parotid gland cancer. Arch Otolaryngol Head Neck Surg. 1991;117:1251–6.
6. Spiro RH. Management of malignant tumors of the salivary glands. Oncology (Williston Park). 1998;12:671–83.
7. Vander Poorten VLM, Balm AJM, Hilgers FJM, Tan IB, Loftus-Coll BM, Keus RB, van Leeuwen FE, Hart AAM. The development of a prognostic score for patients with parotid carcinoma. Cancer. 1999;85:2057–67.
8. Vander Poorten V, Hart A, Vauterin T, Jeunen G, Schoenaers J, Hamoir M, Balm A, Stennert E, Guntinas-Lichius O, Delaere P. Prognostic index for patients with parotid carcinoma: international external validation in a Belgian-German database. Cancer. 2009;115:540–50.
9. Vander Poorten VL, Hart AA, van der Laan BF, Baatenburg de Jong RJ, Manni JJ, Marres HA, Meeuwis CA, Lubsen H, Terhaard CH, Balm AJ. Prognostic index for patients with parotid carcinoma: external validation using the nationwide 1985–1994 Dutch head and neck oncology cooperative group database. Cancer. 2003;97:1453–63.
10. Zbaren P, Vander Poorten V, Witt RL, Woolgar JA, Shaha AR, Triantafyllou A, Takes RP, Rinaldo A, Ferlito A. Pleomorphic adenoma of the parotid: formal parotidectomy or limited surgery? Am J Surg. 2013;205:109–18.
11. UICC. Major salivary glands. In: Brierley JD, Gospodarowicz M, Wittekind C, editors. TNM classification of malignant tumours. Oxford: Wiley-Blackwell; 2017. p. 47–51.
12. Vander Poorten V, Bradley PJ, Takes RP, Rinaldo A, Woolgar JA, Ferlito A. Diagnosis and management of parotid carcinoma with a special focus on recent advances in molecular biology. Head Neck. 2012;34:429–40.
13. Spiro RH. Salivary neoplasms: overview of a 35-year experience with 2,807 patients. Head Neck. 1986;8:177–84.
14. Spiro RH, Armstrong J, Harrison L, Geller NL, Lin SY, Strong EW. Carcinoma of major salivary glands. Recent trends. Arch Otolaryngol Head Neck Surg. 1989;115:316–21.
15. Kane WJ, McCaffrey TV, Olsen KD, Lewis JE. Primary parotid malignancies. A clinical and pathologic review. Arch Otolaryngol Head Neck Surg. 1991;117:307–15.
16. Pedersen D, Overgaard J, Sogaard H, Elbrond O, Overgaard M. Malignant parotid tumors in 110 consecutive patients: treatment results and prognosis. Laryngoscope. 1992;102:1064–9.
17. Poulsen MG, Pratt GR, Kynaston B, Tripcony LB. Prognostic variables in malignant epithelial tumors of the parotid. Int J Radiat Oncol Biol Phys. 1992;23:327–32.
18. Renehan AG, Gleave EN, Slevin NJ, McGurk M. Clinico-pathological and treatment-related factors influencing survival in parotid cancer. Br J Cancer. 1999;80:1296–300.
19. Spiro IJ, Wang CC, Montgomery WW. Carcinoma of the parotid gland. Analysis of treatment results and patterns of failure after combined surgery and radiation therapy. Cancer. 1993;71:2699–705.

20. Therkildsen MH, Christensen M, Andersen LJ, Schiodt T, Hansen HS. Salivary gland carcinomas—prognostic factors. Acta Oncol. 1998;37:701–13.
21. Leverstein H, van der Wal JE, Tiwari RM, Tobi H, van der Waal I, Mehta DM, Snow GB. Malignant epithelial parotid gland tumours: analysis and results in 65 previously untreated patients. Br J Surg. 1998;85:1267–72.
22. Harbo G, Bundgaard T, Pedersen D, Sogaard H, Overgaard J. Prognostic indicators for malignant tumours of the parotid gland. Clin Otolaryngol. 2002;27:512–6.
23. Godballe C, Schultz JH, Krogdahl A, Moller-Grontved A, Johansen J. Parotid carcinoma: impact of clinical factors on prognosis in a histologically revised series. Laryngoscope. 2003;113:411–1417.
24. Mendenhall WM, Morris CG, Amdur RJ, Werning JW, Villaret DB. Radiotherapy alone or combined with surgery for salivary gland carcinoma. Cancer. 2005;103:2544–50.
25. Lima RA, Tavares MR, Dias FL, Kligerman J, Nascimento MF, Barbosa MM, Cernea CR, Soares JR, Santos IC, Salviano S. Clinical prognostic factors in malignant parotid gland tumors. Otolaryngol Head Neck Surg. 2005;133:702–8.
26. Bartels S, Talbot JM, Di Tomasso J, Everts EC, Andersen PE, Wax MK, Cohen JI. The relative value of fine-needle aspiration and imaging in the preoperative evaluation of parotid masses. Head Neck. 2000;22:781–6.
27. Yabuuchi H, Matsuo Y, Kamitani T, Setoguchi T, Okafuji T, Soeda H, Sakai S, Hatakenaka M, Nakashima T, Oda Y, Honda H. Parotid gland tumors: can addition of diffusion-weighted MR imaging to dynamic contrast-enhanced MR imaging improve diagnostic accuracy in characterization? Radiology. 2008;249:909–16.
28. Horiuchi C, Tsukuda M, Taguchi T, Ishiguro Y, Okudera K, Inoue T. Correlation between FDG-PET findings and GLUT1 expression in salivary gland pleomorphic adenomas. Ann Nucl Med. 2008;22:693–8.
29. Cohen EG, Patel SG, Lin O, Boyle JO, Kraus DH, Singh B, Wong RJ, Shah JP, Shaha AR. Fine-needle aspiration biopsy of salivary gland lesions in a selected patient population. Arch Otolaryngol Head Neck Surg. 2004;130:773–8.
30. Klijanienko J, Vielh P. Introduction. In: Klijanienko J, Vielh P, editors. Salivary gland tumours. Basel: Karger; 2000. p. 1–4.
31. Zbaren P, Guelat D, Loosli H, Stauffer E. Parotid tumors: fine-needle aspiration and/or frozen section. Otolaryngol Head Neck Surg. 2008;139:811–5.
32. Vander Poorten VLM, Balm AJM, Hilgers FJM. Management of cancer of the parotid gland. Curr Opin Otolaryngol Head Neck Surg. 2002;10:134–44.
33. Brennan PA, Davies B, Poller D, Mead Z, Bayne D, Puxeddu R, Oeppen RS. Fine needle aspiration cytology (FNAC) of salivary gland tumours: repeat aspiration provides further information in cases with an unclear initial cytological diagnosis. Br J Oral Maxillofac Surg. 2010;48:26–9.
34. Haldar S, Mandalia U, Skelton E, Chow V, Turner SS, Ramesar K, Tighe D, Williams M, Howlett D. Diagnostic investigation of parotid neoplasms: a 16-year experience of freehand fine needle aspiration cytology and ultrasound-guided core needle biopsy. Int J Oral Maxillofac Surg. 2015;44:151–7.
35. Howlett DC, Skelton E, Moody AB. Establishing an accurate diagnosis of a parotid lump: evaluation of the current biopsy methods - fine needle aspiration cytology, ultrasound-guided core biopsy, and intraoperative frozen section. Br J Oral Maxillofac Surg. 2015;53:580–3.
36. Barnes L, Eveson JW, Reichart P, Sidranski P. Pathology and genetics of head and neck tumours. World Health classification of tumours. Lyon: IARC Press; 2005. p. 210.
37. Quer M, Guntinas-Lichius O, Marchal F, Vander Poorten V, Chevalier D, Leon X, Eisele D, Dulguerov P. Classification of parotidectomies: a proposal of the European Salivary Gland Society. Eur Arch Otorhinolaryngol. 2016;273:3307–12.
38. Lim YC, Lee SY, Kim K, Lee JS, Koo BS, Shin HA, Choi EC. Conservative parotidectomy for the treatment of parotid cancers. Oral Oncol. 2005;41:1021–7.
39. Garatea-Crelgo J, Gay-Escoda C, Bermejo B, Buenechea-Imaz R. Morphological study of the parotid lymph nodes. J Craniomaxillofac Surg. 1993;21:207–9.

40. McKean ME, Lee K, McGregor IA. The distribution of lymph nodes in and around the parotid gland: an anatomical study. Br J Plast Surg. 1985;38:1–5.
41. Pisani P, Ramponi A, Pia F. The deep parotid lymph nodes: an anatomical and oncological study. J Laryngol Otol. 1996;110:148–50.
42. Armstrong JG, Harrison LB, Thaler HT, Friedlander-Klar H, Fass DE, Zelefsky MJ, Shah JP, Strong EW, Spiro RH. The indications for elective treatment of the neck in cancer of the major salivary glands. Cancer. 1992;69:615–9.
43. Klussmann JP, Ponert T, Mueller RP, Dienes HP, Guntinas-Lichius O. Patterns of lymph node spread and its influence on outcome in resectable parotid cancer. Eur J Surg Oncol. 2008;34:932–7.
44. Boahene DK, Olsen KD, Lewis JE, Pinheiro AD, Pankratz VS, Bagniewski SM. Mucoepidermoid carcinoma of the parotid gland: the Mayo clinic experience. Arch Otolaryngol Head Neck Surg. 2004;130:849–56.
45. Stennert E, Kisner D, Jungehuelsing M, Guntinas-Lichius O, Schroder U, Eckel HE, Klussmann JP. High incidence of lymph node metastasis in major salivary gland cancer. Arch Otolaryngol Head Neck Surg. 2003;129:720–3.
46. Chen AM, Garcia J, Lee NY, Bucci MK, Eisele DW. Patterns of nodal relapse after surgery and postoperative radiation therapy for carcinomas of the major and minor salivary glands: what is the role of elective neck irradiation? Int J Radiat Oncol Biol Phys. 2007;67:988–94.
47. Herman MP, Werning JW, Morris CG, Kirwan JM, Amdur RJ, Mendenhall WM. Elective neck management for high-grade salivary gland carcinoma. Am J Otolaryngol. 2013;34:205–8.
48. Kirkbride P, Liu FF, O'Sullivan B, Payne D, Warde P, Gullane P, Pintilie M, Keane TJ, Cummings B. Outcome of curative management of malignant tumours of the parotid gland. J Otolaryngol. 2001;30:271–9.
49. O'Brien CJ, McNeil EB, McMahon JD, Pathak I, Lauer CS, Jackson MA. Significance of clinical stage, extent of surgery, and pathologic findings in metastatic cutaneous squamous carcinoma of the parotid gland. Head Neck. 2002;24:417–22.
50. Thom JJ, Moore EJ, Price DL, Kasperbauer JL, Starkman SJ, Olsen KD. The role of total parotidectomy for metastatic cutaneous squamous cell carcinoma and malignant melanoma. JAMA Otolaryngol Head Neck Surg. 2014;140:548–54.
51. Chiesa F, Giugliano G, Ostuni A. Is it necessary to resect the facial nerve in all cases of parotid cancer? In: Mc Gurk M, Combes J, editors. Controversies in the management of salivary gland disease. Oxford: Oxford University Press; 2013. p. 203–9.
52. Charabi S, Balle V, Charabi B, Nielsen P, Thomsen J. Surgical outcome in malignant parotid tumours. Acta Otolaryngol Suppl. 2000;120(543):251–3.
53. O'Brien CJ, Adams JR. Surgical management of the facial nerve in the presence of malignancy about the face. Curr Opin Otolaryngol Head Neck Surg. 2001;9:90–4.
54. Guntinas-Lichius O, Streppel M, Stennert E. Postoperative functional evaluation of different reanimation techniques for facial nerve repair. Am J Surg. 2006;191:61–7.
55. Coca-Pelaz A, Rodrigo JP, Bradley PJ, Vander Poorten V, Triantafyllou A, Hunt JL, Strojan P, Rinaldo A, Haigentz M Jr, Takes RP, Mondin V, Teymoortash A, Thompson LD, Ferlito A. Adenoid cystic carcinoma of the head and neck - an update. Oral Oncol. 2015;51:652–61.
56. Stennert E. Facial nerve reconstruction. In: Myers EN, Ferris RL, editors. Salivary gland disorders. Berlin: Springer; 2007. p. 407–19.
57. Brown PD, Eshleman JS, Foote RL, Strome SE. An analysis of facial nerve function in irradiated and unirradiated facial nerve grafts. Int J Radiat Oncol Biol Phys. 2000;48:737–43.
58. Reddy PG, Arden RL, Mathog RH. Facial nerve rehabilitation after radical parotidectomy. Laryngoscope. 1999;109:894–9.
59. Guntinas-Lichius O. The facial nerve in the presence of a head and neck neoplasm: assessment and outcome after surgical management. Curr Opin Otolaryngol Head Neck Surg. 2004;12:133–41.
60. Lee MC, Kim DH, Jeon YR, Rah DK, Lew DH, Choi EC, Lee WJ. Functional outcomes of multiple sural nerve grafts for facial nerve defects after tumor-ablative surgery. Arch Plast Surg. 2015;42:461–8.

61. House JW, Brackmann DE. Facial nerve grading system. Otolaryngol Head Neck Surg. 1985;93:46–147.
62. Hontanilla B, Qiu SS, Marre D. Effect of postoperative brachytherapy and external beam radiotherapy on functional outcomes of immediate facial nerve repair after radical parotidectomy. Head Neck. 2014;36:113–9.
63. Ch'ng S, Ashford BG, Gao K, McGuinness J, Clark JR. Reconstruction of post-radical parotidectomy defects. Plast Reconstr Surg. 2012;129:275e–87e.
64. May M, Sobol SM, Mester SJ. Hypoglossal-facial nerve interpositional-jump graft for facial reanimation without tongue atrophy. Otolaryngol Head Neck Surg. 1991;104:818–25.
65. Volk GF, Pantel M, Streppel M, Guntinas-Lichius O. Reconstruction of complex peripheral facial nerve defects by a combined approach using facial nerve interpositional graft and hypoglossal-facial jump nerve suture. Laryngoscope. 2011;121:2402–5.
66. Hadlock TA, Greenfield LJ, Wernick-Robinson M, Cheney ML. Multimodality approach to management of the paralyzed face. Laryngoscope. 2006;116:1385–9.
67. Sobol SM, Alward PD. Early gold weight lid implant for rehabilitation of faulty eyelid closure with facial paralysis: an alternative to tarsorrhaphy. Head Neck. 1990;12:149–53.
68. Rose EH. Autogenous fascia lata grafts: clinical applications in reanimation of the totally or partially paralyzed face. Plast Reconstr Surg. 2005;116:20–32.
69. Tan ST. Anterior belly of digastric muscle transfer: a useful technique in head and neck surgery. Head Neck. 2002;24:947–54.
70. Vander Poorten V, Hunt J, Bradley PJ, Haigentz M Jr, Rinaldo A, Mendenhall WM, Suarez C, Silver C, Takes RP, Ferlito A. Recent trends in the management of minor salivary gland carcinoma. Head Neck. 2014;36:444–55.
71. Terhaard CH, Lubsen H, Rasch CR, Levendag PC, Kaanders HH, Tjho-Heslinga RE, van Den Ende PL, Burlage F. The role of radiotherapy in the treatment of malignant salivary gland tumors. Int J Radiat Oncol Biol Phys. 2005;61:103–11.
72. Revenaugh PC, Knott PD, Scharpf J, Fritz MA. Simultaneous anterolateral thigh flap and temporalis tendon transfer to optimize facial form and function after radical parotidectomy. Arch Facial Plast Surg. 2012;14:104–9.
73. Liu FY, Xu ZF, Li P, Sun CF, Li RW, Ge SF, Li JL, Huang SH, Tan X. The versatile application of cervicofacial and cervicothoracic rotation flaps in head and neck surgery. World J Surg Oncol. 2011;9:135.
74. Moore BA, Wine T, Netterville JL. Cervicofacial and cervicothoracic rotation flaps in head and neck reconstruction. Head Neck. 2005;27:1092–101.
75. Behan FC, Lo CH, Sizeland A, Pham T, Findlay M. Keystone island flap reconstruction of parotid defects. Plast Reconstr Surg. 2012;130:36e–41e.
76. Emerick KS, Herr MW, Lin DT, Santos F, Deschler DG. Supraclavicular artery island flap for reconstruction of complex parotidectomy, lateral skull base, and total auriculectomy defects. JAMA Otolaryngol Head Neck Surg. 2014;140:861–6.
77. Epps MT, Cannon CL, Wright MJ, Chaffin AE, Newsome RE, Friedlander PL, Chiu ES. Aesthetic restoration of parotidectomy contour deformity using the supraclavicular artery island flap. Plast Reconstr Surg. 2011;127:1925–31.
78. Barton FE Jr, Spicer TE, Byrd HS. Head and neck reconstruction with the latissimus dorsi myocutaneous flap: anatomic observations and report of 60 cases. Plast Reconstr Surg. 1983;71:199–204.
79. Ahmad QG, Navadgi S, Agarwal R, Kanhere H, Shetty KP, Prasad R. Bipaddle pectoralis major myocutaneous flap in reconstructing full thickness defects of cheek: a review of 47 cases. J Plast Reconstr Aesthet Surg. 2006;59:166–73.
80. Elliott RM, Weinstein GS, Low DW, Wu LC. Reconstruction of complex total parotidectomy defects using the free anterolateral thigh flap: a classification system and algorithm. Ann Plast Surg. 2011;66:429–37.
81. Wong CH, Wei FC. Anterolateral thigh flap. Head Neck. 2010;32:529–40.
82. Higgins KM, Erovic BM, Ravi A, Yeung R, Lee JW, Yao C, Enepekides DJ. Volumetric changes of the anterolateral thigh free flap following adjuvant radiotherapy in total parotidectomy reconstruction. Laryngoscope. 2012;122:767–72.

83. Upton J, Albin RE, Mulliken JB, Murray JE. The use of scapular and parascapular flaps for cheek reconstruction. Plast Reconstr Surg. 1992;90:959–71.
84. Deleyiannis FW, Rogers C, Lee E, Russavage J, Gastman B, Dunklebarger J, Lai S, Ferris R, Myers EN, Johnson J. Reconstruction of the lateral mandibulectomy defect: management based on prognosis and location and volume of soft tissue resection. Laryngoscope. 2006;116:2071–80.
85. Jones NF, Vogelin E, Markowitz BL, Watson JP. Reconstruction of composite through-and-through mandibular defects with a double-skin paddle fibular osteocutaneous flap. Plast Reconstr Surg. 2003;112:758–65.
86. Wallace CG, Tsao CK, Wei FC. Role of multiple free flaps in head and neck reconstruction. Curr Opin Otolaryngol Head Neck Surg. 2014;22:140–6.
87. Wei FC, Yazar S, Lin CH, Cheng MH, Tsao CK, Chiang YC. Double free flaps in head and neck reconstruction. Clin Plast Surg. 2005;32(3):303–8.
88. Clark J, Wang S. Metastatic cancer to the parotid. Adv Otorhinolaryngol. 2016;78:95–103.
89. Vauterin TJ, Veness MJ, Morgan GJ, Poulsen MG, O'Brien CJ. Patterns of lymph node spread of cutaneous squamous cell carcinoma of the head and neck. Head Neck. 2006;28:785–91.
90. Andruchow JL, Veness MJ, Morgan GJ, Gao K, Clifford A, Shannon KF, Poulsen M, Kenny L, Palme CE, Gullane P, Morris C, Mendenhall WM, Patel KN, Shah JP, O'Brien CJ. Implications for clinical staging of metastatic cutaneous squamous carcinoma of the head and neck based on a multicenter study of treatment outcomes. Cancer. 2006;106:1078–83.
91. Hinerman RW, Indelicato DJ, Amdur RJ, Morris CG, Werning JW, Vaysberg M, Kirwan J, Mendenhall WM. Cutaneous squamous cell carcinoma metastatic to parotid-area lymph nodes. Laryngoscope. 2008;118:1989–96.
92. Palme CE, O'Brien CJ, Veness MJ, McNeil EB, Bron LP, Morgan GJ. Extent of parotid disease influences outcome in patients with metastatic cutaneous squamous cell carcinoma. Arch Otolaryngol Head Neck Surg. 2003;129:750–3.
93. Ebrahimi A, Moncrieff MD, Clark JR, Shannon KF, Gao K, Milross CG, O'Brien CJ. Predicting the pattern of regional metastases from cutaneous squamous cell carcinoma of the head and neck based on location of the primary. Head Neck. 2010;32:1288–94.
94. Veness MJ, Morgan GJ, Palme CE, Gebski V. Surgery and adjuvant radiotherapy in patients with cutaneous head and neck squamous cell carcinoma metastatic to lymph nodes: combined treatment should be considered best practice. Laryngoscope. 2005;115:870–5.
95. Medina JE. Neck dissection in the treatment of cancer of major salivary glands. Otolaryngol Clin N Am. 1998;31:815–22.
96. Ali S, Palmer FL, Dilorenzo M, Shah JP, Patel SG, Ganly I. Treatment of the neck in carcinoma of the parotid gland. Ann Surg Oncol. 2014;21:3042–8.
97. Yoo SH, Roh JL, Kim SO, Cho KJ, Choi SH, Nam SY, Kim SY. Patterns and treatment of neck metastases in patients with salivary gland cancers. J Surg Oncol. 2015;111:1000–6.
98. Ali S, Palmer FL, Yu C, Dilorenzo M, Shah JP, Kattan MW, Patel SG, Ganly I. A predictive nomogram for recurrence of carcinoma of the major salivary glands. JAMA Otolaryngol Head Neck Surg. 2013;139:698–705.
99. Hong HR, Roh JL, Cho KJ, Choi SH, Nam SY, Kim SY. Prognostic value of lymph node density in high-grade salivary gland cancers. J Surg Oncol. 2015;111:784–9.
100. Suzuki H, Hanai N, Hirakawa H, Nishikawa D, Hasegawa Y. Lymph node density is a prognostic factor in patients with major salivary gland carcinoma. Oncol Lett. 2015;10:3523–8.
101. Armstrong JG, Harrison LB, Spiro RH, Fass DE, Strong EW, Fuks ZY. Malignant tumors of major salivary gland origin. A matched-pair analysis of the role of combined surgery and postoperative radiotherapy. Arch Otolaryngol Head Neck Surg. 1990;116:290–3.
102. Kelley DJ, Spiro RH. Management of the neck in parotid carcinoma. Am J Surg. 1996;172:695–7.
103. Terhaard CH, Lubsen H, Van Der Tweel I, Hilgers FJ, Eijkenboom WM, Marres HA, Tjho-Heslinga RE, de Jong JM, Roodenburg JL. Salivary gland carcinoma: independent prognostic factors for locoregional control, distant metastases, and overall survival: results of the Dutch head and neck oncology cooperative group. Head Neck. 2004;26:681–93.

104. Kawata R, Koutetsu L, Yoshimura K, Nishikawa S, Takenaka H. Indication for elective neck dissection for N0 carcinoma of the parotid gland: a single institution's 20-year experience. Acta Otolaryngol. 2010;130:286–92.
105. Regis de Brito Santos I, Kowalski LP, Cavalcante de Araujo V, Flavia Logullo A, Magrin J. Multivariate analysis of risk factors for neck metastases in surgically treated parotid carcinomas. Arch Otolaryngol Head Neck Surg. 2001;127:56–60.
106. Zbaren P, Schupbach J, Nuyens M, Stauffer E. Elective neck dissection versus observation in primary parotid carcinoma. Otolaryngol Head Neck Surg. 2005;132:387–91.
107. Frankenthaler RA, Byers RM, Luna MA, Callender DL, Wolf P, Goepfert H. Predicting occult lymph node metastasis in parotid cancer. Arch Otolaryngol Head Neck Surg. 1993;119:517–20.
108. Lau VH, Aouad R, Farwell DG, Donald PJ, Chen AM. Patterns of nodal involvement for clinically N0 salivary gland carcinoma: refining the role of elective neck irradiation. Head Neck. 2014;36:1435–9.
109. Bhattacharyya N, Fried MP. Nodal metastasis in major salivary gland cancer: predictive factors and effects on survival. Arch Otolaryngol Head Neck Surg. 2002;128:904–8.
110. Spitz MR, Batsakis JG. Major salivary gland carcinoma. Descriptive epidemiology and survival of 498 patients. Arch Otolaryngol. 1984;110:45–9.
111. Hellquist H, Skalova A, Barnes L, Cardesa A, Thompson LD, Triantafyllou A, Williams MD, Devaney KO, Gnepp DR, Bishop JA, Wenig BM, Suarez C, Rodrigo JP, Coca-Pelaz A, Strojan P, Shah JP, Hamoir M, Bradley PJ, Silver CE, Slootweg PJ, Vander Poorten V, Teymoortash A, Medina JE, Robbins KT, Pitman KT, Kowalski LP, de BR, Mendenhall WM, Eloy JA, Takes RP, Rinaldo A, Ferlito A. Cervical lymph node metastasis in high-grade transformation of head and neck adenoid cystic carcinoma: a collective international review. Adv Ther. 2016;33:357–68.
112. Gomez DR, Katabi N, Zhung J, Wolden SL, Zelefsky MJ, Kraus DH, Shah JP, Wong RJ, Ghossein RA, Lee NY. Clinical and pathologic prognostic features in acinic cell carcinoma of the parotid gland. Cancer. 2009;115:2128–37.
113. Vander Poorten V, Triantafyllou A, Thompson LD, Bishop J, Hauben E, Hunt J, Skalova A, Stenman G, Takes RP, Gnepp DR, Hellquist H, Wenig B, Bell D, Rinaldo A, Ferlito A. Salivary acinic cell carcinoma: reappraisal and update. Eur Arch Otorhinolaryngol. 2016;273:3511–31.
114. Stenner M, Molls C, Luers JC, Beutner D, Klussmann JP, Huettenbrink KB. Occurrence of lymph node metastasis in early-stage parotid gland cancer. Eur Arch Otorhinolaryngol. 2012;269:643–8.
115. Zbaren P, Schupbach J, Nuyens M, Stauffer E, Greiner R, Hausler R. Carcinoma of the parotid gland. Am J Surg. 2003;186:57–62.
116. Eisele DW, Kleinberg LR, O'Malley BB. Management of malignant salivary gland tumors. In: Harrison LB, Sessions RB, Hong KH, editors. Head and neck cancer. A multidisciplinary approach. Philadelphia: Lippincott-Raven; 1999. p. 721–48.
117. Westra WH. The surgical pathology of salivary gland neoplasms. Otolaryngol Clin N Am. 1999;32:919–43.
118. Zbaren P, Nuyens M, Loosli H, Stauffer E. Diagnostic accuracy of fine-needle aspiration cytology and frozen section in primary parotid carcinoma. Cancer. 2004;100:1876–83.
119. Korkmaz H, Yoo GH, Du W, Hocwald E, Otero-Garcia JE, Volkan AN, Shibuya T, Jacobs JR. Predictors of nodal metastasis in salivary gland cancer. J Surg Oncol. 2002;80:186–9.
120. Medina J, Zbaren P, Bradley PJ. Management of regional metastases of malignant salivary gland neoplasms. Adv Otorhinolaryngol. 2016;78:132–40.
121. Nobis CP, Rohleder NH, Wolff KD, Wagenpfeil S, Scherer EQ, Kesting MR. Head and neck salivary gland carcinomas—elective neck dissection, yes or no? J Oral Maxillofac Surg. 2014;72:205–10.

Surgery for Parapharyngeal Tumors

5

Orlando Guntinas-Lichius

5.1 Introduction

Parapharyngeal tumors are located in the parapharyngeal space. Most parapharyngeal tumors are benign and for a long time asymptomatic. Malignant tumors are rarely considered, which may delay making the correct diagnosis. Salivary gland cancer is rare but the most frequent malignant tumor in the parapharyngeal space. It is important to understand the anatomy of the parapharyngeal space in order to understand why different types of tumors are located in different parts of the parapharyngeal space. Furthermore, the topography helps to realize the advantages and limitations of the different surgical approaches. The most characteristic feature is that the tumor may be asymptomatic for a long time. Parapharyngeal salivary gland cancer normally exceeds already the parapharyngeal space when it presents unspecific symptoms, most of all as a cervical or intraoral mass. The necessary preoperative diagnostics including cross-sectional imaging and the important role of fine-needle aspiration cytology are presented. The main focus of this chapter is on the surgical approaches to the parapharyngeal space in case of salivary gland cancer. The transcervical route is the cornerstone of all surgical approaches and is with all its important modifications at the center of attention.

5.2 Anatomy of the Parapharyngeal Space

The parapharyngeal space is located in the upper cervical region reaching from the inferior surface of the temporal bone to the hyoid (Fig. 5.1). The parapharyngeal space is a virtual inverted pyramidal-shaped space. More precisely, its superior

O. Guntinas-Lichius (✉)
Department of Otorhinolaryngology, Jena University Hospital, Jena, Germany
e-mail: orlando.guntinas@med.uni-jena.de

© Springer Nature Switzerland AG 2019

L. Licitra, L. D. Locati (eds.), *Salivary Gland Cancer*,
https://doi.org/10.1007/978-3-030-02958-6_5

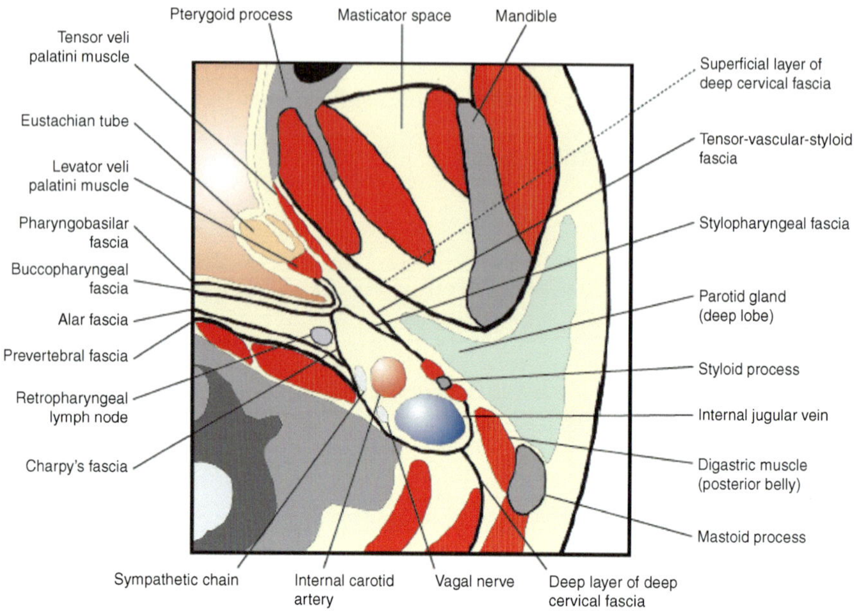

Fig. 5.1 Topographical anatomy of the parapharyngeal space in the axial plane, including the different fascial layers at this level. From: [1]

border is an area of the temporal and sphenoid bones including the carotid canal, the jugular foramen, and the hypoglossal foramen. The superior border ends laterally at the fascia covering the medial pterygoid muscle and medially at the attachment of the pharyngobasilar fascia and posteriorly at the prevertebral fascia. The relevant structures of the inferior boundary are the greater horn of the hyoid, the facial attachments of the posterior belly of the digastric muscle, and the sheath of the submandibular gland. The prevertebral fascia is the posterior boundary along its entire length. Its medial limit is formed by the pharyngobasilar fascia overlying the superior constrictor muscle. The tonsil also lies directly medial to the parapharyngeal space. Important lateral landmarks are the ramus of the mandible, the fascia of the medial pterygoid muscle, the retromandibular portion of the deep lobe of the parotid gland, and most inferiorly the fascia overlying the posterior belly of the digastric muscle. Finally, the pterygomandibular raphe and the submandibular space form the anterior border of the parapharyngeal space.

The parapharyngeal space has two compartments: the anterior muscular compartment (also known as the true parapharyngeal space or prestyloid space) and the posterior neurovascular compartment (formerly retrostyloid or poststyloid space). Most of the anterior compartment is covered by musculature. It contains fat and parotid tissue. It also contains the inferior alveolar, lingual, and auriculotemporal nerves as well as the maxillary artery. Therefore, all primary salivary

Table 5.1 Comparison of the anterior and posterior compartment of the parapharyngeal space

	Anterior compartment (prestyloid)	Posterior compartment (poststyloid)
Anatomic structures	Deep lobe of parotid gland, minor salivary glands, lymph nodes, and parapharyngeal fat	Carotid artery, jugular vein, cranial nerves IX, X, XI, and XII, lymph nodes, cervical sympathetic chain and glomus tissue
Tumors	Salivary gland tumors, lymphomas, and lipomas	Paragangliomas, nerve sheath tumors, lymphomas, connective tissue tumors, and ganglion tumors

gland tumors within the parapharyngeal space originate from the anterior compartment (Table 5.1). Other tumors of the anterior compartment are lipomas and rarely neurogenic tumors.

All primary malignant salivary gland tumors within the parapharyngeal space originate from the anterior compartment of the parapharyngeal space.

5.3 Types of Tumors and Epidemiology

Parapharyngeal tumors are rare. About 0.5–0.8% of all head and neck tumors are parapharyngeal tumors. About 50–77% of the tumors are salivary gland tumors, and pleomorphic adenoma is the most frequent histology [2–4]. Salivary gland tumors can arise from the deep lobe of the parotid gland or from a minor salivary gland. Conversely, this does not mean that all deep lobe parotid tumors are parapharyngeal space tumors. Due to the tumor size at the time of diagnosis it is most often not possible to clarify the origin. For the differential diagnosis of malignant salivary gland cancer in the parapharyngeal space, it is important to realize that about two thirds of the parapharyngeal salivary gland tumors are benign tumors and one third are malignant salivary gland tumors. Neurogenic tumors are the second most entity with up to 25% of all cases. Paragangliomas account for about 15% of the cases.

About two thirds of the parapharyngeal salivary gland tumors are benign tumors and one third are malignant salivary gland tumors.

All types of salivary gland cancer can also occur as parapharyngeal tumors. Due to casuistic reports, the most frequent histological subtypes in the parapharyngeal space are adenoid cystic carcinoma and mucoepidermoid carcinoma. Squamous cell carcinoma, carcinoma ex pleomorphic adenoma, adenocarcinoma, or myoepithelial carcinoma is much rarer [4]. Hence, the distribution of histological subtypes of malignant salivary gland tumors is not different to other regions like parotid or submandibular gland cancer. Other malignant tumors than salivary glands are very rare. Unspecified malignant peripheral nerve sheath tumors, malignant paraganglioma, different types of sarcoma, lymphomas, undifferentiated carcinoma, and metastasis of other primary origin have been found casuistically.

5.4 Symptoms

Like salivary gland cancer at other locations, most tumors may behave like benign tumors for long time. Due to their location, parapharyngeal tumors can grow even to a gigantic size without causing any symptoms. Hence, when symptomatic, parapharyngeal salivary gland cancer already exceeds the parapharyngeal space. All symptoms are unspecific. The most frequent presenting symptom is a cervical or intraoral mass in about half of the patients (Fig. 5.2). The tumor mass may put pressure onto the pharynx, and therefore lead to dysphagia and trismus. Compression of the eustachian tube leads to hearing loss. Pain, facial weakness or facial palsy, dysphonia, and Horner syndrome as signs of neural invasion are indirect but nevertheless unspecific signs of malignancy.

Even malignant salivary gland tumors of the parapharyngeal space are asymptomatic for a long time or the symptoms are unspecific. Pain, trismus, dysphagia, and cranial nerve dysfunction are already symptoms of a larger, advanced tumor.

5.5 Preoperative Diagnostics

A very important part of the clinical examination is the palpation. Parapharyngeal tumors are usually only palpable as a neck lump when the mass is at least larger than 2.5 cm [6]. Bimanual palpation of the tumor is important to assess size and mobility. It might be helpful during bimanual palpation to place the intraoral finger against the

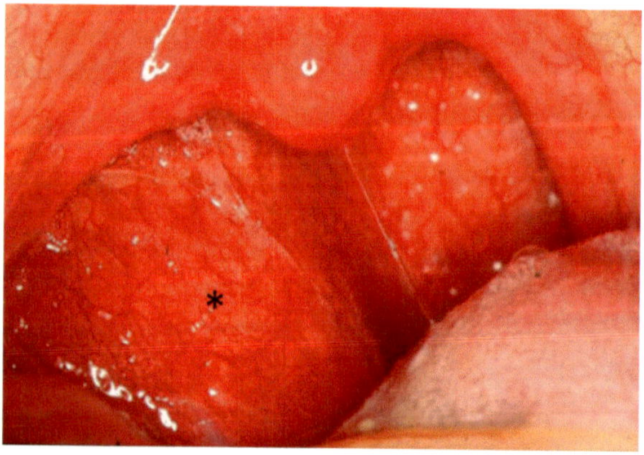

Fig. 5.2 Parapharyngeal salivary gland tumor presenting as intraoral mass (*asterisks*) with protrusion of the lateral pharyngeal wall. From: [5]

tonsil or in the tonsillar fossa if the patient is tonsillectomized. Advanced salivary gland cancer may present with limited mobility and fixation. Lesions of the anterior compartment rather displace the tonsil than lesions of the posterior compartment. The medial enlargement results in an asymmetric intraoral swelling and is sometimes discovered accidently by a dentist. The intraoral mass is typically smooth and not ulcerated for a long time. Only a very advanced parapharyngeal salivary gland cancer shows typical intraoral cancerous ulceration. The inferior pole of the tumor may be palpable as a mass in the angle of the mandible. If a parotid mass and an intraoral mass in the tonsillar fossa can be palpated, this is a sign of a dumbbell-shaped deep lobe parotid tumor and not a sign of a parapharyngeal tumor in the narrower sense.

A negative ultrasound of the neck does not rule out a parapharyngeal tumor. Cross-sectional imaging with CT or MRI scan is necessary to define the relationship of the tumor to other structures in the parapharyngeal space and adjacent structures (Fig. 5.3). As the salivary gland cancer originates from the anterior compartment, it displaces the internal carotid artery posteriorly (Fig. 5.4). In case of salivary gland cancer an angiography is normally not required. An angiography might only be helpful if the differential diagnosis of an angioma or a neuroectodermal tumor has to be ruled out. If the parapharyngeal salivary gland cancer arose from a minor salivary gland, a fat plane between the parotid and the tumor might be maintained in smaller tumors.

If a pathologist experienced in salivary gland cytology is available, transcervical fine-needle aspiration cytology (FNAC) is ideal to confirm or rule out salivary gland cancer. Ultrasound-guidance improves the accuracy if the tumor can be visualized by ultrasound. CT guidance is an alternative, but rarely performed for parapharyngeal

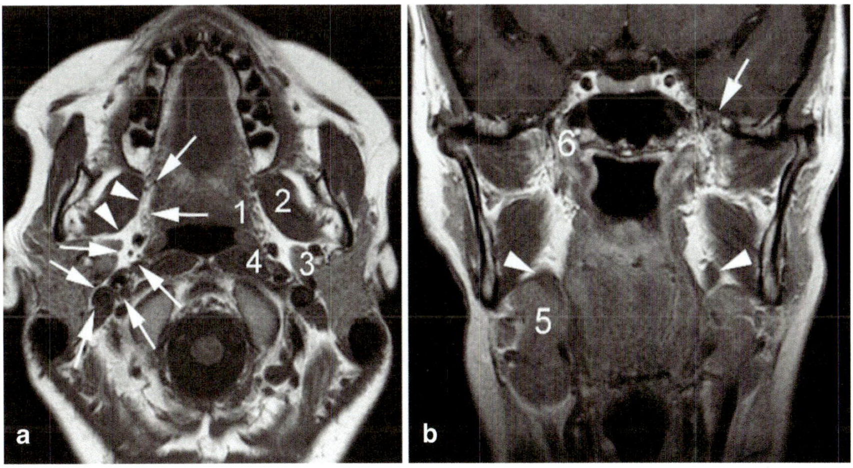

Fig. 5.3 Axial T1-weighted spin-echo image (**a**) at the level of the soft palate. The boundaries of the parapharyngeal space (PPS) (including prestyloid and retrostyloid compartment) are indicated by *arrows* and *arrowheads* on the right. On the left, the adjacent spaces are labeled: 1, pharyngeal mucosal space; 2, masticator space; 3, parotid space; 4, retropharyngeal/prevertebral space. (**b**) Coronal T1-weighted spin-echo images through prestyloid compartment of the PPS. Inferiorly, this space is closed by the submandibular gland (5), while superiorly, it reaches the skull base (6). The foramen ovale (*arrow*), through which the mandibular nerve passes, communicates with the masticator space. The styloglossal muscles run through the PPS (*arrowheads*). From [1]

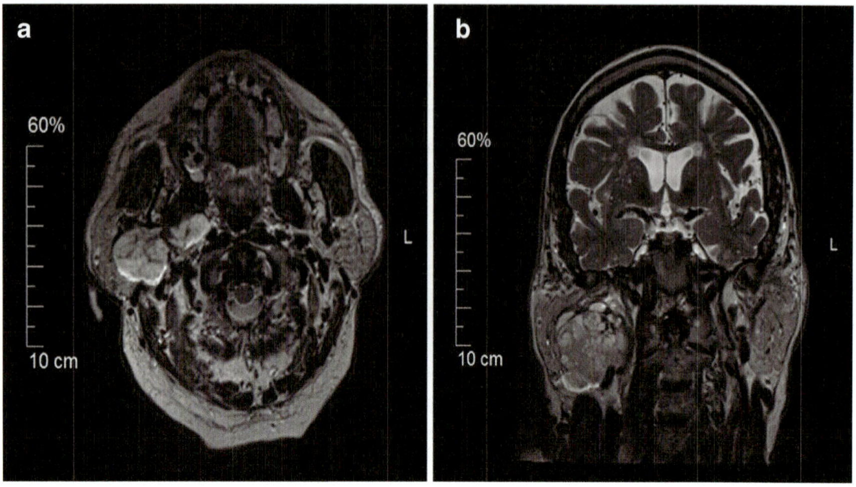

Fig. 5.4 Axial (**a**) and coronal (**b**) MRI showing a large mucoepidermoid cancer of the parapharyngeal space on the right side

tumors. If the mass is palpable transorally in the tonsillar fossa, a transoral FNAC is much easier. Core-needle biopsy becomes more popular as an alternative to FNAC, as standard histology can be performed on the core samples. Although core-needle biopsy is as safe as FNAC, still it is a matter of debate [7, 8].

It is recommended to use cross-sectional imaging with CT or MRI to define the relationship of the tumor to other structures of the parapharyngeal and adjacent structures. Transcervical fine-needle aspiration cytology (FNAC) is recommended to confirm or rule out salivary gland cancer.

Of course, if the patient has a preoperative facial palsy due to tumor infiltration, facial nerve diagnostics is mandatory to plan rehabilitation of the facial nerve [9]. Patients with parapharyngeal salivary gland cancer need a standard tumor staging as other salivary gland cancer patients including complete head and neck examination, CT/MRI imaging of the neck and CT of the thorax, if clinically indicated in advanced cancer (NCCI guidelines Version 1.2016).

5.6 Operative Setting/Intraoperative Neuromonitoring

Nasotracheal intubation and muscle relaxation are important to improve the visualization of the surgical field independent from the approach chosen. Intraoperative neuromonitoring is also recommended especially for the assessment of facial nerve and vagus nerve function. Additionally, monitoring of other cranial nerves like the glossopharyngeal, accessory, and hypoglossus nerve is feasible [10]. Intraoperative neuromonitoring is most important to have an additional tool to protect the facial nerve. Especially, when a parotid-sparing approach is used, facial neuromonitoring is the only way to get information on the facial nerve without surgical identification of the nerve. Finally, even with the widest approach, the parapharyngeal space can have hidden corners. This is especially hindering when confronted with a large tumor. Most important is to understand the relation of the tumor to the internal carotid artery. Patients should be considered at high risk of internal carotid artery injury if lesion surrounds the vessel for more than half of its circumference; if there is evidence of stenosis or irregularity of the vessel wall [11]. If the internal carotid artery is involved, subadventitial dissection, i.e. the separation of the muscular from the adventitial layer of the vessel, might be possible in individual cases [11]. In high risk patients, preoperative internal carotid artery endovascular stenting and/or permanent balloon occlusion is also an option [12]. Intraoperative Doppler imaging can help to locate the internal carotid artery.

Nasotracheal intubation, muscle relaxation, and neuromonitoring are important intraoperative measures to support the resection of the tumor.

5.7 Approaches to the Parapharyngeal Space

Table 5.2 gives an overview about the common approaches and routes to the parapharyngeal space. The most frequent approaches are the transcervical, transcervical–transparotid with or without mandibulotomy, and/or the infratemporal access. Most of the salivary cancer cases are approached via a transcervical or transcervical–transparotid route [13]. There are some novel possibilities alone or in

Table 5.2 Overview of the surgical approaches to parapharyngeal salivary gland cancer

Surgical approach	Comment
Transcervical	Standard approach for most benign parapharyngeal space tumors, but normally not sufficient for malignant tumors as a better overview is needed
Transcervical–transparotid	This is the minimal standard approach for malignant salivary gland tumors of the parapharyngeal space. If the facial nerve is not infiltrated, a total parotidectomy is included. If the facial nerve is infiltrated by the tumor, a radical parotidectomy is performed
Transoral	This approach cannot be recommended for malignant salivary gland tumors of the parapharyngeal space
Infratemporal	For tumors with extension into the infratemporal fossa, complex approach, endoscopic approach also possible
Mandibulotomy	A mandibulotomy might be necessary in addition to the transcervical–transparotid approach to enlarge the exposure of the parapharyngeal space
Transcervical endoscopic	This new technique can be combined with the transcervical–transparotid approach to get a better view into parapharyngeal space and around the tumor to control the large vessels and the cranial nerves
Transcervical robotic	Today certainly an experimental approach even for benign tumors. This approach cannot be recommended currently for malignant tumors in clinical routine

s. Otherwise, closure (of reconstruction) is performed by approximation of the transected muscles. If a mandibulotomy was performed, an osteosynthesis is performed now.
t. Finally, the subcutaneous layers and the skin are closed.

Different maneuvers have been introduced to increase the exposure:

- Resection of the styloid process with surrounding musculature and the posterior belly of the digastric muscle;
- Mobilization or resection of the submandibular gland;
- Division of the stylomandibular ligament to move the mandible;
- Check if the muscle relaxation still is effective.

A mandibulotomy should be considered in all cases of malignant tumors, as a wide view of the operating field is essential for tumor resection and vascular control. Several mandibulotomy techniques have been described [15]. Osteotomies at the mandibular symphysis or close to the mandibular angle are the oldest techniques. Disadvantages are inferior aesthetic results, higher risk of malocclusion, and damage of the mental nerve. A lateral mandibulotomy does not help sufficiently to widen the exposure of the parapharyngeal space. The double mandibular osteotomy technique enlarges the access to the parapharyngeal space significantly [16]. Due to two lesion sites at the mandible there is a higher risk of later mandibular instability. Modified midline mandibular osteotomy with transient intraoperative mandibular swing offers an excellent view into the parapharyngeal space in case of large parapharyngeal tumors [15, 17].

If the transcervical–transparotid approach does not allow a safe control over the large vessels within the parapharyngeal space, an additional mandibulotomy is recommended.

5.9 Transoral Approach and Transoral Robotic Approach

In case of malignant salivary gland tumors of the parapharyngeal space, the classical transoral approach cannot be recommended. Control over the neurovascular structures is very limited or the vessels can even not be seen when resecting the tumor. An extension of the tumor into the deep lobe of the parotid gland cannot be controlled. There is a much higher risk of tumor spillage than via the transcervical approach. Theoretically, the transoral route might be feasible for very small malignant lesion not extending to the styloid process when there is a contraindication against the transcervical route. The introduction of transoral robotic surgery (TORS) brought a revival of this approach mainly, of course, for benign tumors. But resection of malignant tumors via this route has been described, too [18]. One should be aware that

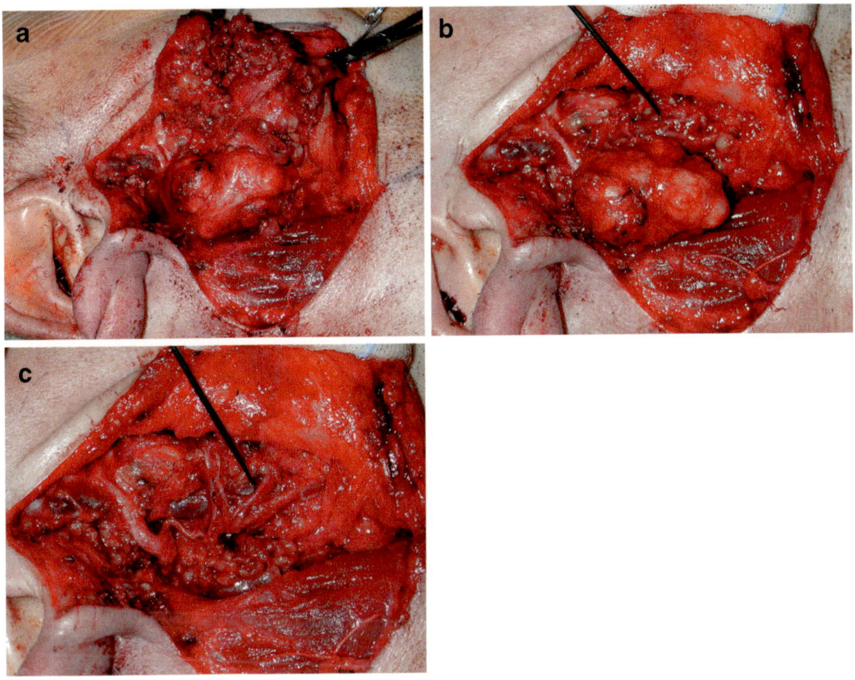

Fig. 5.6 Transcervical–transparotid approach used in the same case as shown in Fig. 5.4. (**a**) Large mucoepidermoid cancer of the parapharyngeal space on the right side. (**b**) After lateral parotidectomy; (**c**) after total parotidectomy and resection of the tumor with preservation of the facial nerve which was not tumor-infiltrated

even in benign tumors a high rate of intraoperative tumor fragmentation was noted when using the TORS approach [19, 20]. Actually, it is less the robotic technique itself but mainly the three-dimensional endoscopic view is providing a much better view around the tumor and better protection of the vessels and nerves. The future will show if the combined transparotid–transoral robot-assisted approach is of help for selected large malignant tumors with unclear medial extension [21] (Fig. 5.6).

5.10 Transcervical Endoscopic and Other New Approaches

To improve the overview of the transcervical approach, especially to improve the exposure of the cranial parts along the skull base, an endoscopic approach using rigid endoscopes was introduced [22, 23]. To use endoscopes might be helpful to confirm successful hemostasis and complete tumor resection. However, case reports describing experiences with endoscopes in patients with malignant salivary gland tumors are lacking so far. Endoscopes can also be used for a combined transnasal–transcervical approach also allowing a better exposure of the cranial portion of the lesion at the skull base [24].

5.11 Adjuvant Measures

If parts of the peripheral facial nerve and its branches have to be resected due to tumor infiltration, a reconstruction of the nerve in the same surgical session gives the best results [9]. Segmental defects of the peripheral facial nerve can be reconstructed by interpositional nerve grafts, for instance using the greater auricular nerve. The greater auricular nerve can be exposed directly without needing to extend the transcervical approach. More complex defects can be reconstructed combining interpositional nerve grafts and, for instance, a hypoglossal-facial jump nerve suture [25]. If a nerve reconstruction is not feasible because most of the peripheral facial nerve has been resected, reanimation of eye closure using an upper lid weight and reconstruction of the zygomatic function using a muscle transfer are alternative options [26].

Treatment of salivary gland cancer in the parapharyngeal space should be not different to parotid gland cancer (for instance, see NCCN guidelines [27]). It is recommended that any patient with cervical lymph node metastases (N+) should receive a neck dissection at best in the same surgical session. Patients with a clinical N0 neck should receive a neck dissection at least if it is a higher-grade and high-stage (T3-T4) primary tumor.

Adjuvant radiotherapy is recommended for any adenoid cystic carcinoma, intermediate or high grade tumors, close or positive margins, neural or perineural invasion, pN+, and lymphatic or vascular invasion. Because of the narrow conditions in the parapharyngeal space and the close relation to the skull base, close margin is typical for resected salivary gland cancer of the parapharyngeal space. Therefore, adjuvant radiotherapy is normally recommended for malignant salivary gland tumors in this location.

> If the facial nerve is tumor-infiltrated, facial nerve reconstruction surgery should be performed as single-stage surgery if possible. Moreover, the neck dissection should also be performed in the same surgical session.

5.12 Complications of Surgery

Cranial nerve injuries (cranial nerves V, VII, IX; X, XI, XII) are the commonest complications. Vagal nerve injury occurs in about 14% of the cases [4]. Other typical complications are Horner's syndrome, first bite syndrome, trismus, vascular injury, dysphagia, dysphonia, and palatal insufficiency [4]. Vascular injury can lead to severe hemorrhage or stroke. If the salivary gland cancer involves the carotid artery or encloses more than half of the artery, the risk of vascular complications is increased.

If a mandibulotomy is performed, sensory disturbances of the neighbored teeth can occur. The inferior alveolar nerve can be damaged. Instability of the mandible, malocclusion and dysfunction of the temporomandibular joint are other possible sequelae of a mandibular osteotomy.

There are special complications associated with the transoral approach. These possible complications are additional arguments against this approach. There is a high risk of tumor rupture and tumor spillage. The unavoidable contamination of the surgical wound with saliva can lead to increased risk of wound infection.

5.13 Follow-Up

Recommendations for the follow-up shall be based on the follow-up recommendations for head and neck cancer treating with curative intent. A follow-up examination should be performed every 1–3 months in the first year, every 2–6 months in the second year, every 4–8 months in the year 3–5, and later every 12 months. Post-treatment baseline imaging with CT or MRI of the primary site is recommended within 6 months of treatment. If osteosynthesis material was used for obturating the transient mandibulotomy, it should not be explanted earlier than 12 months after surgery. If facial nerve reconstruction surgery is performed, the final results can be evaluated not earlier than 12 months after surgery. Some patients need additional minor procedures or botulinum toxin treatment against synkinesis to optimize the functional result.

5.14 Conclusions

Although salivary gland cancer of the parapharyngeal space is rare, the treatment, especially the surgical treatment is based on well-defined and established surgical approaches. The transcervical–transparotid approach still is and probably will be far into the future the approach of first choice. The combination with endoscopic techniques without or with a robotic system mainly will help to expand the possibilities of the transcervical approach and will help to preserve critical structures, especially large vessels and important cranial nerves in the parapharyngeal space. There is a high risk of cranial nerve injury for patients treated for salivary gland cancer in the parapharyngeal space. Therefore, it is important for the head and neck surgeon dealing with the tumor to offer treatments to overcome the functional deficits related to cranial nerve injury.

References

1. Hermans R, Farina D. Parapharyngeal space neoplasms. In: Hermans R, editor. Head and neck cancer imaging. Heidelberg: Springer; 2006.
2. Cassoni A, Terenzi V, Della Monaca M, Bartoli D, Battisti A, Rajabtork Zadeh O, Valentini V. Parapharyngeal space benign tumours: our experience. J Craniomaxillofac Surg. 2014;42(2):101–5. https://doi.org/10.1016/j.jcms.2013.03.002.

3. Locketz GD, Horowitz G, Abu-Ghanem S, Wasserzug O, Abergel A, Yehuda M, Fliss DM. Histopathologic classification of parapharyngeal space tumors: a case series and review of the literature. Eur Arch Otorhinolaryngol. 2016;273(3):727–34. https://doi.org/10.1007/s00405-015-3545-5.
4. Riffat F, Dwivedi RC, Palme C, Fish B, Jani P. A systematic review of 1143 parapharyngeal space tumors reported over 20 years. Oral Oncol. 2014;50(5):421–30. https://doi.org/10.1016/j.oraloncology.2014.02.007.
5. Bootz F, Greschus S, van Bremen T. Diagnosis and treatment of parapharyngeal space tumors. HNO. 2016;64(11):815–21. https://doi.org/10.1007/s00106-016-0259-y.
6. Carrau RL, Myers EN, Johnson JT. Management of tumors arising in the parapharyngeal space. Laryngoscope. 1990;100(6):583–9. https://doi.org/10.1288/00005537-199006000-00006.
7. Douville NJ, Bradford CR. Comparison of ultrasound-guided core biopsy versus fine-needle aspiration biopsy in the evaluation of salivary gland lesions. Head Neck. 2013;35(11):1657–61. https://doi.org/10.1002/hed.23193.
8. Eom HJ, Lee JH, Ko MS, Choi YJ, Yoon RG, Cho KJ, Nam SY, Baek JH. Comparison of fine-needle aspiration and core needle biopsy under ultrasonographic guidance for detecting malignancy and for the tissue-specific diagnosis of salivary gland tumors. Am J Neuroradiol. 2015;36(6):1188–93. https://doi.org/10.3174/ajnr.A4247.
9. Volk GF, Pantel M, Guntinas-Lichius O. Modern concepts in facial nerve reconstruction. Head Face Med. 2011;6:25.
10. Singh R, Husain AM. Neurophysiologic intraoperative monitoring of the glossopharyngeal and vagus nerves. J Clin Neurophysiol. 2011;28(6):582–6. https://doi.org/10.1097/WNP.0b013e31823e9b00.
11. Paderno A, Piazza C, Nicolai P. Recent advances in surgical management of parapharyngeal space tumors. Curr Opin Otolaryngol Head Neck Surg. 2015;23(2):83–90. https://doi.org/10.1097/MOO.0000000000000134.
12. Prasad SC, Piccirillo E, Chovanec M, La Melia C, De Donato G, Sanna M. Lateral skull base approaches in the management of benign parapharyngeal space tumors. Auris Nasus Larynx. 2015;42(3):189–98. https://doi.org/10.1016/j.anl.2014.09.002.
13. Chang SS, Goldenberg D, Koch WM. Transcervical approach to benign parapharyngeal space tumors. Ann Otol Rhinol Laryngol. 2012;121(9):620–4. https://doi.org/10.1177/000348941212100910.
14. Presutti L, Molteni G, Malve L, Marchioni D, Ghidini A, Tassi S, Chiarini L, Alicandri-Ciufelli M. Parapharyngeal space tumors without mandibulotomy: our experience. Eur Arch Otorhinolaryngol. 2012;269(1):265–73. https://doi.org/10.1007/s00405-011-1594-y.
15. Jungehuelsing M, Guntinas-Lichius O, Klussmann JP, Eckel HE, Stennert E. Modifications of the midline mandibulotomy for access to the parapharyngeal space. Laryngoscope. 2010;120(8):1557–62. https://doi.org/10.1002/lary.20872.
16. Attia EL, Bentley KC, Head T, Mulder D. A new external approach to the pterygomaxillary fossa and parapharyngeal space. Head Neck Surg. 1984;6(4):884–91.
17. Jungehülsing M, Guntinas-Lichius O, Klussmann JP, Schröder U. Surgical exposure of the mesopharynx. HNO. 2003;51:931–49.
18. Park YM, De Virgilio A, Kim WS, Chung HP, Kim SH. Parapharyngeal space surgery via a transoral approach using a robotic surgical system: transoral robotic surgery. J Laparoendosc Adv Surg Tech A. 2013;23(3):231–6. https://doi.org/10.1089/lap.2012.0197.
19. Chan JY, Tsang RK, Eisele DW, Richmon JD. Transoral robotic surgery of the parapharyngeal space: a case series and systematic review. Head Neck. 2015;37(2):293–8. https://doi.org/10.1002/hed.23557.
20. O'Malley BW Jr, Quon H, Leonhardt FD, Chalian AA, Weinstein GS. Transoral robotic surgery for parapharyngeal space tumors. ORL J Otorhinolaryngol Relat Spec. 2010;72(6):332–6. https://doi.org/10.1159/000320596.
21. De Virgilio A, Park YM, Kim WS, Byeon HK, Lee SY, Kim SH. Transoral robotic surgery for the resection of parapharyngeal tumour: our experience in ten patients. Clin Otolaryngol. 2012;37(6):483–8. https://doi.org/10.1111/j.1749-4486.2012.02525.x.

22. Beswick DM, Vaezi A, Caicedo-Granados E, Duvvuri U. Minimally invasive surgery for parapharyngeal space tumors. Laryngoscope. 2012;122(5):1072–8. https://doi.org/10.1002/lary.23244.
23. Pilolli F, Giordano L, Galli A, Bussi M. Parapharyngeal space tumours: video-assisted minimally invasive transcervical approach. Acta Otorhinolaryngol Ital. 2016;36(4):259–64. https://doi.org/10.14639/0392-100X-709.
24. Wasano K, Yamamoto S, Tomisato S, Kawasaki T, Ogawa K. Modified endoscopic transnasal-transmaxillary-transpterygoid approach to parapharyngeal space tumor resection. Head Neck. 2016;38(6):933–8. https://doi.org/10.1002/hed.24399.
25. Volk GF, Pantel M, Streppel M, Guntinas-Lichius O. Reconstruction of complex peripheral facial nerve defects by a combined approach using facial nerve interpositional graft and hypoglossal-facial jump nerve suture. Laryngoscope. 2011;121(11):2402–5. https://doi.org/10.1002/lary.22357.
26. Jungehülsing M, Guntinas-Lichius O. Muscle flaps and static procedures. In: Guntinas-Lichius O, Schaitkin BM, editors. Facial nerve disorders and diseases: diagnosis and management. Stuttgart: Thieme; 2016.
27. NCCN Guidelines for Head and Neck Cancers V.2.2016. 2016. https://www.nccn.org/Common/FileManager.ashx?fileManagerId=d52f51d0-bf44-4ce0-9f60-0c02f668eea6

Surgery for Submandibular and Sublingual Malignant Tumors

6

Natalie L. Silver and Randal S. Weber

6.1 Introduction

Salivary gland tumors may originate in either major or minor salivary glands, and the proportion of benign to malignant salivary gland neoplasms is dependent on location. A mass in the submandibular gland or a minor salivary gland is more likely to be malignant. In a review of more than 2000 salivary gland tumor cases, 73% of the tumors were found in the parotid with only 15% found to be malignant, while 11% were found in the submandibular gland with 37% found to be malignant [1]. Tumors of the sublingual gland are extremely rare and comprise 0.5–1% of all salivary tumors, and 80–90% are malignant [2, 3].

It is imperative for the physician to distinguish a chronic benign process, such as sialadenitis, from a submandibular gland neoplasm, and then further determine if a neoplasm is benign or malignant. This is done through careful history and physical exam, as well as utilization of preoperative imaging and fine needle aspiration.

Management of submandibular gland malignancy can be challenging due the relative rarity of the disease and the diversity of its behavior due to a variety of histologic subtypes and grades. Adenoid cystic carcinoma is the most common subtype in the submandibular gland, followed by mucoepidermoid carcinoma and then adenocarcinoma. Table 6.1 displays the histologic spectrum of malignancy for tumors of the submandibular gland at our institution [4, 5]. Adenoid cystic carcinoma is also the most common malignant sublingual gland tumor (71%) followed by mucoepidermoid carcinoma (18%) [6].

N. L. Silver
University of Florida, Department of Otolaryngology, Division of Head and Neck Surgical Oncology, Gainesville, FL, USA
e-mail: Natalie.silver@ent.ufl.edu

R. S. Weber (✉)
MD Anderson Cancer Center, Department of Head and Neck Surgery, Houston, TX, USA
e-mail: rsweber@mdanderson.org

© Springer Nature Switzerland AG 2019
L. Licitra, L. D. Locati (eds.), *Salivary Gland Cancer*,
https://doi.org/10.1007/978-3-030-02958-6_6

Table 6.1 Histology of malignant submandibular gland tumors

Histologic type	Number of patients (% total)
Adenoid cystic	57 (66%)
Mucoepidermoid carcinoma	15 (17%)
Adenocarcinoma	5 (6%)
Undifferentiated	3 (3%)
Acinic cell	2 (2%)
Lymphoepithelioma	2 (2%)
Squamous cell	1 (1%)
Carcinoma ex pleomorphic adenoma	1 (1%)
Other	1 (1%)
Total	87

6.2 Clinical Presentation

Most often, a tumor of the submandibular gland presents as a mass or swelling. For patients with chronic sialadenitis, the typical symptoms include intermittent swelling of the submandibular gland that is associated with eating or drinking. The gland may become firm and painful. Benign and malignant tumors of the submandibular gland can both present as a painless mass. However, when a neoplasm is accompanied with pain, it suggests malignancy. In up to 20% of patients with malignant tumors, pain may be constant and progressive, while benign neoplasms rarely present with pain [7]. Gradual enlargement is also more common in patients with submandibular neoplasia, and progressive enlargement over a short period of time suggests malignancy (Fig. 6.1a–c). Tumors of the sublingual gland present as a submucosal mass in the floor of mouth and usually at an advanced stage due to the late onset of symptoms and less noticed location.

Physical examination includes inspection and palpation of the neck as well as the oral cavity. Bimanual palpation should be performed to determine if the gland is fixated to adjacent structures such as the mandible or skin. It is important to determine sensation of the tongue (indicating lingual nerve involvement), tongue fasciculations or weakness (indicating hypoglossal nerve involvement), and lip weakness (indicating marginal mandibular nerve involvement), all of which indicate perineural spread of the tumor. The presence or absence of trismus should be assessed and, if present, indicates invasion of the medial pterygoid muscle.

Careful examination of the neck is critical to identify lymphadenopathy, particularly in level I, because adenopathy with an enlarged submandibular or sublingual gland is highly suspicious for malignancy. At initial presentation, the presence of lymph node metastasis from a submandibular gland malignancy ranges from 8 to 35% of patients [7–9].

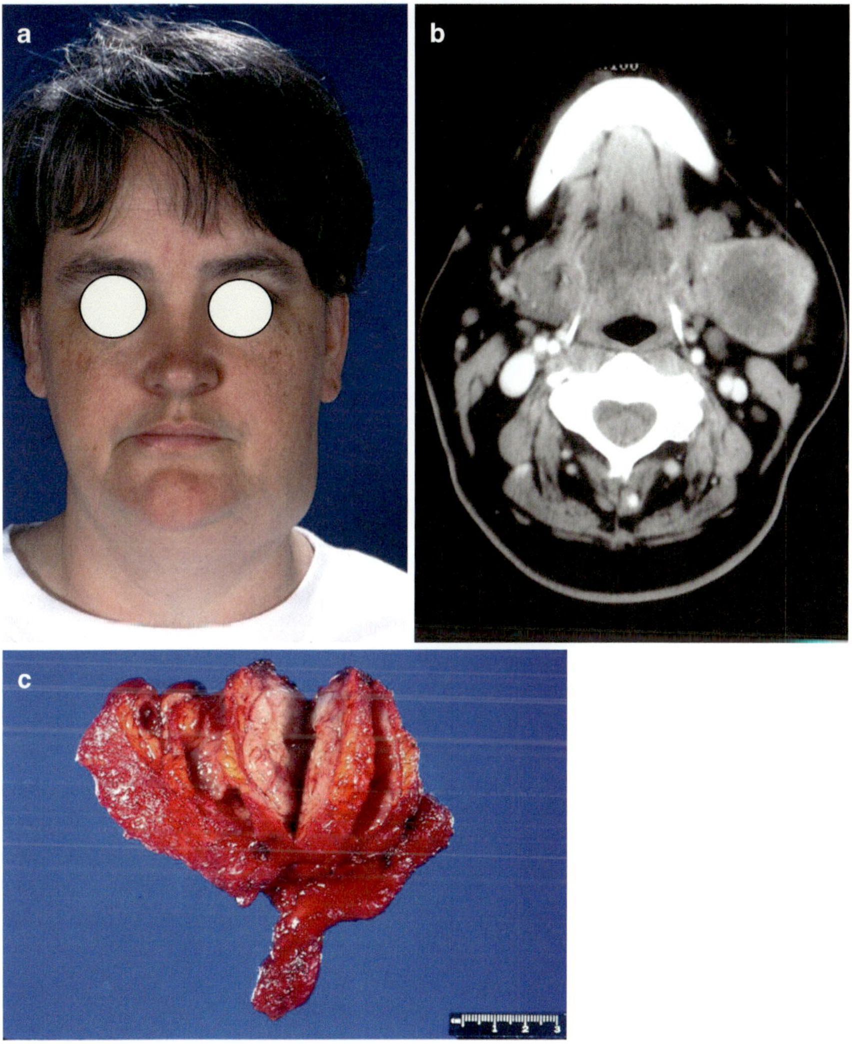

Fig. 6.1 (**a**) The patient presented with an enlarging submandibular mass suspicious for malignancy. (**b**) CT scan with contrast revealed a heterogeneously enhancing mass of the submandibular gland that did not appear to be locally invasive. (**c**) The tumor was completely excised with a level I lymph node dissection, and final pathology revealed carcinosarcoma of the submandibular gland with no positive lymph nodes or perineural invasion

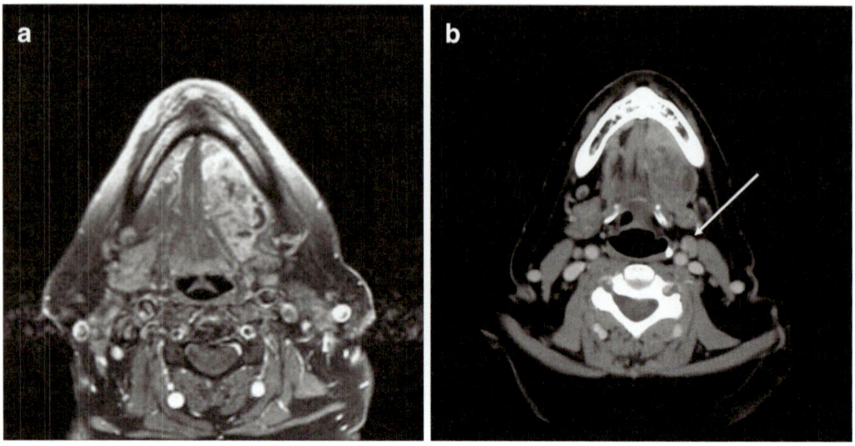

Fig. 6.2 Adenoid cystic carcinoma of the sublingual gland imaged using both MRI (**a**) and CT scan with contrast (**b**). Arrow pointing to a metastatic level II lymph node

6.3 Imaging Studies

Imaging for submandibular and sublingual gland lesions augments the physical exam and aids in the following: determining if a lesion is intrinsic or extrinsic to the gland, evaluating the extent of the lesion with respect to local invasion, establishing perineural involvement, and determining if there is metastatic disease. All of these are important to delineate prior to surgical management so that the appropriate procedures are discussed and planned for [10].

Although imaging lacks the specificity to determine benign from malignant tumors, a computed tomography (CT) scan with contrast can provide valuable information regarding mandibular bone invasion, the local extent of the tumor, and the presence or absence of pathologic lymphadenopathy (Fig. 6.1b, c). Magnetic resonance imaging (MRI) can provide superior soft tissue detail to CT scans and can help assess perineural spread (Fig. 6.2a, b).

Positron emission tomography (PET)-CT in salivary gland disease can help rule out distant metastasis if the primary cancer has enhanced fluorodeoxyglucose (FDG) uptake. In FDG-avid cancers, PET-CT may be useful in initial staging, in histologic grading, and in monitoring for recurrence [11, 12]. However, an inflamed or infected submandibular gland may also uptake FDG and enhance on PET-CT.

6.4 Fine Needle Aspiration Biopsy

The role of preoperative fine needle aspiration (FNA) as a diagnostic test is a vital part of the clinical management algorithm for submandibular gland disease. For inflammatory causes of salivary gland enlargement, nonsurgical management can often be used, or a simple submandibular gland excision may be planned without a level I neck dissection. Therefore, when properly combined with clinical-radiologic findings, FNA results (which typically demonstrate the presence of acute and chronic inflammatory cells) can aid in surgical planning; and cultures for suspected infectious masses could be obtained. Regarding malignancy, if the histopathologic type can be determined in advance, this information may be used for preoperative counseling regarding the extent of surgery, primarily regarding the necessity of a neck dissection. This is also true for sublingual gland masses. Differentiating between benign and malignant salivary gland tumors can be difficult with FNA. Nonetheless, with experienced cytopathologists, FNA is accurate in over 90–95% of patients [13]. The use of fine needle aspiration (FNA) in working up salivary tumors is also cost-effective. Layfield et al. demonstrated that routine FNA in the work-up of salivary gland lesions saves up to $70,000 per 100 patients and FNA reduces the operative intervention by 65% in submandibular masses and by 35% in parotid masses [14].

Ultrasound-guided biopsy can be useful in a heterogeneous gland that is suspicious. Also, core needle biopsy is more sensitive and specific than FNA in diagnosing malignant lesions and can therefore be used as an additional diagnostic tool in uncertain lesions, especially for patients who may require extensive surgery to be discussed in advance [15].

6.5 Histopathology

Salivary gland malignancies are extraordinarily heterogeneous and complex in histology. This results in variable clinical behavior and therefore clinical management. The 2005 WHO classification described 24 different salivary gland phenotypes, and the same TNM staging classification is used for all histologic types of salivary gland cancer arising in the major salivary glands [16]. It is essential for treating physicians to understand the spectrum of clinical progression and biological aggressiveness of the most common histological types.

6.6 Adenoid Cystic Carcinoma

Adenoid cystic carcinoma is the most common type of malignant tumor of the submandibular and sublingual gland. It is characterized by locally infiltrative growth pattern with perineural invasion and high rates of local recurrences and delayed distant metastasis [17, 18]. For submandibular gland cancers, perineural invasion can be seen in up to 75% of cases and can affect the extent of surgery, requiring sacrifice of nerves if involved by tumor, most often the lingual and hypoglossal nerves [19]. Perineural spread may also involve the marginal mandibular nerve or the cervical branch of the facial nerve. Adenoid cystic carcinoma is more aggressive in the minor salivary glands than in the parotid. Solid tumor subtype, lymphovascular invasion, and positive margins also correlate with a poorer prognosis [20, 21]. Despite the ability to achieve good initial local control, adenoid cystic carcinoma is the most common type of salivary gland carcinoma associated with distant metastasis and can develop many years after initial diagnosis [22]. And, although the majority of patients with clinically early-stage adenoid cystic carcinoma of the salivary glands have a favorable prognosis, a significant percentage (20%) will develop distant metastasis and therefore need to be monitored carefully over longer periods of time [23].

6.7 Mucoepidermoid Carcinoma

Mucoepidermoid carcinoma is the second most common malignant tumor of the submandibular and sublingual gland and can be low, intermediate, or high grade in histology. High-grade lesions, advanced stage, perineural invasion, positive margins, and submandibular/sublingual gland location are all associated with a worse prognosis. There is a higher proportion of intermediate- or high-grade lesions in patients presenting with a submandibular gland primary, and up to 50% of mucoepidermoid carcinoma cases in this region will have cervical metastasis compared to 28% for the parotid gland [24]. High-grade tumors are more aggressive, can invade locally, and are also more likely to have nodal metastasis [25]. However, even low-grade mucoepidermoid carcinomas of the submandibular gland can recur and metastasize more frequently than those of the parotid or minor salivary glands, necessitating aggressive resection of any mucoepidermoid carcinoma primary in this location [24, 26].

6.8 Adenocarcinoma

Adenocarcinoma of the salivary glands represents a wide array of histopathologic entities such as salivary duct carcinoma, adenocarcinoma not otherwise specified (NOS), polymorphous low-grade adenocarcinoma, and basal cell carcinoma. It is generally differentiated into low- and high-grade histologies with salivary duct carcinoma and about half of adenocarcinoma NOS representing high-grade entities. Overall survival is low at 43% over 5 years and is associated with several clinicopathologic factors such as a fixed mass or rapid tumor growth, a diagnosis of adenocarcinoma NOS, and positive surgical margins [27].

6.9 Surgical Management

Surgery is the primary treatment for patients with resectable submandibular and sublingual salivary gland cancer. The minimal procedure performed should be complete excision of the affected gland and a level IA and IB lymph node dissection with careful attempt to spare uninvolved nerves. Generally, this is an acceptable treatment for tumors that are low grade and early stage (i.e., no clinical or radiographic neck disease). High-grade, advanced stage tumors will require more extensive surgery involving an ipsilateral selective neck dissection in addition to excision of the sublingual gland and/or submandibular gland. Excision of sublingual gland tumors less than 2 cm in size may be removed transorally, but the ipsilateral submandibular gland should also be excised as the ductal system can be compromised. Sublingual tumors that are larger than 2 cm in size should be removed en bloc using a pull-through technique [28]. When a tumor is locally advanced, resection of adjacent structures such as the mandible, involved nerves, or skin may be necessary (Fig. 6.3a, b). In these cases, reconstruction may be required with local, regional, or free microvascular flaps [7, 10].

There are several clinicopathologic factors that are considered when recommending adjuvant treatment. Indications are positive surgical margins, high-grade histology, locally advanced disease (perineural/bone invasion), and advanced stage. Postoperative treatment generally consists of ipsilateral neck irradiation and can significantly increase local control as compared with surgery alone [29]. Garden et al. treated patients with adenoid cystic carcinoma of the submandibular gland and suspected microscopic residual disease with postoperative radiotherapy and achieved a 10-year survival of ~60% [20]. Currently under investigation is the role for adjuvant chemoradiotherapy for resected high-risk salivary gland lesions (Radiation Therapy Oncology Group, Protocol #1008).

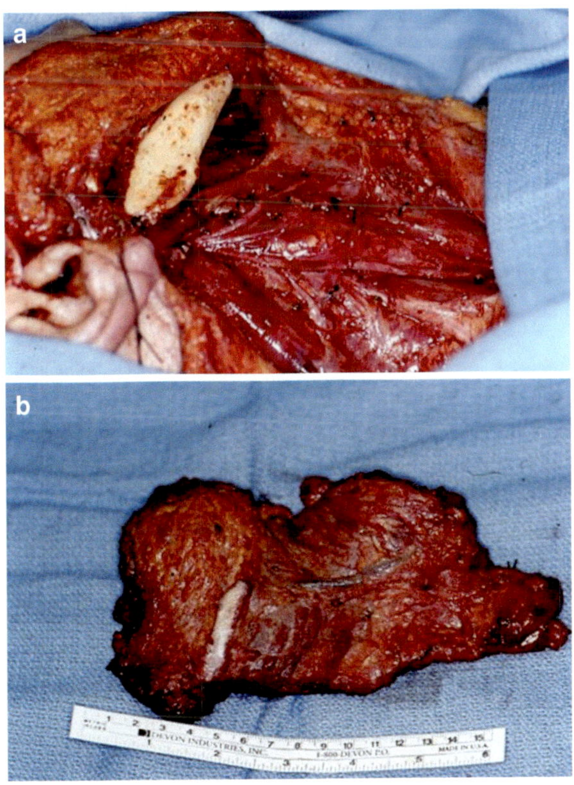

Fig. 6.3 (**a**) The patient presented with recurrent high-grade mucoepidermoid carcinoma of the submandibular gland requiring wide local excision of the gland with removal of tissues from the floor of mouth and previous scar; a radical neck dissection was also performed. (**b**) The entire specimen was removed en bloc

At our institution, in 86 patients with submandibular gland malignancy treated initially with surgery, 45% developed recurrences. Half of those patients recurred locoregionally and the other half at distant sites. The 2- and 5-year survival was 82% and 69%, respectively [7]. Locoregional control was enhanced by adjuvant radiation.

6.10 Surgical Technique for Excision of Malignant Submandibular Gland Tumors

The patient is placed supine and general endotracheal anesthesia is induced. A shoulder roll is placed extending the neck. The neck and face are prepped and draped with adequate exposure of the submental area and corner of the mouth. An incision is marked in a natural skin crease at least two fingerbreadths below the edge of the mandible to protect the marginal mandibular nerve (Fig. 6.4a). The incision should extend from the anterior boarder of the sternocleidomastoid muscle to the submental region. The skin and platysma are incised, and the superior flap is

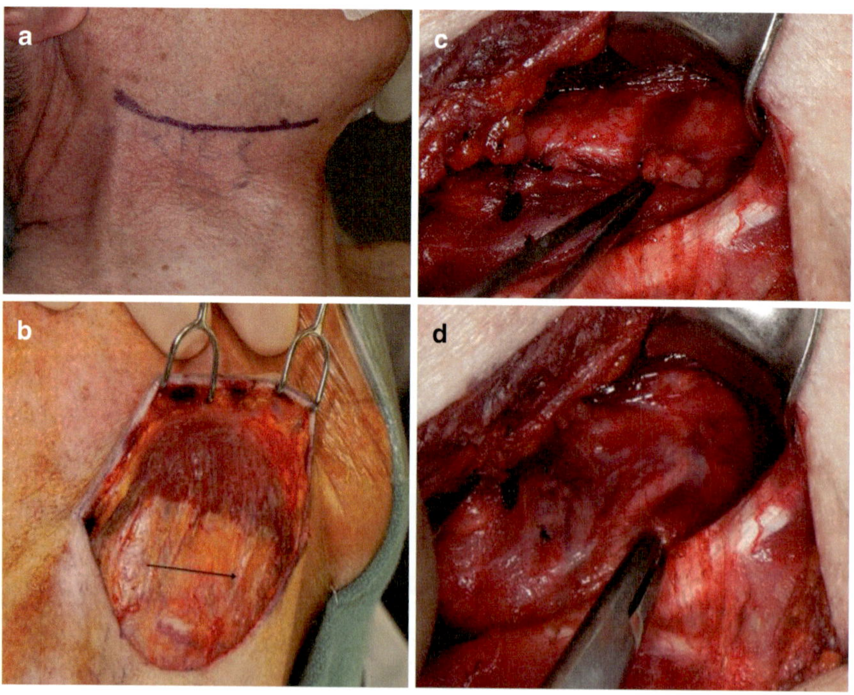

Fig. 6.4 (**a**) An incision is marked at least two fingerbreadths below the edge of the mandible. (**b**) Subplatysmal flaps are elevated. Arrow pointing to marginal mandibular nerve. (**c**) The lingual nerve is visible. The submandibular ganglion and duct have been ligated. (**d**) The hypoglossal nerve here is visible deep to the ligated submandibular duct. Rights to reprint these pictures have been obtained from Wolters Kluwer Health. License#3677830789655

elevated to the inferior boarder of the mandible, and the inferior flap is elevated below the submandibular gland (Fig. 6.4b). If the platysma is infiltrated with tumor, flap elevation should be in a supraplatysmal plane with excision of the involved muscle. The marginal mandibular nerve is identified, traced over the mandible, and elevated superiorly. The facial artery and vein are clamped and ligated inferior to the marginal mandibular nerve. The perifacial lymph nodes, proximal facial vessels, and the lateral aspects of the submandibular gland are reflected inferiorly and anteriorly. The mylohyoid muscle is skeletonized to its inferior edge about the digastric tendon including all of the fatty areolar tissue. If a tumor is fixed to the mandible without evidence of invasion, then a rim of the mandible may be excised. Frank invasion necessitates a mandibulectomy.

Next, the submental region is dissected. The medial edge of the contralateral anterior belly of the digastric muscle is first skeletonized. The submental lymph nodes are reflected inferiorly off of the underlying mylohyoid muscle. If any muscle is infiltrated with tumor, it is resected with the gland. The specimen is reflected toward the ipsilateral anterior belly of the digastric and also skeletonized. The level IA specimen should be continuous with the level IB contents. The mylohyoid muscle is then retracted, exposing the lingual nerve and the deeper portion of the submandibular gland. When perineural invasion is suspected, frozen section samples may be sent intraoperatively, and if nerves are positive for tumor, they are resected with the gland. The nerves should be followed in a retrograde fashion until clear margins can be obtained. Of note, adenoid cystic carcinoma often has skip metastasis, making frozen section analysis less reliable when attempting to clear margins.

The submandibular ganglion is next clamped, cut, and ligated (Fig. 6.4c). The submandibular duct is identified and followed. The duct is ligated, and the surrounding portion of the submandibular gland is reflected inferiorly with the attached specimen. Prior to ligating the duct, the hypoglossal nerve should be identified deep to the duct and preserved if uninvolved by tumor (Fig. 6.4d). The specimen is reflected posteriorly, where it remains tethered by the proximal portion of the facial artery. The artery is clamped, cut, and ligated. The wound is irrigated and a suction drain is placed. The wound is closed in several layers [5].

6.11 Surgical Management of the Neck

A clinically positive neck should be treated with an ipsilateral neck dissection including all grossly involved nodes while attempting to spare vital structures. The most common involved nodes from carcinoma of the submandibular gland are levels I–III, but it can skip levels; therefore a comprehensive neck dissection is recommended in the setting of clinically positive disease [25].

The management of the N0 neck is controversial. Options include observation, elective neck dissection, or radiation. As mentioned previously, all malignant tumors in the submandibular gland mandate a level IA and IB dissection. However, elective neck dissection is typically reserved for tumors with a high propensity for occult metastasis.

6.12 Conclusion

Submandibular and sublingual gland malignancies are rare and present both a treatment and diagnostic challenge due to their histologic heterogeneity and aggressiveness. Complete submandibular gland excision with a regional dissection of the submental lymph nodes is the primary treatment for malignant submandibular gland tumors. Sublingual gland tumors should also be completely excised with a complete level I neck dissection. The neck should be surgically addressed based on pathology and nodal status. Adjuvant radiotherapy can decrease local recurrence rates and improve survival in patients with adverse features, while adjuvant chemotherapy is being investigated. It is imperative to follow patients long after initial treatment due to the high likelihood of distant metastasis.

References

1. Eveson JW, Cawson RA. Salivary gland tumours. A review of 2410 cases with particular reference to histological types, site, age and sex distribution. J Pathol. 1985;146:51–8.
2. Nishijima W, Tokita N, Takooda S, Tsuchiya S, Watanabe I. Adenocarcinoma of the sublingual gland: case report and 50 year review of the literature. Laryngoscope. 1984;94:96–101.
3. Lombardi D, McGurk M, Vander Poorten V, et al. Surgical treatment of salivary malignant tumors. Oral Oncol. 2017;65:102–13.
4. Kaszuba SM, Zafereo ME, Rosenthal DI, El-Naggar AK, Weber RS. Effect of initial treatment on disease outcome for patients with submandibular gland carcinoma. Arch Otolaryngol Head Neck Surg. 2007;133:546–50.
5. Weber R. Excision of the submandibular gland. In: Ferris RL, editor. Master techniques in otolaryngology head and neck surgery. Philadelphia: Lippincot Williams and Wilkins; 2013. p. 261–9.
6. Liu Y, Li H, Qin L, Huang X, Su M, Han Z. Prognostic factors in malignant sublingual salivary gland tumors. J Oral Maxillofac Surg. 2017;75:1542.
7. Weber RS, Byers RM, Petit B, Wolf P, Ang K, Luna M. Submandibular gland tumors. Adverse histologic factors and therapeutic implications. Arch Otolaryngol Head Neck Surg. 1990;116:1055–60.
8. Spiro RH. Salivary neoplasms: overview of a 35-year experience with 2,807 patients. Head Neck Surg. 1986;8:177–84.
9. Bhattacharyya N. Survival and prognosis for cancer of the submandibular gland. J Oral Maxillofac Surg. 2004;62:427–30.
10. Dias F. Management of tumors of the submandibular and sublingual glands. In: Myers E, editor. Salivary gland disorders. New York: Springer; 2007. p. 339–74.
11. Razfar A, Heron DE, Branstetter BF, Seethala RR, Ferris RL. Positron emission tomography-computed tomography adds to the management of salivary gland malignancies. Laryngoscope. 2010;120:734–8.
12. Roh JL, Ryu CH, Choi SH, et al. Clinical utility of 18F-FDG PET for patients with salivary gland malignancies. J Nucl Med. 2007;48:240–6.
13. Stewart CJ, MacKenzie K, McGarry GW, Mowat A. Fine-needle aspiration cytology of salivary gland: a review of 341 cases. Diagn Cytopathol. 2000;22:139–46.
14. Layfield LJ, Gopez E, Hirschowitz S. Cost efficiency analysis for fine-needle aspiration in the workup of parotid and submandibular gland nodules. Diagn Cytopathol. 2006;34:734–8.
15. Novoa E, Gurtler N, Arnoux A, Kraft M. Diagnostic value of core-needle biopsy and fine-needle aspiration in salivary gland lesions. Head Neck. 2016;38:E346.

16. Eveson JW. WHO histological classification of tumours of the salivary glands. In: Barnes L, editor. World Health Organization classification of tumours: pathology and genetics of head and neck tumours. Lyon: IARC Press; 2005. p. 210.
17. Sung MW, Kim KH, Kim JW, et al. Clinicopathologic predictors and impact of distant metastasis from adenoid cystic carcinoma of the head and neck. Arch Otolaryngol Head Neck Surg. 2003;129:1193–7.
18. Spiro RH. Distant metastasis in adenoid cystic carcinoma of salivary origin. Am J Surg. 1997;174:495–8.
19. Spiro RH, Huvos AG, Strong EW. Adenoid cystic carcinoma of salivary origin. A clinicopathologic study of 242 cases. Am J Surg. 1974;128:512–20.
20. Garden AS, Weber RS, Morrison WH, Ang KK, Peters LJ. The influence of positive margins and nerve invasion in adenoid cystic carcinoma of the head and neck treated with surgery and radiation. Int J Radiat Oncol Biol Phys. 1995;32:619–26.
21. Cohen AN, Damrose EJ, Huang RY, Nelson SD, Blackwell KE, Calcaterra TC. Adenoid cystic carcinoma of the submandibular gland: a 35-year review. Otolaryngol Head Neck Surg. 2004;131:994–1000.
22. Bradley PJ. Distant metastases from salivary glands cancer. ORL J Otorhinolaryngol Relat Spec. 2001;63:233–42.
23. Bhayani MK, Yener M, El-Naggar A, et al. Prognosis and risk factors for early-stage adenoid cystic carcinoma of the major salivary glands. Cancer. 2012;118:2872–8.
24. Spiro RH, Huvos AG, Berk R, Strong EW. Mucoepidermoid carcinoma of salivary gland origin. A clinicopathologic study of 367 cases. Am J Surg. 1978;136:461–8.
25. McHugh CH, Roberts DB, El-Naggar AK, et al. Prognostic factors in mucoepidermoid carcinoma of the salivary glands. Cancer. 2012;118:3928–36.
26. Luna MA. Salivary mucoepidermoid carcinoma: revisited. Adv Anat Pathol. 2006;13:293–307.
27. Huang AT, Tang C, Bell D, et al. Prognostic factors in adenocarcinoma of the salivary glands. Oral Oncol. 2015;51:610–5.
28. Bradley PJ, Ferris RL. Surgery for malignant sublingual and minor salivary gland neoplasms. Adv Otorhinolaryngol. 2016;78:113–9.
29. Terhaard CHJ, Lubsen H, Rasch CRN, et al. The role of radiotherapy in the treatment of malignant salivary gland tumors. Int J Radiat Oncol Biol Phys. 2005;61:103–11.

Surgery for Malignant Tumors of the Minor Salivary Glands

7

Davide Lombardi, Remo Accorona, Davide Lancini, Vittorio Rampinelli, Anna Bozzola, and Piero Nicolai

7.1 Introduction

The incidence of malignant tumors of the minor salivary glands (MiSGMTs) ranges from 14 to 20 cases per million/year, with the majority of patients in the fifth to sixth decade of life [1–3]. Up to 80% of these lesions are located in the oral cavity (the most frequent primary site is the hard palate) and oropharynx; the sinonasal tract and nasopharynx are affected in 20% of the cases, with the hypopharynx, larynx, and trachea considered together in about 2% [1–5].

The literature is rich in studies on MiSGMT. However, for different reasons it is difficult to extrapolate specific information on the different histologies, especially with regard to the different anatomic sites and subsites. Many studies cover very long frames with a change in histologic taxonomy, focus on mixed heterogeneous histologic subtypes, and/or group together minor and major salivary gland tumors.

In most reports, adenoid cystic carcinoma (AdCC) accounts for the majority of cases, ranging from 32 to 71%, followed by mucoepidermoid carcinoma (MEC), which represents 15–38% of MiSGMT [6–11]. However, other 22 malignant salivary tumor types have been described in the literature, some of which have a non-negligible incidence: i.e., adenocarcinoma not otherwise specified (ACNOS) accounts for 9–28% of the cases and acinic cell carcinoma (ACN) for 1–9%, while all the other histologic subtypes considered together range from 0 to 16% [3, 12–27].

D. Lombardi (✉) · D. Lancini · V. Rampinelli · P. Nicolai
Department of Otorhinolaryngology – Head and Neck Surgery, University of Brescia, Brescia, Italy
e-mail: davinter@libero.it

R. Accorona
Department of Otorhinolaryngology, General Hospital of Bolzano, Bolzano, Italy

A. Bozzola
Section of Pathology, Department of Molecular and Translational Medicine, University of Brescia, Brescia, Italy

© Springer Nature Switzerland AG 2019

L. Licitra, L. D. Locati (eds.), *Salivary Gland Cancer*, https://doi.org/10.1007/978-3-030-02958-6_7

Typically, the signs and symptoms of MiSGMT depend on the anatomic site of origin. The classical presentation consists in a painless submucosal fixed swelling, associated with obstructive symptoms when the tumor is located in the sinonasal cavities, pharynx, and laryngotracheal axis. According to Vander Poorten et al. [3], pain and nerve impairment are present in up to 26% of patients and strongly suggest a diagnosis of AdCC.

The management of MiSGMT poses specific problems related to histology, as well as to the site of origin. For this reason, preoperative histologic diagnosis, together with assessment of local and regional extension, is essential for surgical planning. Of note, the indications and treatment strategies in MiSGMT overlap with those of other epithelial malignancies, with the exception of AdCC, which presents peculiar biological features that will be discussed afterward.

In preoperative workup, the first step is to assess the disease with radiologic imaging such as computed tomography (CT) and/or magnetic resonance imaging (MRI) with contrast medium [28, 29]. The second step is to perform an incisional biopsy that does not interfere with the definitive treatment. Indeed, an adequate tissue sample makes it easier for the pathologist to accurately classify the tumor or, at least, to provide an indication of the tumor grade [30]. All the other information such as the presence of perineural growth and lymphovascular invasion can usually be obtained only from the definitive specimen. When the pathologist poses a preoperative suspect of high-grade malignant tumor, positron emission tomography (PET) and ultrasonography (US) of the neck are recommended to rule out systemic and regional spread, respectively. It is worth remembering that in AdCC PET scan has a low sensitivity and preoperative assessment is better performed using CT scan with contrast enhancement of the chest and abdomen together with bone scintigraphy.

As a general rule, surgery followed by adjuvant radiotherapy is commonly indicated as the treatment of choice for MiSGMT [3, 31]. Resectability is preoperatively determined based on staging workup, site of origin of the lesion, histology, and surgical expertise. A challenging scenario is offered by cases in which preoperative imaging anticipates that macroscopic disease will be left behind in critical anatomic areas (i.e., cavernous sinus). Up to now, no data supporting radiotherapy with state-of-the-art technology as an alternative to incomplete surgery followed by radiotherapy are available in the literature [31].

The goal of surgery is to achieve radical resection with clear margins: in all series, margin status is an important prognostic factor [20, 21, 32, 33]. However, there are specific problems to be considered when planning intervention: AdCC is characterized by a peculiar tendency to perineural, submucosal, and subperiosteal/perichondral spread, all features which need to be accurately identified by preoperative imaging and intraoperative frozen sections. All the named nerves adjacent to the tumor should be carefully inspected and, in case of doubtful invasion, should be biopsied; in case of positivity, they should be resected until clear margins are obtained proximally and distally, if possible [31, 34]. Among the different localizations, the sinonasal tract and the nasopharynx are probably the most critical in relation to the potential of the lesion to involve vital anatomical structures and, consequently, to the difficulty of resecting the lesion with adequate margins. Another characteristic of AdCC, which has an impact on treatment outcome, is that the lesion is diagnosed at an advanced stage in the majority of patients. This is especially true for the sinonasal tract and nasopharynx, where T3–T4 lesions account for up to 78% of cases [7, 32, 35, 36]. The oral cavity and oropharynx (up to 70%) and laryngotracheal axis (up to 60%) follow [4, 5, 37, 38].

Non-adenoid cystic carcinomas (NAdCC) are diagnosed at relatively earlier stage compared to AdCC [39]. In spite of the high degree of histologic heterogeneity, in NAdCC tumor grade is probably the most important prognostic factor. Low- and intermediate-grade lesions display indolent growth, low tendency to spread along nerves and subperiosteal/perichondral planes, and favorable prognosis [33, 40–42]; usually a less aggressive policy of surgical resection is advised in these lesions. As a general rule, a margin greater than 1 cm is considered adequate [39]. Conversely, high-grade tumors can display a more aggressive and rapid pattern of growth with perineural and lymphovascular spread, and thus more aggressive surgical treatment is generally required.

In addition, surgical planning for both AdCC and NAdCC tumors needs to consider the possibility of a reconstructive phase; in fact, although in recent years there has been an evolving trend of surgical techniques in favor of approaches that tend to minimize morbidity and optimize both functional and esthetic results (i.e., endoscopic transnasal surgery for sinonasal and nasopharyngeal tumors, transoral robotic surgery for base of the tongue tumors), extensive surgical resection can be still required.

Once the tumor is staged and graded, adjuvant radiotherapy is recommended for most patients. Going into detail, in case of AdCC, the indications include all patients with exclusion of pT1 tumors without histologic risk factors (perineural and/or lymphovascular spread, solid variant); in case of NAdCC, adjuvant radiotherapy is recommended for all high-grade tumors, pT3–T4 low-grade tumors, and pT2 low-grade tumors in the presence of aggressive features (involved margins and/or proximity to vital structures) [3, 31]. Of note, an improved locoregional control does not invariably translate in higher survival rates; this is especially true for high-grade tumors, which are characterized by a high rate of distant failure [3, 14].

In view of the peculiarities of the different subsites in terms of surgical requirements, we will provide a separate discussion. Furthermore, all the main pathways of spread typically involved in AdCC, in view of its tendency to spread along nerves and subperiosteal/perichondral planes, will be reviewed.

7.2 Oral Cavity

Pathways of spread:

1. Spaces: sublingual, submandibular, pterygopalatine fossa (palate lesions), masticatory, parapharyngeal
2. Nerves: lingual, hypoglossal, inferior alveolar (oral floor and tongue lesions), greater and lesser palatine, nasopalatine, Vidian (trigone and palate lesions), maxillary, and mandibular

Minor salivary gland tumors arising in the oral cavity are rare, accounting for about 10% of all salivary gland tumors, with a malignancy rate generally superior to

50% [12, 22, 30]. The hard palate is the most frequently involved site, followed by buccal mucosa and retromolar trigon, with AdCC and MEC being the most frequently encountered histologies [3, 25, 27, 30]. The tumor often presents as a slow-growing, submucosal mass; ulceration and pain are rare, especially at presentation [26, 30]. The importance of histologic type and grading on treatment planning and outcome emphasizes the need, whenever possible, for an incisional biopsy to obtain a representative tissue sample [26, 27, 30, 43].

When dealing with salivary gland cancer of the oral cavity, it is a matter of debate if all the tumors necessarily require resection of the bone. For low-grade MEC, some authors advocate less aggressive treatment than that used in oral squamous cell carcinoma or more aggressive salivary histologies [41], in view of the limited biologic aggressiveness and slow growth of the tumor. When the lesion does not directly involve the bone, careful intraoperative assessment of the periosteum with frozen sections should be performed, and, in the absence of infiltration, sparing the bone is considered an adequate choice (Fig. 7.1). Conversely, whenever a low-grade tumor shows bone involvement, bony removal could be modulated according to the site of origin of the lesion and entity of bone invasion; thus, limited palatectomy and partial or total maxillectomy may be performed, accordingly (Fig. 7.2) [27]. The same conservative philosophy does not apply to more aggressive neoplasms with a tendency to spread along subperiosteal and submucosal planes, such as AdCC or

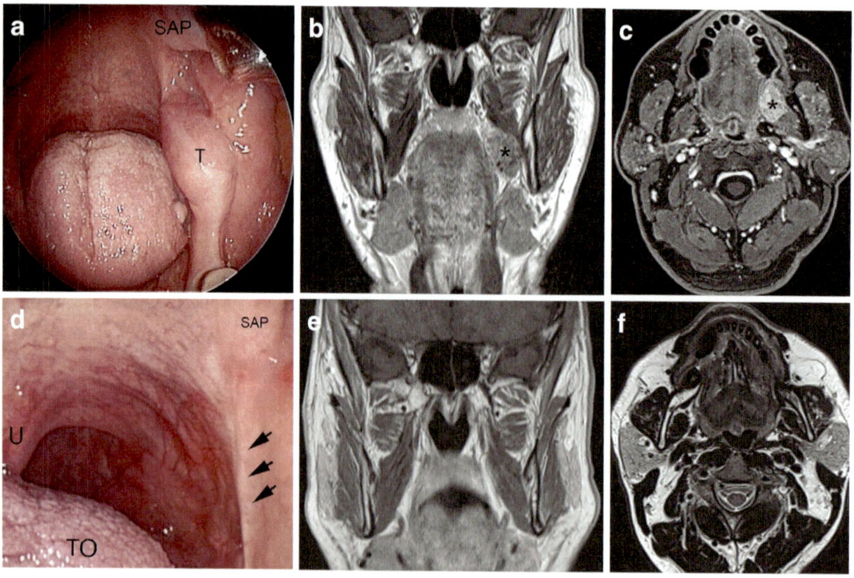

Fig. 7.1 Small submucosal mass involving the left retromolar trigone (**a**). Preoperative MRI in coronal (**b**) and axial (**c**) planes shows that the lesion (asterisk) had no bone involvement. Preoperative biopsy was consistent with low-grade MEC. The lesion was excised through a transoral approach; frozen sections on the mandibular periosteum were negative, and bony removal was not required. Postsurgical endoscopy (**d**) showed a perfectly healed mucosal incision (arrows); MRI on coronal (**e**) and axial (**f**) planes confirmed the absence of local relapse at 3 years after surgery (*SAP* superior alveolar process, *T* tumor, *TO* tongue, *U* uvula)

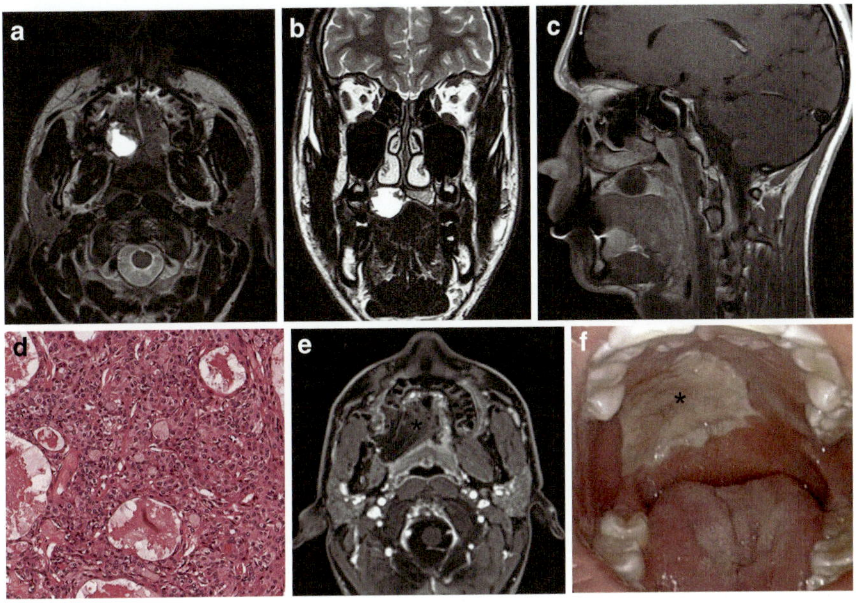

Fig. 7.2 MRI on axial (**a**), coronal (**b**), and sagittal (**c**) planes of a slow-growing lesion involving the full thickness of the right hard palate in a 19-year-old man. Incisional biopsy was consistent with low-grade MEC, and definitive histology confirmed the diagnosis (**d**) (hematoxylin-eosin [H–E]). After transoral inferior maxillectomy, palatal reconstruction was performed by fascio-cutaneous forearm free flap. MRI (**e**) and oral endoscopy (**f**) show the absence of local recurrence and optimal results of palatal reconstruction (asterisk, flap)

high-grade lesions, therefore reducing the possibility of limited surgical approaches. Li et al. presented a series of 103 patients with a salivary gland tumor of the hard palate [27]. The authors clearly demonstrated that AdCC is the histology with the highest risk of positive margins and recurrence that, in this site, is mainly local; their results are perfectly in agreement with those published by other authors [30]. In AdCC, therefore, every effort should be directed toward intraoperatively assessing the status of surgical margins as well as all possible pathways of spread in order to obtain complete resection and minimize the risk of recurrence.

In the presence of tumors extensively involving the hard palate, oral tongue, and/or the floor of the mouth, the surgeon should follow the same principles applied in squamous cell carcinoma. Moreover, after ablative surgery, different options, ranging from prosthetic obturator to pedicled and free flaps, are available [44, 45].

It is worth remembering that the oral cavity, along with the oropharynx, is the preferential site of origin of a recently described salivary cancer, namely, cribriform adenocarcinoma (Fig. 7.3) [46–48]. As pointed out by Skalova et al. [49], in addition to a peculiar cytologic profile and PRKD gene alterations, this tumor is characterized by a relatively indolent growth of the primary lesion and early neck involvement; all these factors contribute in differentiating cribriform adenocarcinoma from "conventional" polymorphous low-grade adenocarcinoma.

Apart from cribriform adenocarcinoma, the risk of nodal involvement at presentation is unexpectedly low. In the series from the MD Anderson Cancer Center, only

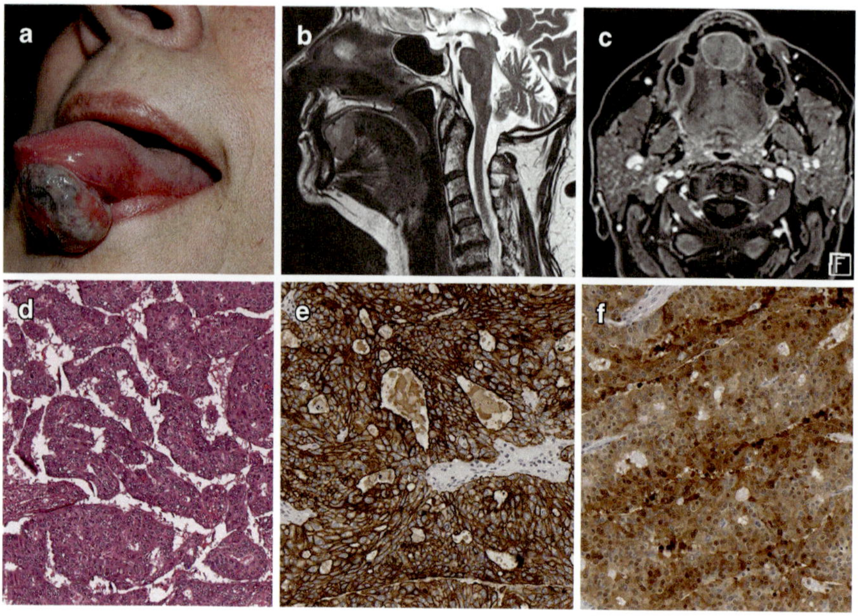

Fig. 7.3 A neoplasm originating from the ventral surface of the oral tongue is clearly visible at clinical (**a**) and MRI evaluation on sagittal (**b**) and axial (**c**) planes. Since preoperative biopsy suggested a diagnosis of cribriform adenocarcinoma, the patient underwent transoral excision with primary closure and bilateral neck dissection. Definitive histology was consistent with the preoperative diagnosis of cribriform adenocarcinoma (H–E staining in **d**, cytocheratin 7 in **e**, S-100 in **f**)

3% of patients had clinically involved cervical lymph nodes at presentation, a rate that was also confirmed in the study from the cancer center in Guangzhou (3.9%) [27, 30]. Kakarala and Bhattacharyya performed a review on 639 cases of oral MiSGMT and found a rate of nodal involvement of 6.6% [25]. Dubal et al., in a SEER database analysis on more than 1000 patients with AdCC of the oral cavity, reported that 6.2% had neck metastasis at presentation [50]. Regarding the risk of occult disease, there are some difficulties in extrapolating specific data since some studies have analyzed oral and oropharyngeal cases together [26], whereas others report only the overall rate of nodal involvement; furthermore, there are studies addressing only the risk in specific subtypes [36]. Mucke et al., in a series of 95 patients with MiSGMT of the oral region in which neck dissection was performed in 57 (66%) cases, detected lymph node positivity in 29 (30.5% overall and 50.9% of those who underwent neck dissection) [43]. Recognizing that their rates were higher than expected, the authors explained the finding with the relatively high number of advanced T-stage lesions in the series. Nobis et al. found occult neck involvement in 13 patients with MiSGMT of the oral cavity (34.2% overall, 37.1% among those who underwent elective neck dissection) [51]. Amit et al., in a multicenter analysis on the role of elective neck dissection in head and neck AdCC, found an overall rate of occult nodal disease of 17%, with the oral cavity being the most frequently involved site (66% of all cases) [36]. Consistently with previous statements, it seems that the risk of occult nodal involvement in MiSGMT is higher in case of advanced T-stage, oral cavity localizations, and high tumor grade. As a consequence, elective treatment of the neck is advised in patients with these risk factors.

7.3 Nasoethmoidal Complex

Pathways of spread:

1. Spaces/areas: the anterior cranial fossa, pterygopalatine fossa, and orbit
2. Nerves: the olfactory phyla (→ anterior cranial fossa), palatine, Vidian (→ ICA), and ethmoidal (→ orbit with possible perineural spread along ophthalmic and/or optic nerve toward the orbital apex and middle cranial fossa)

The most common salivary histologies are AdCC and MEC [52, 53]. Presenting complaints may be scarce and non-specific, thus leading to delayed diagnosis in a relevant proportion of cases [7, 53].

Surgery with possible adjuvant radiotherapy may be considered as the best treatment strategy available in sinonasal salivary cancer [7]. Different from nasopharyngeal tumors, sinonasal MiSGMT does not require a different treatment strategy from non salivary cancers: salivary and non-salivary tumors share the same indications and contraindications for surgery; regardless of the approach, the surgical technique is the same. The most important difference in terms of surgical indications and technique is between AdCC and NAdCC carcinomas due to the specific pattern of growth of AdCC with a natural tendency toward perineural spread and subperiosteal diffusion [31].

For many decades craniofacial resection (CFR), combining a transfacial with a subfrontal approach, has been considered the gold standard for treating naso-ethmoidal malignancies [54, 55]. From the end of the last century, the use of transnasal endoscopic surgery was advocated even for treatment of very selected sinonasal malignancies [56]. In the following years, due to increased surgical expertise and more sophisticated surgical tools, the number of patients treated and the oncologic results led to consider this minimally invasive approach a valid alternative to CFR [57–62]. Endoscopy allows to operate within a magnified surgical field, avoiding any facial incision; moreover, this approach has been demonstrated to be very useful in lesions such as AdCC since it allows to precisely assess the status of all the sites and structures potentially involved by the tumor [31]. Indications and contraindications to a purely endoscopic excision of naso-ethmoidal malignant tumors along with surgical technique have been widely described [57–59, 61, 62]. Far from including a single technique valid for all tumors, the endoscopic approach entails a spectrum of surgical options modulated according to the local extension and biology of the neoplasm. Endoscopic resection (ER) is performed for naso-ethmoidal lesions without extrasinusal extension and no critical relationship with the orbit and skull base (Fig. 7.4). Lesions with focal contact with the skull base, conversely, may require resection of the overlying bone. In the presence of olfactory niche or skull base involvement (with or without dura infiltration) or when microscopic involvement of the dura along olfactory phila is suspected (wide area of contact by tumors with a known propensity for perineural or subperiosteal spread),

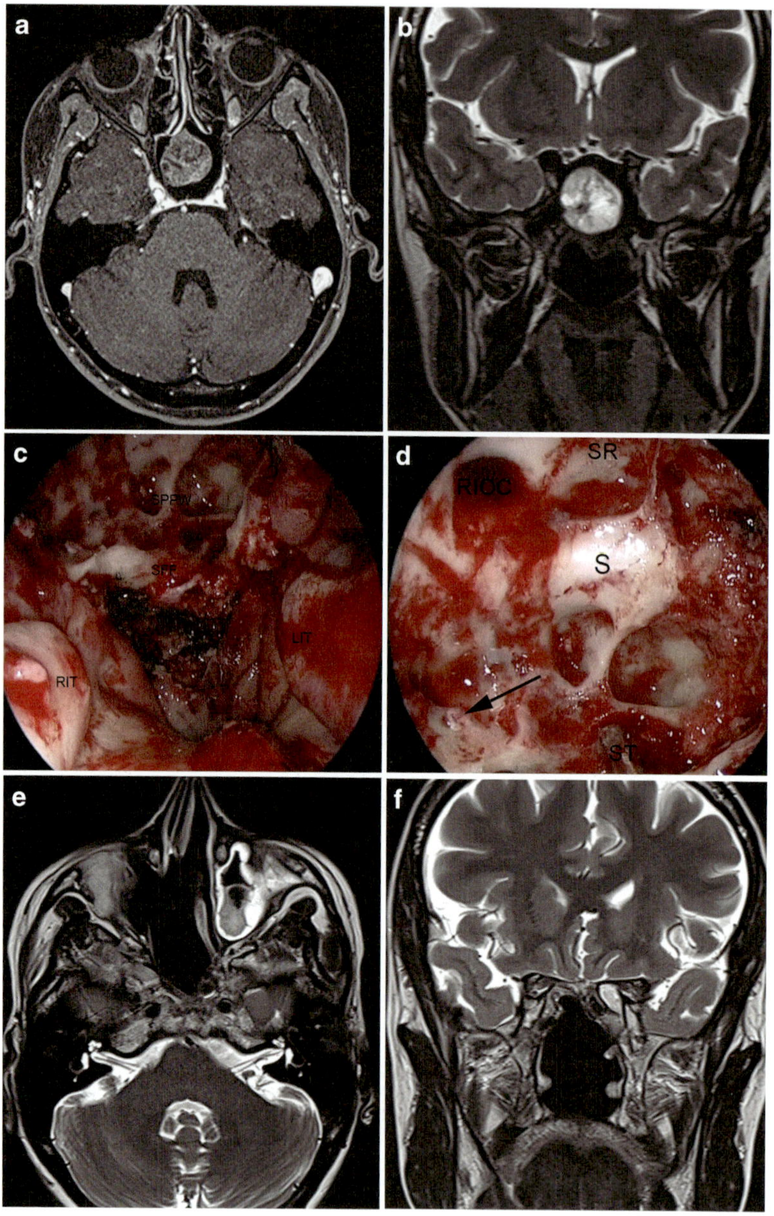

Fig. 7.4 AdCC (mixed tubular-cribriform pattern of growth) involving the sphenoetmhoidal region with no evidence of perineural spread or intracranial extension at preoperative MRI evaluation on axial (**a**) and coronal plane (**b**). A transnasal endoscopic resection without craniectomy was planned; intraoperatively (**c** and **d**), no involvement of the Vidian nerve (arrow in **d**) and sphenoid bone was found. The patient underwent postoperative radiotherapy. MRI on axial (**e**) and coronal (**f**) planes shows no sign of local recurrence at 5 years after treatment. (*LIT* left inferior turbinate, *RIOC* right interoptic-carotid recess, *RIT* right inferior turbinate, *S* sellar region, *SFF* sphenoid sinus floor, *SR* sphenoid roof, *SSPW* sphenoid sinus posterior wall, *ST* suction tube)

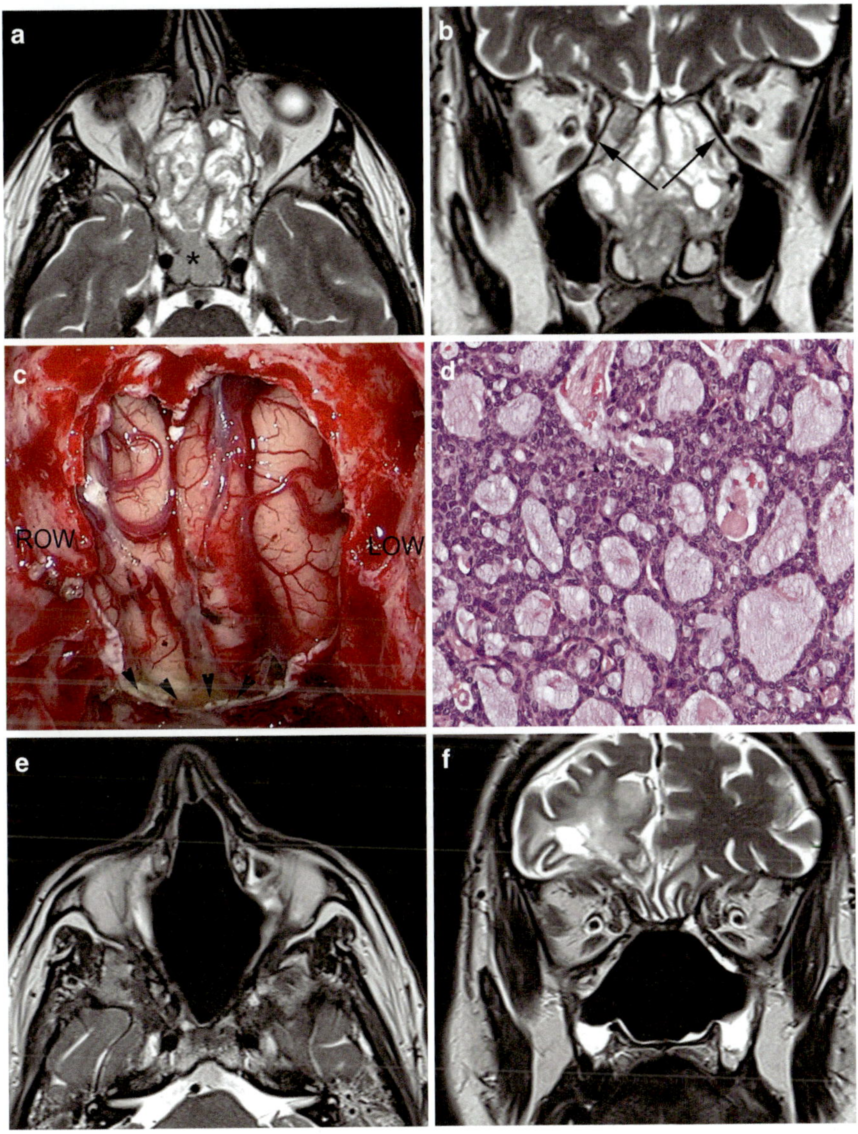

Fig. 7.5 MRI on axial (**a**) and coronal (**b**) planes shows a naso-ethmoidal AdCC with a large area of contact with both orbital walls (arrows) and the anterior skull base; the sphenoid sinus was not involved and filled with mucus (asterisk in **a**). An endoscopic resection with transnasal craniectomy was performed (**c**); the arrowheads point to the posterior dural resection margin. Definitive histology confirmed a mainly cribriform AdCC (**d**) with microscopic dural involvement; adjuvant radiotherapy was therefore performed. MRI on axial (**e**) and coronal (**f**) planes showed no local recurrence at 4 years after treatment; brain post-actinic damage was also visible (*LOW* left orbital wall, *ROW* right orbital wall)

endoscopic resection with transanal craniectomy (ERTC) should be utilized. In this regard, in AdCC abutting the anterior skull base, a more liberal use of ERTC than in NAdCC is recommended (Fig. 7.5). Especially in tumors (AdCC) whose precise local extension may be assessed only at surgery, informed consent should be conceived to enable the surgeon to intraoperatively switch to a more extended procedure in case of involvement of critical structures.

An endoscopic transnasal approach may be combined with a classic subfrontal approach (cranio-endoscopic approach [CER]) in the presence of macroscopic dural involvement of the orbital roof going beyond the vertical plane crossing the eyeball, frontal sinus invasion (with the exception of marginal infiltration of the posterior wall), or massive brain infiltration. Involvement of the hard palate, maxillary sinus walls (except the medial one), orbital content, lacrimal pathway (with the exception of the nasolacrimal duct), or nasal bones may be still considered as contraindications to an endoscopic approach. In these cases, a classic transfacial approach is indicated. When reconstruction of the skull is required, a variety of options are available: pedicled flaps such as the pericranial or nasoseptal flap, autologous material (the fascia lata or iliotibial tract) with a multilayer reconstruction technique [59, 63]; allogenic material is preferably used in combination with a vascularized flap. Lesions with encasement of the ICA, bilateral macroscopic orbit infiltration, optic chiasm involvement, and massive brain infiltration with surrounding edema are deemed unresectable. The management of the orbit will be discussed in the section on maxillary sinus neoplasms.

The risk of nodal involvement in naso-ethmoidal lesions is traditionally considered low, and this statement may also be applied to non-salivary sinonasal tumors. Cantù et al., indeed, in a pivotal paper on the risk of nodal involvement in sinonasal cancer, found nodal involvement in only 5 of 305 (1.6%) patients with naso-ethmoidal lesions [64]. Neck recurrence occurred in 15 (4.9%) patients; notably, no regional relapse was observed in patients with AdCC ($n = 24$) or MEC ($n = 1$). The authors concluded that elective treatment on the neck for naso-ethmoidal lesions is required only for undifferentiated carcinoma (UC).

7.4 Maxillary Sinus

Pathways of spread:

1. Spaces/sites: the pterygopalatine fossa (→ orbit, via the inferior orbital fissure), masticatory space, infratemporal fossa, and middle cranial fossa.
2. Nerves: infraorbital with centripetal (along the maxillary and mandibular nerve toward Gasser's ganglion and Meckel's cave) and centrifugal (premaxillary soft tissues) extension, ophthalmic (→ other orbit nerves), palatine, Vidian. The pathway mandibular-auriculotemporal nerve may lead to facial nerve involvement.

AdCC is the most common salivary cancer affecting the maxillary sinus, whereas ADC and MEC are less frequent [52, 65–67]; among sinonasal primary sites, the maxillary sinus is the most frequently involved by salivary malignant tumors [7, 53]. Presenting complaints are usually non-specific (nasal obstruction, epistaxis) and, along with the slow growth of the majority of salivary cancers, explain why diagnosis is often reached at an advanced stage of the disease when other signs and symptoms (facial numbness, pain or swelling, visual disturbances) suggest invasion of surrounding spaces, nerves, or structures.

Surgery followed by adjuvant radiotherapy is considered the mainstay of treatment for resectable maxillary salivary cancer [7, 66, 67]; nevertheless, some critical issues in surgical planning and crucial differences with treatment of the most frequent maxillary tumors, i.e., squamous cell carcinoma (SCC), need to be reviewed.

In maxillary sinus malignancies, an endoscopic approach should be limited to small lesions exclusively involving the medial wall; this very restrictive indication explains why it is feasible in only a small minority of cases [57]. For all other lesions, different types of maxillectomies (partial, total, and extended total) are available [52]. The specific patterns of growth of AdCC imply that all the possible pathways of spread (perineural, submucosal, and subperiosteal) should be evaluated by preoperative imaging and intraoperatively by multiple frozen sections, even in the absence of macroscopic evidence of involvement. It is inherent that, especially in AdCC, the final resection is often larger than that expected on the basis of preoperative diagnostic workup. In this regard, the pterygopalatine fossa, a real crossroad for AdCC toward surrounding spaces and structures, may be involved in multiple ways: with a direct extension through the maxillary posterior bony wall (Fig. 7.6) or via perineural spread, mainly along the infraorbital and maxillary nerves (Fig. 7.7). It is therefore of utmost importance that this space, even in the absence of macroscopic involvement, is accurately exposed and cleared whenever necessary; the status of the periosteum and nerves should also be checked. In the presence of perineural invasion, the nerve should be resected under the guidance of frozen sections until the residual stumps (proximal and distal) show the absence of neoplastic infiltration [31].

Similarly to naso-ethmoidal lesions, another critical point is the management of the orbital content. As a general rule, orbital clearance is required whenever the periorbit has been crossed and a macroscopic infiltration of fat or muscles is detected (Fig. 7.8). For lesions only in contact with or minimally infiltrating the orbit wall, removal of bone and possibly of the adjacent periorbit is deemed an adequate solution. Notably, AdCC may extend directly to the orbit through adjacent spaces (i.e., the pterygopalatine fossa and inferior orbit fissure), thus reaching critical areas such as the orbital apex. Tumors involving the orbital apex, due to their poorly accessible location as well as a relevant risk of middle cranial fossa extension through dural and perineural spread, may require an aggressive surgical treatment entailing not only orbital clearance but also resection of the surrounding skull base and dura [68].

In addition, management of skull base is crucial. Maxillary sinus tumors require resection of the adjacent skull base whenever there is involvement of the overlying mucosa or soft tissues. In the presence of spread along the olfactory phyla and/or bone invasion, the resection should include also the dura. Nishio et al. reviewed a series of 40 patients with T4 maxillary cancer (only a minority with salivary origin) involving the anterior skull base who received anterolateral craniofacial resection [69]. They reported encouraging oncologic results (5-year overall survival of 62.7%) with a dismal prognosis for patients ($n = 5$) with cavernous sinus involvement; notably, all these five cases experienced CNS complications. They concluded that, in the presence of

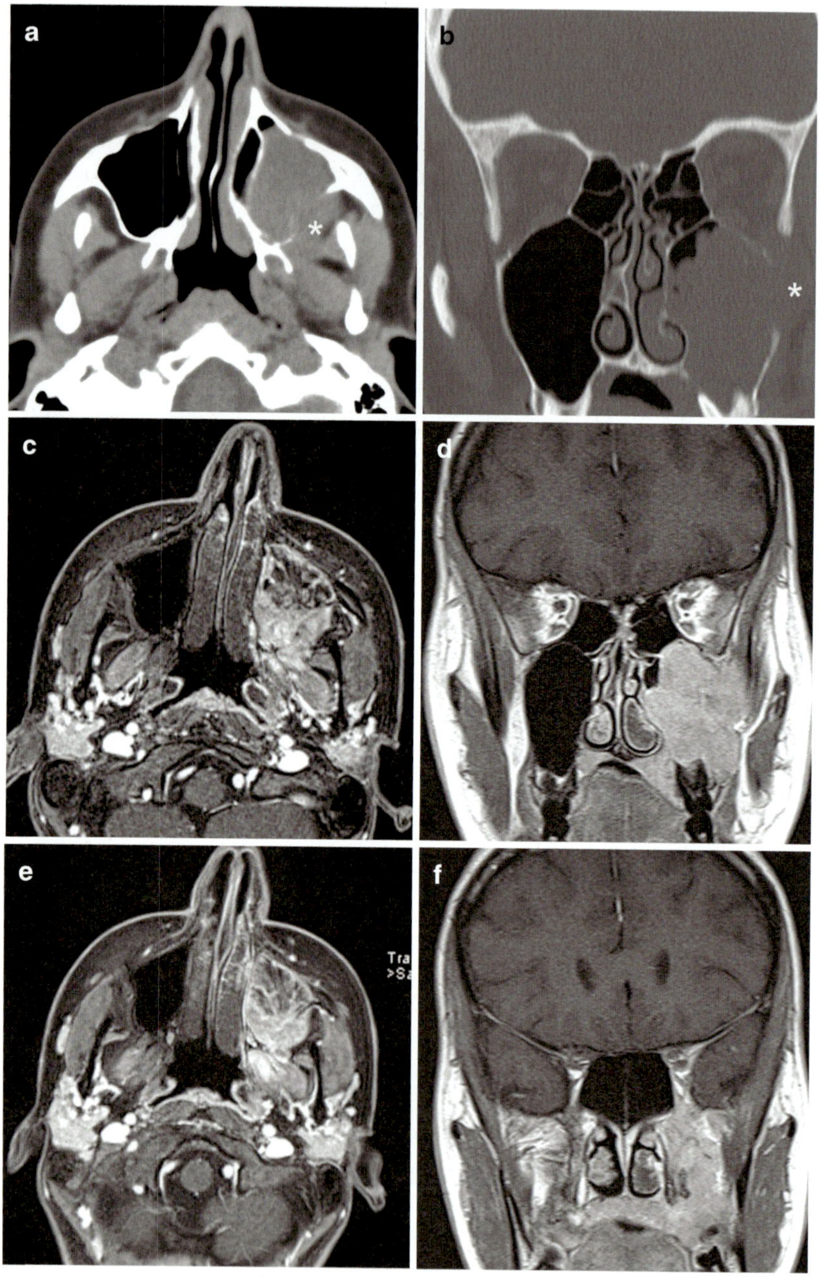

Fig. 7.6 Serendipitous finding of an otherwise asymptomatic left maxillary lesion in a 24-year-old girl at plain CT on axial (**a**) and coronal (**b**) planes; erosion of the posterior wall of the sinus with possible extension (asterisk) into the surrounding spaces is evident. MRI on axial (**c**, **e**) and coronal (**d**, **f**) planes better depicts the presence of a malignant tumor (later revealed to be AdCC), infiltrating the posterior wall of the maxillary sinus and massively involving the pterygoid root, pterygopalatine fossa, and masticatory space

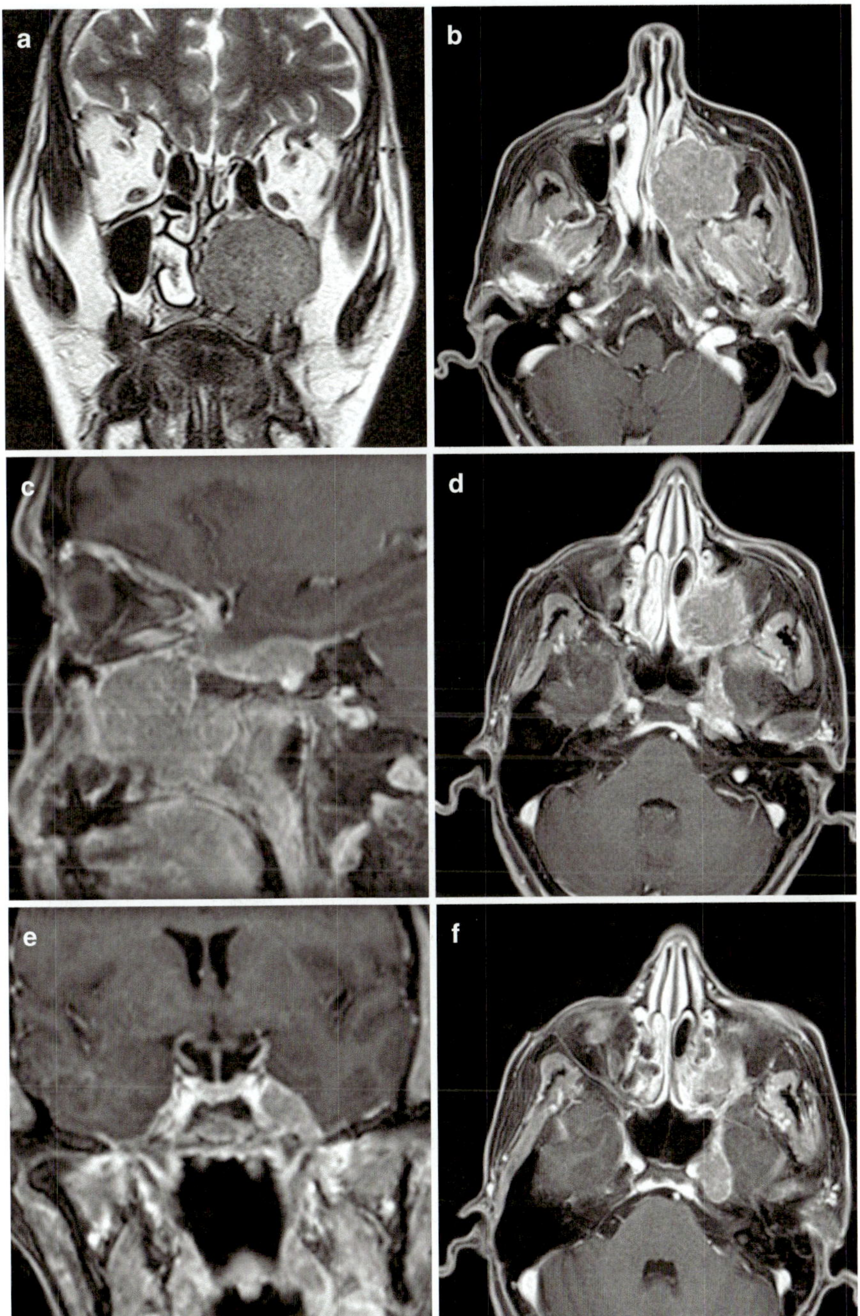

Fig. 7.7 A 65-year-old woman with facial numbness lasting 6 months. MRI on coronal (**a**, **e**), axial (**b**, **d**, **f**), and sagittal (**c**) planes shows a maxillary AdCC involving nearly the entire sinus with marked perineural spread along maxillary nerve causing massive cavernous sinus involvement

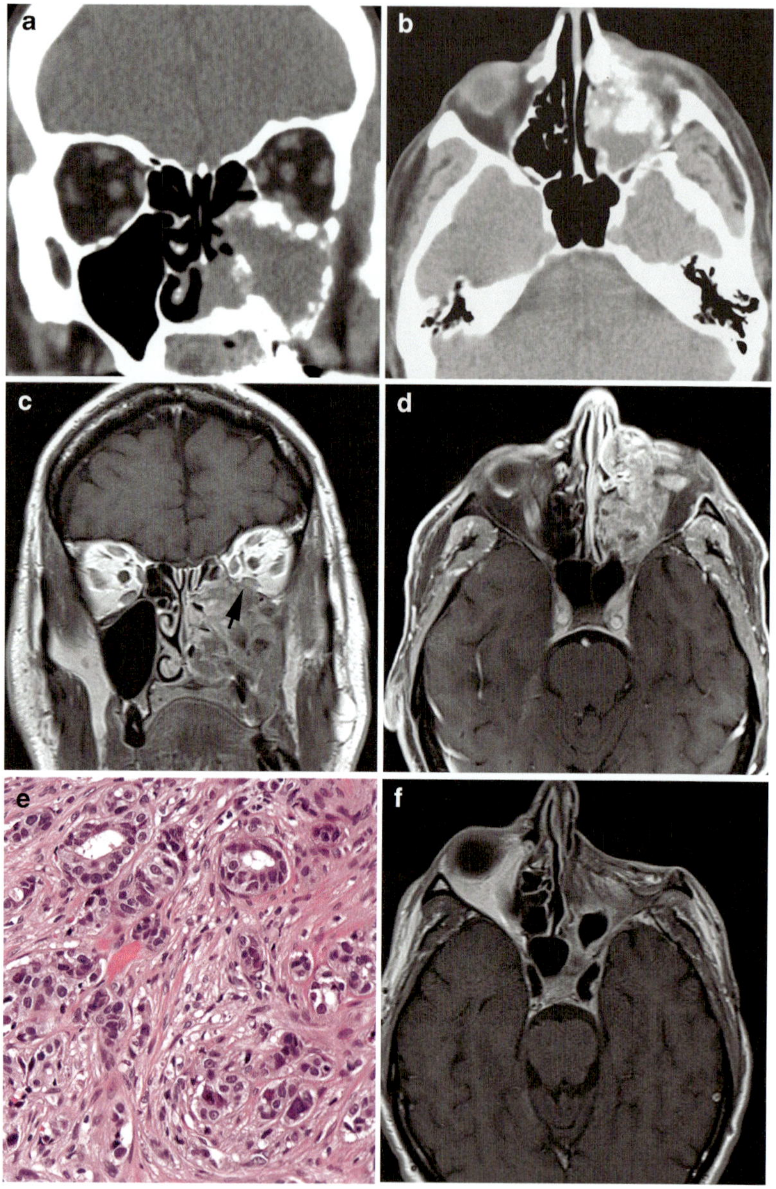

Fig. 7.8 Left maxillary sinus lesion in a 72-year-old patient; pre-treatment CT (**a**, **b**) and MRI (**c**, **d**) on coronal and axial planes, respectively, show a maxillary neoplasm extensively invading the bone and with a critical relationship with the orbital content (arrows). Incisional biopsy was consistent with high-grade, not otherwise specified, salivary cancer. The patient underwent radical maxillectomy with orbital clearance (orbit invasion confirmed by frozen sections), selective neck dissection (I–III), and reconstruction with the rectus abdominis free flap. Definitive histology was consistent with salivary duct cancer (H–E staining in **e**) (pT4a N0 M0). Twenty-four months after the end of adjuvant radiotherapy, no signs of local relapse were identified at MRI (**f**), and PET-CT showed multiple lung metastases

involvement of the cavernous sinus, due to surgical morbidity as well as poor prognosis, surgical resection should no longer be justified. The authors' statement emphasized the concept that aggressive surgery with possible disfiguring mutilation may be considered justified only if R0 or R1 surgical margins may be obtained, especially in tumors where free surgical margins are reached in a relatively low percentage of patients [7, 52]. Whenever macroscopic residual disease is expected, the possibility of nonsurgical treatment should also be discussed with the patient. In this scenario, promising data on heavy-ion therapy (carbon and proton) for treatment of resectable and unresectable AdCC have been reported [70, 71]. It is worth remembering that currently there is no general consensus about the ideal treatment strategy of advanced AdCC (surgery with adjuvant radiotherapy vs. partial removal with planned residual disease and radiotherapy vs. exclusive radiotherapy). Tumor involvement of critical areas and structures, the efficacy and morbidity of each treatment, specific expertise of the surgical and radiation oncology team, and patient's willingness are all factors that must be balanced and which all contribute to the final treatment decision [31].

One of the most striking differences between maxillary SCC and salivary tumors is the risk of nodal involvement. Dooley and Shah, in a review on the risk of nodal involvement in maxillary SCC, mention some papers that report an overall incidence of N+ at diagnosis of about 15% [72–75]. The risk of neck involvement in maxillary sinus salivary cancer seems to be lower. Cantù et al. found neck metastases in 33 of 399 (8.3%) patients with maxillary sinus malignancies: nodal disease was found in 16/156 (10.6%) cases with SCC and in 4 additional cases with UC [64]. No details on histology in the remaining 13 cases were provided, but the overall rate of nodal disease in non-SCC, non-UC carcinoma was 6% [64]. Moreover, neck recurrences (51/399, 12.5%) from maxillary sinus primary lesions were more frequent in the SCC-UC (35/156, 22.4%) than in the non-SCC-UC (16/243, 6.6%) subgroup. Pantvaidya et al., in a review on 163 patients with sinonasal salivary malignancies, reported that 7.9% of patients were cN+ at presentation, with equal distribution between AdCC, ADC, and MEC [52]. On the other hand, Lupinetti et al. found that only 2% of patients with sinonasal AdCC were N+ [7]. These low rates of involvement apparently do not justify the need for elective treatment of the neck, apart from aggressive, high-grade tumors.

After major surgical ablation, there is the need to plan an adequate reconstruction, whose main aims are to divide the sinonasal cavities from the intracranial content and the oral cavity, allow dental prosthetic rehabilitation, and restore facial contour. Several options are available, namely, prosthetic obturator, pedicled flaps (the temporalis muscle), and free flaps (see chapter on reconstruction).

7.5 Nasopharynx

Pathways of spread:

1. Spaces: the pterygopalatine fossa, parapharyngeal space, and masticatory space
2. Nerves: Vidian, maxillary, mandibular, and oculomotor

AdCC and MEC are, by far, the two most frequent histologies affecting the nasopharynx [3, 76]. The treatment of nasopharyngeal MiSGMT can substantially differ from that of the more frequent "classic" non-salivary nasopharyngeal carcinomas (NPC). While there is general consensus that radiotherapy, with or without chemotherapy, is the gold standard for primary NPC, the treatment of tumors of salivary origin is more controversial [77]. This striking difference may be explained by the greater radio-chemosensitivity of NPC in comparison with salivary cancers. NPC is also characterized by a very high risk of clinical involvement (cN+) of retro-lateropharyngeal and lateral neck nodes that therefore need to be treated concomitantly with the primary lesion. The risk of clinically involved lymph nodes (cN+) in nasopharyngeal salivary tumors is considered lower. Notably, Schramm and Imola reported a 47% rate of occult nodal metastasis in a series of 23 patients with MiSGMT of the nasopharynx [76]; however, this rate was calculated only among the 15 patients who underwent elective neck dissection. The scarce radiosensitivity of the primary tumor and lower risk of clinical nodal metastasis explain why nasopharyngeal salivary malignant neoplasms may be effectively treated with radical intent by surgery, with different techniques according to tumor location and extent.

For many years, only external approaches have been adopted for the treatment of recurrent NPC or primary non-NPC tumors; nasopharyngectomy was and may still be performed through trans-maxillary [78], trans-palatal, infratemporal [76], trans-mandibular, or maxillary swing procedures [79]. All these approaches, however, are burdened with significant sequelae and complications related to osteotomies and soft tissue incisions, such as nasopalatal fistulas, trigeminal branch numbness, temporomandibular joint dysfunction, or osteitis.

In the last decade, the development of angled scopes and dedicated surgical instruments as well as increased surgical experience has allowed to effectively treat selected cases of nasopharyngeal salivary cancer using a minimally invasive, transnasal endoscopic approach [77]. As pointed out by Castelnuovo et al. [77], who extensively described surgical techniques and indications, the critical points for a purely endoscopic nasopharyngectomy are the dura of the posterior cranial fossa and the parapharyngeal-paraclival tract of the internal carotid artery (ICA). One of the major advantages with a transnasal endoscopic approach is the possibility to modulate the approach according to the site of origin and local extension of the tumor. For lesions limited to the posterior wall of the nasopharynx, a simple resection of the posterior nasopharyngeal wall is performed (NER type 1) [77, 80]. Whenever the lesion extends to involve the roof of the nasopharynx, the resection should be extended to the overlying floor of the sphenoid sinus (NER type 2). When the tumor extends laterally to the eustachian tube and the lateral wall of the nasopharynx, the surgical procedure required is more complex (NER type 3) and requires a trans-pterygoid trans-maxillary approach (Fig. 7.9). The posterior wall of the maxillary sinus along with the content of the pterygopalatine fossa and the pterygoid process is removed in order to expose the cartilaginous portion of the eustachian tube.

Tumors with a critical relationship with the ICA, macroscopic posterior cranial fossa dural involvement, and/or intracranial extension should not be treated by a

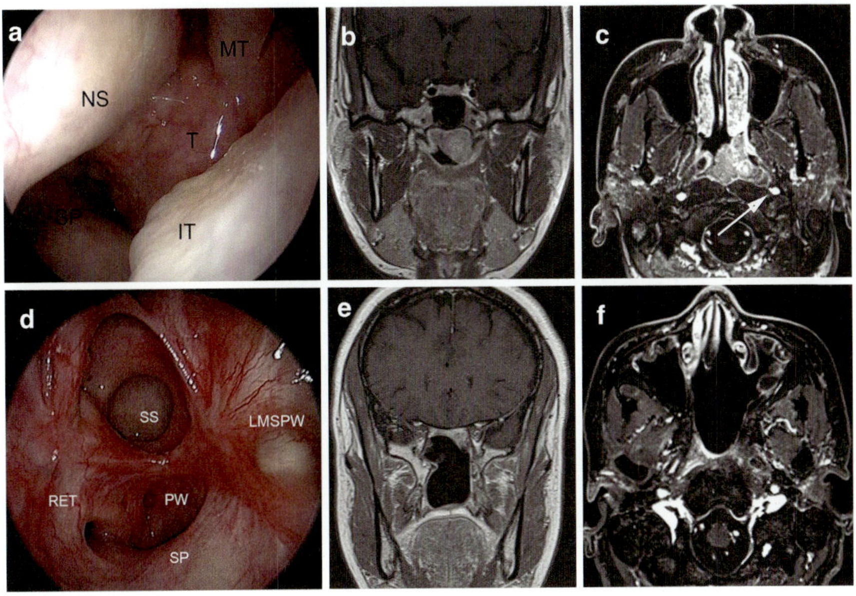

Fig. 7.9 Pre-treatment nasal endoscopy (**a**) and MRI in coronal (**b**) and axial (**c**) planes showing a nasopharyngeal AdCC with no critical relationship with the left ICA (arrow in **c**) and no intracranial extension. The patient was treated by transnasal endoscopic nasopharyngectomy (NER Type 3) [77] and adjuvant radiotherapy. Nasal endoscopy (**d**) and MRI on coronal (**e**) and axial (**f**) planes show no signs of local recurrence at 7 years after treatment (*IT* inferior turbinate, *LMSPW* left maxillary sinus posterior wall, *MT* middle turbinate, *NS* nasal septum, *PW* posterior nasopharyngeal wall, *RET* right eustachian tube, *SP* soft palate, *SS* sphenoid sinus, *T* tumor)

purely transnasal endoscopic approach [77]. In these cases a combined procedure (i.e., endoscopic and infratemporal) or a purely external approach is required.

The group from the Queen Mary Hospital in Hong Kong demonstrated that the maxillary swing approach, mainly conceived for treatment of recurrent NPC, may warrant good oncologic and functional outcomes with a reasonable rate of complications [81–83]. This approach allows, whenever necessary, to extend the resection to the skull base, and even the ICA may be resected; in these cases an extracranial-intracranial vascular bypass may be accomplished [82]. In recent years, some preclinical and clinical experiences have advocated the use of robotic surgery for the treatment of nasopharyngeal tumors, although this approach appears to have several limitations (it is cumbersome and does not include the possibility to use drills and chisel) and seems therefore to be far from definitive validation [84, 85]. Finally, different reconstructive options are available with the main intent to reconstruct the dura and cover the ICA and bone, thus minimizing the risk of postoperative hemorrhage and/or osteitis/osteonecrosis. The reconstructive choice may vary from locally harvested flaps (pericranium, nasoseptal flap, temporoparietal fascial flap, temporalis muscle) to free flaps (rectus abdominis, lateral thigh, radial forearm) according to the different situations [81, 86, 87].

The delayed diagnosis of nasopharyngeal neoplasms with possible locally advanced disease at presentation, the risk of occult nodal involvement, and the specific biology of MiSGMT concur in defining a definitive role for adjuvant radiotherapy [88], whereas exclusive radiotherapy, especially with heavy particles, is presently considered a viable choice in the treatment of unresectable lesions (Fig. 7.10) [89].

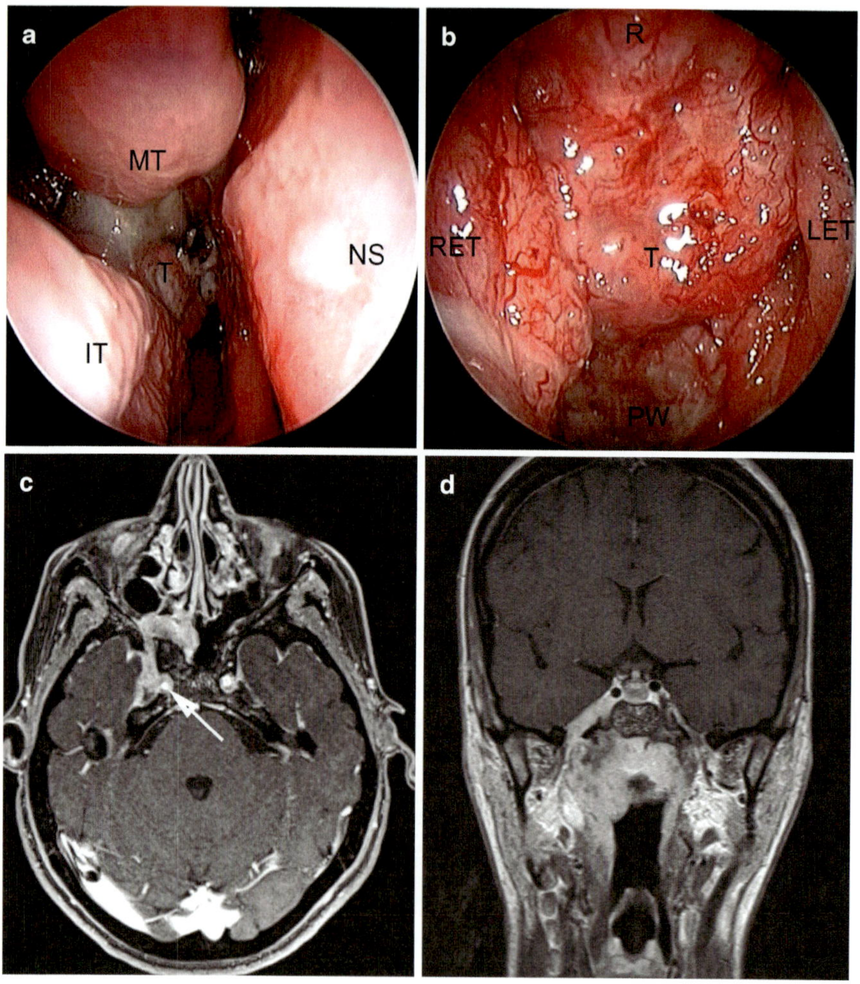

Fig. 7.10 Nasal endoscopy shows an AdCC reaching the right choanal region (**a**) and involving the entire nasopharyngeal surface with mucosal spreading over the right eustachian tube (**b**). At MRI (**c**, **d**), the lesion is found to have macroscopic intracranial extension along trigeminal branches with right ICA encasement (arrow in **c**) and cavernous sinus involvement. The lesion was deemed not suitable for surgical treatment, and the patient underwent exclusive radiotherapy (*IT* inferior turbinate, *LET* left eustachian tube, *MT* middle turbinate, *NS* nasal septum, *PW* posterior nasopharyngeal wall, *RET* right eustachian tube, *T* tumor)

7.6 Oropharynx

Pathways of spread:

1. Spaces/sites: the parapharyngeal space, masticatory space, mobile tongue, and floor of the mouth
2. Nerves: hypoglossal, lingual, glossopharyngeal

MiSGMT rarely affects the oropharynx, and the base of the tongue is the most commonly involved subsite, followed by the soft palate and palatine tonsil [90]; even in this site, MEC and AdCC are the most frequently encountered histologies. Surgery, which is considered the mainstay of treatment, includes a large spectrum of approaches: transoral, transcervical, and transmandibular (with or without mandibulectomy) [90]. The latter is classically considered to provide the best exposure, though at the expense of possible sequelae and complications (i.e., malocclusion, osteitis, or osteonecrosis) [91]. Iyer et al. reported that, even if an open-neck approach was used in 67% of 61 patients undergoing primary surgery for oropharyngeal MiSGMT, positive margins were observed in 28 (46%) cases; not surprisingly, the majority of involved margins were found in base of tongue tumors [90].

In the last decade, the introduction of robotic surgery has added a new tool for the treatment of oropharyngeal tumors. Villanueva et al. reported a preliminary experience in the treatment of ten cases of oropharyngeal MiSGMT by this approach [91]. Functional and quality-of-life outcomes were excellent; moreover, only one of the ten patients had positive margins at definitive histology. Notably, the authors reported a complication rate that was less than in traditional open-neck approaches to the oropharynx. This finding is completely in agreement with data reported in papers comparing robotic and open surgery for oropharyngeal SCC [92]. However, the authors recognized the inherent limitations of the study, namely, the low number of cases and preliminary functional evaluation. Moreover, it is clearly stated that transoral robotic surgery should be considered as an appropriate tool for the treatment of early-stage lesions [91].

As a general rule, oropharyngeal primary tumors are considered at high risk of nodal involvement, especially when the tongue base is involved [93]. While there is no doubt that cN+ patients, whenever deemed operable, are candidates for therapeutic neck dissection, elective treatment of the neck is more controversial. On the one hand, it is difficult to retrieve data on a specific site/subsite, and, on the other, the impact of elective treatment of the neck in MiSGMT is less relevant in view of a very high risk of distant failure [93].

7.7 Larynx

Pathways of spread:

1. Sites: the hypopharynx and esophagus, thyroid gland, and trachea
2. Nerves: recurrent laryngeal, superior laryngeal

Tumors of salivary origin are extremely rare in the larynx, since they account for less than 1% of all malignancies in this anatomic site [3, 4, 94]. The subglottis is the most involved subsite followed by the glottis and supraglottis [3, 95]; AdCC and MEC are the most frequent histologies [4, 94], whereas other subtypes such as ACNOS are extremely rare [96]. Hoarseness and dyspnea are the most frequent presenting complaints, even if diagnosis, mainly as a consequence of a slow growth, is often delayed [94, 95].

The mainstay of treatment of salivary laryngeal cancer is surgical excision, possibly followed by radiotherapy [97]. Due to the frequent subglottic origin and late diagnosis at an advanced stage, conservative surgery is only occasionally feasible [98], and therefore total laryngectomy is the surgical option that is most frequently reported in the literature [95].

In supraglottic tumors, conservative options include horizontal supraglottic laryngectomy by a transoral endoscopic or conventional cervicotomic approach; the former should be performed in the absence of massive involvement of the pre-epiglottic space and tongue base invasion (Fig. 7.11) [99, 100]. Among lesions involving the glottic plane, only those without cartilage and posterior paraglottic space involvement and with limited subglottic extension may be effectively treated by transoral excision with CO_2 laser; in all other cases, a cervicotomic approach is required. Supracricoid laryngectomy (with crico-hyoid- or crico-hyoid-epiglottopexy) is considered a valid surgical option, provided that at least one functional cricoarytenoid unit may be spared and no critical extension toward the inter-aritenoid space and the subglottis is demonstrated [101, 102]. In AdCC the indications for conservative surgery are further decreased by its well-known propensity

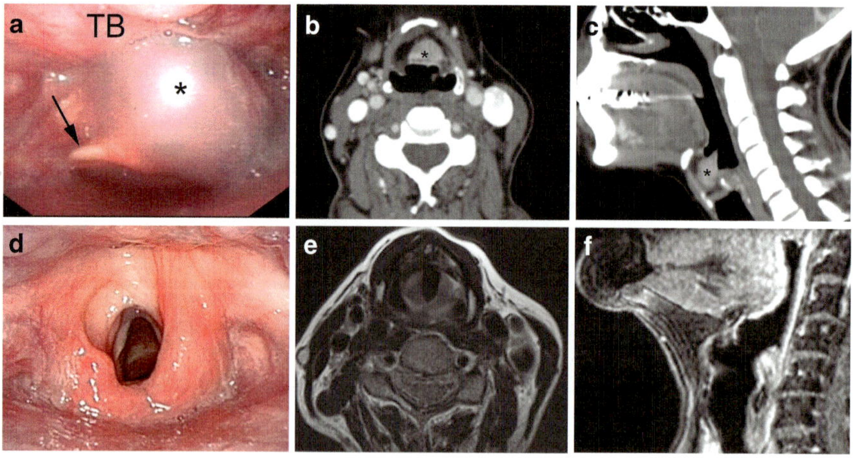

Fig. 7.11 A well-defined lesion (asterisk) was found on the lingual surface of the epiglottis (arrow) (**a**). Preoperative CT on axial (**b**) and sagittal (**c**) planes shows a mildly enhancing lesion (asterisk) with marginal pre-epiglottic space involvement and no extension into the tongue base. A transoral supraglottic laryngectomy was performed. Definitive histology was consistent with AdCC (cribriform type, no solid component). Resection margins were clear, and perineural spread was absent; no adjuvant radiotherapy was therefore planned. Seven years after treatment, laryngoscopy (**d**) and MRI on axial (**e**) and sagittal (**f**) planes are negative for recurrence (*TB* tongue base)

for perineural and submucosal spread, thus confirming total laryngectomy as the only therapeutic option in the majority of cases [95, 103].

Subglottic lesions are commonly diagnosed at an advanced stage, thus requiring total laryngectomy extending to the first tracheal rings. In rare cases with limited cricoid arch involvement, at least one functioning cricoarytenoid unit, and longitudinal tracheal involvement less than 4.5–5 cm, a conservative approach (crico-tracheal resection and anastomosis) may be performed [104].

The risk of nodal disease in laryngeal salivary cancer is difficult to assess, since most of the investigations report on low number of patients and/or the risk is detailed for specific histologies only, such as AdCC [4, 94, 105]. The risk of cN+ in laryngeal salivary cancer is about 25–27% [4, 94]; when only AdCC is analyzed, the rate drops to 13.3–15.4% [95, 97, 105]. Marchiano et al. in a systematic review on 89 cases of laryngeal AdCC reported neck involvement in 13 of 89 (14.6%) patients [95]. Coca-Pelaz et al. completed a multicenter analysis on the risk of nodal involvement in laryngeal AdCC: they were able to assess the status of cervical lymph nodes in 156 patients, and only 24 (15.4%) showed disease in the neck [105]. All the aforementioned authors concur in considering neck dissection mandatory in cN+ patients, whereas the role of elective treatment of the neck is more controversial. Hellquist et al. highlighted that, in the presence of a high transformation of head and neck AdCC, the risk of nodal metastasis is 5–10 times higher than conventional AdCC and therefore elective neck dissection is strongly advised in patients with this highly aggressive variant [106]. Even in laryngeal MEC, there is general consensus about the need for elective treatment of the neck in the presence of high-grade lesions [107, 108].

References

1. Albeck H, Nielsen NH, Hansen HE, et al. Epidemiology of nasopharyngeal and salivary gland carcinoma in Greenland. Arctic Med Res. 1992;51:189–95.
2. Ellis GL, Auclair P. The normal salivary glands. In: Ellis GL, Auclair P, editors. Tumors of the salivary glands. Washington, DC: Armed Forces Institute of Pathology; 1996. p. 1–23.
3. Vander Poorten V, Hunt J, Bradley PJ, et al. Recent trends in the management of minor salivary gland carcinoma. Head Neck. 2014;36:444–55.
4. Ganly I, Patel SG, Coleman M, Ghossein R, Carlson D, Shah JP. Malignant minor salivary gland tumors of the larynx. Arch Otolaryngol Head Neck Surg. 2006;132:767–70.
5. Nielsen TK, Bjorndal K, Krogdahl A, et al. Salivary gland carcinomas of the larynx: a national study in Denmark. Auris Nasus Larynx. 2012;39:611–4.
6. Kim KH, Sung MW, Chung PS, Rhee CS, Park CI, Kim WH. Adenoid cystic carcinoma of the head and neck. Arch Otolaryngol Head Neck Surg. 1994;120:721–6.
7. Lupinetti AD, Roberts DB, Williams MD, et al. Sinonasal adenoid cystic carcinoma: the M. D. Anderson Cancer Center experience. Cancer. 2007;110:2726–31.
8. Sanghvi S, Patel NR, Patel CR, Kalyoussef E, Baredes S, Eloy JA. Sinonasal adenoid cystic carcinoma: comprehensive analysis of incidence and survival from 1973 to 2009. Laryngoscope. 2013;123:1592–7.
9. Li N, Xu L, Zhao H, El-Naggar AK, Sturgis EM. A comparison of the demographics, clinical features, and survival of patients with adenoid cystic carcinoma of major and minor salivary glands versus less common sites within the Surveillance, Epidemiology, and End Results registry. Cancer. 2012;118:3945–53.

10. Marcinow A, Ozer E, Teknos T, et al. Clinicopathologic predictors of recurrence and overall survival in adenoid cystic carcinoma of the head and neck: a single institutional experience at a tertiary care center. Head Neck. 2014;36:1705–11.
11. Coca-Pelaz A, Rodrigo JP, Bradley PJ, et al. Adenoid cystic carcinoma of the head and neck—an update. Oral Oncol. 2015;51:652–61.
12. Spiro RH, Thaler HT, Hicks WF, Kher UA, Huvos AH, Strong EW. The importance of clinical staging of minor salivary gland carcinoma. Am J Surg. 1991;162:330–6.
13. Sadeghi A, Tran LM, Mark R, Sidrys J, Parker RG. Minor salivary gland tumors of the head and neck: treatment strategies and prognosis. Am J Clin Oncol. 1993;16:3–8.
14. Garden AS, Weber RS, Ang KK, Morrison WH, Matre J, Peters LJ. Postoperative radiation therapy for malignant tumors of minor salivary glands. Outcome and patterns of failure. Cancer. 1994;73:2563–9.
15. Anderson JN Jr, Beenken SW, Crowe R, et al. Prognostic factors in minor salivary gland cancer. Head Neck. 1995;17:480–6.
16. Parsons JT, Mendenhall WM, Stringer SP, Cassisi NJ, Million RR. Management of minor salivary gland carcinomas. Int J Radiat Oncol Biol Phys. 1996;35:443–54.
17. Chou C, Zhu G, Luo M, Xue G. Carcinoma of the minor salivary glands: results of surgery and combined therapy. J Oral Maxillofac Surg. 1996;54:448–53.
18. Jones AS, Beasley NJ, Houghton DJ, Helliwell TR, Husband DJ. Tumours of the minor salivary glands. Clin Otolaryngol Allied Sci. 1998;23:27–33.
19. Le QT, Birdwell S, Terris DJ, et al. Postoperative irradiation of minor salivary gland malignancies of the head and neck. Radiother Oncol. 1999;52:165–71.
20. Vander Poorten VL, Balm AJ, Hilgers FJ, Tan IB, Keus RB, Hart AA. Stage as major long term outcome predictor in minor salivary gland carcinoma. Cancer. 2000;89:1195–204.
21. Terhaard CH, Lubsen H, Van der Tweel I, et al. Salivary gland carcinoma: independent prognostic factors for locoregional control, distant metastases, and overall survival: results of the Dutch head and neck oncology cooperative group. Head Neck. 2004;26:681–92; discussion 692-683.
22. Pires FR, Pringle GA, de Almeida OP, Chen SY. Intra-oral minor salivary gland tumors: a clinicopathological study of 546 cases. Oral Oncol. 2007;43:463–70.
23. Loh KS, Barker E, Bruch G, et al. Prognostic factors in malignancy of the minor salivary glands. Head Neck. 2009;31:58–63.
24. Kruse AL, Gratz KW, Obwegeser JA, Lubbers HT. Malignant minor salivary gland tumors: a retrospective study of 27 cases. Oral Maxillofac Surg. 2010;14:203–9.
25. Kakarala K, Bhattacharyya N. Survival in oral cavity minor salivary gland carcinoma. Otolaryngol Head Neck Surg. 2010;143:122–6.
26. Carrillo JF, Maldonado F, Carrillo LC, et al. Prognostic factors in patients with minor salivary gland carcinoma of the oral cavity and oropharynx. Head Neck. 2011;33:1406–12.
27. Li Q, Zhang XR, Liu XK, et al. Long-term treatment outcome of minor salivary gland carcinoma of the hard palate. Oral Oncol. 2012;48:456–62.
28. Matsuzaki H, Yanagi Y, Hara M, et al. Minor salivary gland tumors in the oral cavity: diagnostic value of dynamic contrast-enhanced MRI. Eur J Radiol. 2012;81:2684–91.
29. Matsuzaki H, Yanagi Y, Hara M, et al. Diagnostic value of dynamic contrast-enhanced MRI for submucosal palatal tumors. Eur J Radiol. 2012;81:3306–12.
30. Beckhardt RN, Weber RS, Zane R, et al. Minor salivary gland tumors of the palate: clinical and pathologic correlates of outcome. Laryngoscope. 1995;105:1155–60.
31. Lombardi D, McGurk M, Vander Poorten V, et al. Surgical treatment of salivary malignant tumors. Oral Oncol. 2017;65:102–13.
32. da Cruz Perez DE, de Abreu Alves F, Nobuko Nishimoto I, de Almeida OP, Kowalski LP. Prognostic factors in head and neck adenoid cystic carcinoma. Oral Oncol. 2006;42:139–46.
33. McHugh CH, Roberts DB, El-Naggar AK, et al. Prognostic factors in mucoepidermoid carcinoma of the salivary glands. Cancer. 2012;118:3928–36.
34. Ramakrishna R, Raza SM, Kupferman M, Hanna E, DeMonte F. Adenoid cystic carcinoma of the skull base: results with an aggressive multidisciplinary approach. J Neurosurg. 2016;124:115–21.

35. Michel G, Joubert M, Delemazure AS, Espitalier F, Durand N, Malard O. Adenoid cystic carcinoma of the paranasal sinuses: retrospective series and review of the literature. Eur Ann Otorhinolaryngol Head Neck Dis. 2013;130:257–62.
36. Amit M, Binenbaum Y, Sharma K, et al. Analysis of failure in patients with adenoid cystic carcinoma of the head and neck. An international collaborative study. Head Neck. 2014;36:998–1004.
37. Bianchi B, Copelli C, Cocchi R, Ferrari S, Pederneschi N, Sesenna E. Adenoid cystic carcinoma of intraoral minor salivary glands. Oral Oncol. 2008;44:1026–31.
38. DeAngelis AF, Tsui A, Wiesenfeld D, Chandu A. Outcomes of patients with adenoid cystic carcinoma of the minor salivary glands. Int J Oral Maxillofac Surg. 2011;40:710–4.
39. Lopes MA, Santos GC, Kowalski LP. Multivariate survival analysis of 128 cases of oral cavity minor salivary gland carcinomas. Head Neck. 1998;20:699–706.
40. Omlie JE, Koutlas IG. Acinic cell carcinoma of minor salivary glands: a clinicopathologic study of 21 cases. J Oral Maxillofac Surg. 2010;68:2053–7.
41. Ord RA, Salama AR. Is it necessary to resect bone for low-grade mucoepidermoid carcinoma of the palate? Br J Oral Maxillofac Surg. 2012;50:712–4.
42. Patel TD, Vazquez A, Marchiano E, Park RC, Baredes S, Eloy JA. Polymorphous low-grade adenocarcinoma of the head and neck: a population-based study of 460 cases. Laryngoscope. 2015;125:1644–9.
43. Mucke T, Robitzky LK, Kesting MR, et al. Advanced malignant minor salivary glands tumors of the oral cavity. Oral Surg Oral Med Oral Pathol Oral Radiol Endod. 2009;108:81–9.
44. Kesting MR, Holzle F, Wales C, et al. Microsurgical reconstruction of the oral cavity with free flaps from the anterolateral thigh and the radial forearm: a comparison of perioperative data from 161 cases. Ann Surg Oncol. 2011;18:1988–94.
45. Piazza C, Paderno A, Taglietti V, Nicolai P. Evolution of complex palatomaxillary reconstructions: the scapular angle osteomuscular free flap. Curr Opin Otolaryngol Head Neck Surg. 2013;21:95–103.
46. Michal M, Skalova A, Simpson RH, et al. Cribriform adenocarcinoma of the tongue: a hitherto unrecognized type of adenocarcinoma characteristically occurring in the tongue. Histopathology. 1999;35:495–501.
47. Michal M, Kacerovska D, Kazakov DV. Cribriform adenocarcinoma of the tongue and minor salivary glands: a review. Head Neck Pathol. 2013;7(Suppl 1):S3–11.
48. Worrall DM, Brant JA, Chai RL, Weinstein GS. Cribriform adenocarcinoma of the tongue and minor salivary gland: transoral robotic surgical resection. ORL J Otorhinolaryngol Relat Spec. 2015;77:87–92.
49. Skalova A, Sima R, Kaspirkova-Nemcova J, et al. Cribriform adenocarcinoma of minor salivary gland origin principally affecting the tongue: characterization of new entity. Am J Surg Pathol. 2011;35:1168–76.
50. Dubal PM, Unsal AA, Chung SY, et al. Population-based trends in outcomes in adenoid cystic carcinoma of the oral cavity. Am J Otolaryngol. 2016;37:398–406.
51. Nobis CP, Rohleder NH, Wolff KD, Wagenpfeil S, Scherer EQ, Kesting MR. Head and neck salivary gland carcinomas—elective neck dissection, yes or no? J Oral Maxillofac Surg. 2014;72:205–10.
52. Pantvaidya GH, Vaidya AD, Metgudmath R, Kane SV, D'Cruz AK. Minor salivary gland tumors of the sinonasal region: results of a retrospective analysis with review of literature. Head Neck. 2012;34:1704–10.
53. Rhee CS, Won TB, Lee CH, et al. Adenoid cystic carcinoma of the sinonasal tract: treatment results. Laryngoscope. 2006;116:982–6.
54. Patel SG, Singh B, Polluri A, et al. Craniofacial surgery for malignant skull base tumors: report of an international collaborative study. Cancer. 2003;98:1179–87.
55. Ganly I, Patel SG, Singh B, et al. Craniofacial resection for malignant paranasal sinus tumors: report of an International Collaborative Study. Head Neck. 2005;27:575–84.
56. Unger F, Walch C, Stammberger H, Papaefthymiou G, Haselsberger K, Pendl G. Olfactory neuroblastoma (esthesioneuroblastoma): report of six cases treated by a novel combination of endoscopic surgery and radiosurgery. Minim Invasive Neurosurg. 2001;44:79–84.

57. Nicolai P, Battaglia P, Bignami M, et al. Endoscopic surgery for malignant tumors of the sinonasal tract and adjacent skull base: a 10-year experience. Am J Rhinol. 2008;22:308–16.
58. Hanna E, DeMonte F, Ibrahim S, Roberts D, Levine N, Kupferman M. Endoscopic resection of sinonasal cancers with and without craniotomy: oncologic results. Arch Otolaryngol Head Neck Surg. 2009;135:1219–24.
59. Villaret AB, Yakirevitch A, Bizzoni A, et al. Endoscopic transnasal craniectomy in the management of selected sinonasal malignancies. Am J Rhinol Allergy. 2010;24:60–5.
60. Lund VJ, Stammberger H, Nicolai P, et al. European position paper on endoscopic management of tumours of the nose, paranasal sinuses and skull base. Rhinol Suppl. 2010;22:1–143.
61. Castelnuovo P, Battaglia P, Turri-Zanoni M, et al. Endoscopic endonasal surgery for malignancies of the anterior cranial base. World Neurosurg. 2014;82:S22–31.
62. Lund VJ, Wei WI. Endoscopic surgery for malignant sinonasal tumours: an eighteen year experience. Rhinology. 2015;53:204–11.
63. Mattavelli D, Schreiber A, Ferrari M, et al. Three-layer reconstruction with iliotibial tract after endoscopic resection of sinonasal tumors: technical note. World Neurosurg. 2017;101:486.
64. Cantù G, Bimbi G, Miceli R, et al. Lymph node metastases in malignant tumors of the paranasal sinuses: prognostic value and treatment. Arch Otolaryngol Head Neck Surg. 2008;134:170–7.
65. Bhattacharyya N. Survival and staging characteristics for non-squamous cell malignancies of the maxillary sinus. Arch Otolaryngol Head Neck Surg. 2003;129:334–7.
66. da Cruz Perez DE, Pires FR, Lopes MA, de Almeida OP, Kowalski LP. Adenoid cystic carcinoma and mucoepidermoid carcinoma of the maxillary sinus: report of a 44-year experience of 25 cases from a single institution. J Oral Maxillofac Surg. 2006;64:1592–7.
67. Andrade MF, de Faria PR, Cardoso SV, et al. Adenoid cystic carcinoma of the maxillary sinus: a clinical-pathological report of 10 years of experience from a single institution. Int J Oral Maxillofac Surg. 2014;43:1313–8.
68. Sugawara T, Aoyagi M, Ogishima T, et al. Extended orbital exenteration for sinonasal malignancy with orbital apex extension: surgical technique and clinical analysis. J Neurosurg. 2015;123:52–8.
69. Nishio N, Fujimoto Y, Fujii M, et al. Craniofacial resection for T4 maxillary sinus carcinoma: managing cases with involvement of the skull base. Otolaryngol Head Neck Surg. 2015;153:231–8.
70. Takagi M, Demizu Y, Hashimoto N, et al. Treatment outcomes of particle radiotherapy using protons or carbon ions as a single-modality therapy for adenoid cystic carcinoma of the head and neck. Radiother Oncol. 2014;113:364–70.
71. Jensen AD, Nikoghosyan AV, Lossner K, et al. COSMIC: a regimen of intensity modulated radiation therapy plus dose-escalated, raster-scanned carbon ion boost for malignant salivary gland tumors: results of the prospective phase 2 trial. Int J Radiat Oncol Biol Phys. 2015;93:37–46.
72. Dooley L, Shah J. Management of the neck in maxillary sinus carcinomas. Curr Opin Otolaryngol Head Neck Surg. 2015;23:107–14.
73. Paulino AC, Fisher SG, Marks JE. Is prophylactic neck irradiation indicated in patients with squamous cell carcinoma of the maxillary sinus? Int J Radiat Oncol Biol Phys. 1997;39:283–9.
74. Le QT, Fu KK, Kaplan MJ, Terris DJ, Fee WE, Goffinet DR. Lymph node metastasis in maxillary sinus carcinoma. Int J Radiat Oncol Biol Phys. 2000;46:541–9.
75. Valentini V, Terenzi V, Battisti A, et al. Management of clinically negative neck in maxillary carcinoma. J Craniofac Surg. 2010;21:759–62.
76. Schramm VL Jr, Imola MJ. Management of nasopharyngeal salivary gland malignancy. Laryngoscope. 2001;111:1533–44.
77. Castelnuovo P, Nicolai P, Turri-Zanoni M, et al. Endoscopic endonasal nasopharyngectomy in selected cancers. Otolaryngol Head Neck Surg. 2013;149:424–30.
78. Brown DH. The Le Fort I maxillary osteotomy approach to surgery of the skull base. J Otolaryngol. 1989;18:289–92.
79. Wei WI, Lam KH, Sham JS. New approach to the nasopharynx: the maxillary swing approach. Head Neck. 1991;13:200–7.

80. Castelnuovo P, Dallan I, Bignami M, et al. Nasopharyngeal endoscopic resection in the management of selected malignancies: ten-year experience. Rhinology. 2010;48:84–9.
81. Chan JY, Chow VL, Tsang R, Wei WI. Nasopharyngectomy for locally advanced recurrent nasopharyngeal carcinoma: exploring the limits. Head Neck. 2012;34:923–8.
82. Chan JY. Surgical management of recurrent nasopharyngeal carcinoma. Oral Oncol. 2014;50:913–7.
83. Chan YW, Chow VL, Wei WI. Quality of life of patients after salvage nasopharyngectomy for recurrent nasopharyngeal carcinoma. Cancer. 2012;118:3710–8.
84. Cho HJ, Kang JW, Min HJ, et al. Robotic nasopharyngectomy via combined endonasal and transantral port: a preliminary cadaveric study. Laryngoscope. 2015;125:1839–43.
85. Tsang RK, Holsinger FC. Transoral endoscopic nasopharyngectomy with a flexible next-generation robotic surgical system. Laryngoscope. 2016;126:2257–62.
86. Chen MY, Wang SL, Zhu YL, et al. Use of a posterior pedicle nasal septum and floor mucoperiosteum flap to resurface the nasopharynx after endoscopic nasopharyngectomy for recurrent nasopharyngeal carcinoma. Head Neck. 2012;34:1383–8.
87. Fortes FS, Carrau RL, Snyderman CH, et al. Transpterygoid transposition of a temporoparietal fascia flap: a new method for skull base reconstruction after endoscopic expanded endonasal approaches. Laryngoscope. 2007;117:970–6.
88. Zeidan YH, Pekelis L, An Y, et al. Survival benefit for adjuvant radiation therapy in minor salivary gland cancers. Oral Oncol. 2015;51:438–45.
89. Gentile MS, Yip D, Liebsch NJ, Adams JA, Busse PM, Chan AW. Definitive proton beam therapy for adenoid cystic carcinoma of the nasopharynx involving the base of skull. Oral Oncol. 2017;65:38–44.
90. Iyer NG, Kim L, Nixon IJ, et al. Factors predicting outcome in malignant minor salivary gland tumors of the oropharynx. Arch Otolaryngol Head Neck Surg. 2010;136:1240–7.
91. Villanueva NL, de Almeida JR, Sikora AG, Miles BA, Genden EM. Transoral robotic surgery for the management of oropharyngeal minor salivary gland tumors. Head Neck. 2014;36:28–33.
92. White H, Ford S, Bush B, et al. Salvage surgery for recurrent cancers of the oropharynx: comparing TORS with standard open surgical approaches. JAMA Otolaryngol Head Neck Surg. 2013;139:773–8.
93. Suarez C, Barnes L, Silver CE, et al. Cervical lymph node metastasis in adenoid cystic carcinoma of oral cavity and oropharynx: a collective international review. Auris Nasus Larynx. 2016;43:477–84.
94. Zhang M, Li KN, Li C, Zhou L, Zhu JX, Wang SY. Malignant minor salivary gland carcinomas of the larynx. ORL J Otorhinolaryngol Relat Spec. 2014;76:222–6.
95. Marchiano E, Chin OY, Fang CH, Park RC, Baredes S, Eloy JA. Laryngeal adenoid cystic carcinoma: a systematic review. Otolaryngol Head Neck Surg. 2016;154:433–9.
96. Spinazzi EF, Abboud MT, Dubal PM, et al. Laryngeal adenocarcinoma not otherwise specified: a population-based perspective. Laryngoscope. 2017;127:424–9.
97. Moukarbel RV, Goldstein DP, O'Sullivan B, et al. Adenoid cystic carcinoma of the larynx: a 40-year experience. Head Neck. 2008;30:919–24.
98. Luna-Ortiz K, Cano-Valdez AM, Chacon AP, Gomez AH. Horizontal partial laryngectomy in mucoepidermoid carcinoma of the larynx after failure of laser surgery followed by radiotherapy: a case report. Cases J. 2009;2:8421.
99. Peretti G, Piazza C, Ansarin M, et al. Transoral CO2 laser microsurgery for Tis-T3 supraglottic squamous cell carcinomas. Eur Arch Otorhinolaryngol. 2010;267:1735–42.
100. Peretti G, Piazza C, Cattaneo A, De Benedetto L, Martin E, Nicolai P. Comparison of functional outcomes after endoscopic versus open-neck supraglottic laryngectomies. Ann Otol Rhinol Laryngol. 2006;115:827–32.
101. Succo G, Crosetti E, Bertolin A, et al. Benefits and drawbacks of open partial horizontal laryngectomies, part A: early- to intermediate-stage glottic carcinoma. Head Neck. 2016;38(Suppl 1):E333–40.
102. Succo G, Crosetti E, Bertolin A, et al. Benefits and drawbacks of open partial horizontal laryngectomies, part B: intermediate and selected advanced stage laryngeal carcinoma. Head Neck. 2016;38(Suppl 1):E649–57.

103. Testa D, Guerra G, Conzo G, et al. Glottic-Subglottic adenoid cystic carcinoma. A case report and review of the literature. BMC Surg. 2013;13(Suppl 2):S48.
104. Piazza C, Del Bon F, Barbieri D, et al. Tracheal and crico-tracheal resection and anastomosis for malignancies involving the thyroid gland and the airway. Ann Otol Rhinol Laryngol. 2016;125:97–104.
105. Coca-Pelaz A, Barnes L, Rinaldo A, et al. Cervical lymph node metastasis in adenoid cystic carcinoma of the larynx: a collective international review. Adv Ther. 2016;33:553–79.
106. Hellquist H, Skalova A, Barnes L, et al. Cervical lymph node metastasis in high-grade transformation of head and neck adenoid cystic carcinoma: a collective international review. Adv Ther. 2016;33:357–68.
107. Ferlito A, Rinaldo A, Devaney KO, Carbone A. Management of the clinically negative cervical lymph nodes in patients with non-conventional squamous carcinoma of the larynx. J Laryngol Otol. 1999;113:619–23.
108. Mokhtari S, Mokhtari S. Clinical features and differential diagnoses in laryngeal mucoepidermoid carcinoma. Clin Med Insights Pathol. 2012;5:1–6.

Surgical Management of Recurrent Disease

8

M. Guzzo

Salivary gland cancers (SGCs) are an uncommon disease including a heterogeneous group of cancer subtypes with different biological behaviors. The relative rarity and the clinical diversity of these tumors require a multidisciplinary management in high-volume head and neck cancer center [1]. Appropriate surgery, followed by radiotherapy when needed, represents the best therapeutic approach to prevent the recurrences of the disease.

Many features have been correlated with the recurrence rate and survival of patients. Some of them have been studied and confirmed only in selected histological subtypes. In general, tumor size (cT3/cT4), tumors with high-grade histology, lymph node metastases, extraparenchymal extension, neural invasion, lymphatic or vascular invasion, and close (<1 mm) or positive resection margins lead to a worse prognosis and to a high risk of local recurrence. Moreover, a group of molecular markers have been correlated with biologic behavior of these tumors with conflicting results. This is the case of Ki67 (MIB1) that when expressed at high level by mucoepidermoid and adenoid cystic carcinomas seems related to a worse prognosis [2].

Patterns of recurrence are heterogeneous. Consequently, the site of relapse and the interval between the primary treatment and recurrence can be different. Most of the patients have recurrence within 5 years. Despite multimodality treatments, the rate of local recurrence ranges from 15% to 80% at 5 years according to tumor stage and histotype. Late recurrences are also possible. The rate of late recurrences (more than 5 years after the treatment of the primary) is close to 20%. Different figures can be found according to diverse histotypes such as adenoid cystic carcinoma (ACC) or high-grade cancers. ACC shows a high risk of recurrence and the unique clinical behavior to recur as late as 30 years after initial treatment. Local recurrence and

M. Guzzo (✉)
Department of Head and Neck Surgery, Fondazione IRCCS
Istituto Nazionale dei Tumori Milano, Milan, Italy
e-mail: marco.guzzo@istitutotumori.mi.it

© Springer Nature Switzerland AG 2019

L. Licitra, L. D. Locati (eds.), *Salivary Gland Cancer*,
https://doi.org/10.1007/978-3-030-02958-6_8

distant metastases have been reported to occur in about 30% and 50% of the cases, respectively [3]. Salivary duct carcinoma (SDC), a very aggressive malignancy, tends to recur earlier (more than 50% of recurrence rate) and with a high rate of tumor-related deaths within 5 years (from 55% to 65%). SGCs are more likely to recur locally or distally, being regional lymph node metastasis less than 10%. Consequently, a complete restaging of the disease including a head and neck MRI and a total body CT scan should be always advised before planning surgery for local/regional recurrences. If distant metastases have been discovered, surgical indication should be carefully balanced. This is also true in the case of ACC with synchronous presence of local relapse and small slow-growing lung metastases. In these patients Wan der Val et al. [4] found an average time between the occurrence of lung metastases and death of 32.3 months which may support a possible indication for surgery in selected cases.

Recurrent SGCs should be considered as high-grade tumors by definition. Accordingly to the site of occurrences (minor or major salivary gland), an open or ultrasound core needle biopsy is always recommended before planning surgery. Biopsy-proven salivary cancer recurrence often needs multimodality treatment; consequently, it is recommended to discuss the case in a multidisciplinary setting. Surgery, where applicable, in combination with postoperative radiotherapy, when feasible, is the treatment of choice also in case of recurrent disease. About 60% of the patients that experienced a recurrence will be suitable for surgery [5] that appears to be appropriate when performed with curative intent.

A comprehensive head and neck examination followed by a proper radiological imaging is mandatory before to manage a recurrent disease. Local-regional recurrence may be sometimes difficult to detect because it is "hidden" by combined side effects of the previous surgery and radiotherapy. The patient could be asymptomatic. Local pain embittered by palpation may be found along with cranial nerve palsy (i.e., CN VII) in the case of deep and infiltrative recurrence. Other clinical signs may vary according to the site of the disease. Nodal recurrence usually appears as a neck lump or swelling. Distant metastases are discovered preferably by imaging. Unresectable disease and patients with poor performance status or distant metastases (except for ACC patients) should be addressed to radiotherapy, chemotherapy, or palliation.

The distortion of anatomy and the posttreatment fibrosis tend to make difficult the surgical dissection putting at risk the functional facial nerve preservation. Kobajashi et al. reported less than 50% of facial nerve preservation after surgery for parotid recurrent tumors. The use of intraoperative facial nerve monitoring (IFNM) is controversial among surgeons. IFNM may help to identify the nerve without complete dissection of the fibrosis that surrounds the branch reducing the manipulation and the risk of nerve injury. Some authors [6, 7] recently reported that IFNM decreases the immediate postoperative facial nerve weakness, reduces the time of surgery, and increases postoperative nerve recovery. Because of the potential presence of scar tissue and neural-perineural spread, intraoperative frozen section is recommended in an attempt to obtain clear margins of resection. Appropriate soft tissue or nerve reconstruction with regional flap or free tissue transfer should be considered. The risks and the benefits of the procedure should be discussed in details as well as the potential extension of the operation, e.g., mandibulectomy, mastoidectomy, skin resection, neck dissection, or nerve sacrifice. The patient should be widely aware about postoperative deficit, and he will be requested to sign a complete informed consent.

Data on the final outcome of these patients are scarce in the literature. However, some reports including a variety of histopathological types suggest that an aggressive treatment including surgery is oncologically sound with a 5-year disease-free survival of 64.1% [5, 8]. The prognosis seems to be related to the presence of lymph node metastases and tumor grade. The 10-year cancer-specific mortality for patients with early and late recurrences was 77.7% and 7.7%, respectively [9].

References

1. Merdad M, Richmon JD, Quon H. Management of recurrent malignant salivary neoplasms. Adv Otorhinolaryngol. 2016;78:168–74.
2. Gllespie MB, Albergotti WG, Eisele DW. Recurrent salivary gland cancer. Curr Treat Options in Oncol. 2012;13:58–70.
3. Hirvonen K, Back L, Saarilahti K, Leivo I, Hagstrom J, Makitie AA. Pattern of recurrent disease in major salivary gland adenocystic carcinoma. Virchows Arch. 2015;467:19–25.
4. Wan der Val J, Becking AG, Snow GB, Van der Waal I. Distant metastases of adenoid cystic carcinoma of the salivary glands and the value of diagnostic examination during follow-up Head Neck. 2002;24:779–83.
5. Kobajashi K, Nakao K, Yoshida M, Ando M, Ebihara Y, Asakage T, Yamasoba T. Recurrent cancer of the parotid gland. How well does salvage surgery work for locoregional failure? ORL J Otorhinolaryngol Relat Spec. 2009;71:239–43.
6. Huawei L, Wen W, Huang H, Liang Y, Tan X, Liu S, Liu C, Hu M. Recurrent Pleomorphic adenoma of the parotid gland: Intraoperative facial monitoring during parotidectomy. Otolaryngol Head Neck Surg. 2014;15:87–91.
7. Sood AJ, Houlton JJ, Nguyen AS, Gillespie MB. Facial nerve monitoring during parotidectomy: a systematic review and meta-analysis. Otolaryngol Head Neck Surg. 2015;152:631–7.
8. Chen AM, Garcia J, Granchi PJ, Johnson J, Eisele DW. Late recurrence from salivary gland cancer: when does 'cure' mean cure? Cancer. 2008;112:340–4.
9. Park CG, Roh JL, Cho KJ, Jin MH, Choi SH, Nam SY, Kim SY. Incidence and risk factors of late recurrence in patients with salivary gland cancer. Clin Otolaryngol. 2017;42:416–24.

Principles of Reconstruction: Reconstruction of the Parotid Area

9

Silvano Ferrari, Andrea Ferri, Bernardo Bianchi, and Enrico Sesenna

Tumours of the major salivary glands are mostly located in the parotid gland, and already mentioned surgical resection with free margins is considered the best treatment in the vast majority of cases. However, the auricular-parotid area is critical for several reasons, both cosmetically and functionally.

The aesthetical impact of a parotid defect is quite evident: facial contour is dramatically impaired in cases of unreconstructed defects, especially if the entire parotid gland is sacrificed. In case of composite resections, when skin is involved, scars and differences in terms of colour match and texture between the face and the tissue used for skin replacement are a major issue as well. Finally, the most critical and challenging point is related, also functionally, to the management of the facial nerve, which is always an issue to consider when approaching a tumour of the parotid gland.

In this context, the role of reconstruction is very important. The goals that need to be achieved are different and depend essentially on the extension of the resection and on the characteristics of the patient in terms of comorbidities, cosmetic expectations, donor site availability and previous surgical or radiation treatments. The ideal reconstruction should provide enough tissue for defect replacement, a skin with the same features of colour, texture and thickness of the resected one, restore facial contour and take consideration of potential facial nerve impairment.

Local flaps, such as the SMAS (superficial muscular aponeurotic system) or SCM (sternocleidomastoid muscle) flaps, regional fasciocutaneous flaps as the cervicofacial/cervicopectoral, supraclavicular or submental flaps, musculocutaneous pedicled flaps as the pectoralis major and the trapezius or even free flaps in case of wide defects as ALT (anterolateral thigh) or latissimus dorsi free flaps, are the main options for the management of this area [1]. Careful selection of the technique is undoubtedly a key point in achievement of the best results.

S. Ferrari · A. Ferri (✉) · B. Bianchi · E. Sesenna
Maxillo-Facial Surgery Division, Head and Neck Department, University Hospital of Parma, Parma, Italy
e-mail: silvano.ferrari@unipr.it; enrico.sesenna@unipr.it

© Springer Nature Switzerland AG 2019
L. Licitra, L. D. Locati (eds.), *Salivary Gland Cancer*,
https://doi.org/10.1007/978-3-030-02958-6_9

Among these options, the auricular-parotid area differs from other sites in the head and neck (such as oral cavity or midface) because its lateral position, very close to the back and shoulder, often makes it reachable by a pedicled flap, dramatically reducing the need for free tissue transfers and the associated technical difficulties of the reconstruction. Therefore, the frequent use of regional flaps, even in the free flap era, should not seem outdated [2, 3]. Furthermore, surgery of this area usually spares impairment of the oral cavity and upper airways, ensuring fast and safe recovery; this aspect together with possible reconstruction with a "low-impact" technique makes surgery feasible even in patients with poor prognosis or with poor general conditions, and even sometimes as palliative treatment.

As alluded to above, defects of the parotid area can be very heterogeneous, but, considering only reconstructive needs, they can be divided as follows:

1. Defects involving only the parotid gland
2. Defects extending to the skin overlying the parotid
3. Composite defects extending to other structures (facial skin, masseter muscle, mastoid, skull base, masticatory space, etc.)
4. Resections that include facial nerve sacrifice (main trunk or branches)

This academic classification can be useful because the purpose of reconstructions is very different in these defects, and therefore the reconstructive technique will also change contextually.

9.1 Reconstruction of Gland Defects

As already discussed, tumours confined to the parotid gland are usually treated by parotidectomies that can be partial, superficial or total, essentially basing the choice of the resection on tumour's histology, size and position (superficial or deep lobe). Concerning the reconstructive perspective, the first point to address is that the sacrifice of a part or the whole parotid gland, if not reconstructed, will lead to a depression in the pre-auricular and/or submandibular area proportional to the amount of parotid tissue resected. When benign tumours are removed, partial parotidectomy or extracapsular dissection allows the use of spared parotid tissue for parotid bed reconstruction, and further reconstructive techniques are usually not necessary.

However these options are rarely usable when malignant tumours are treated, since total parotidectomies are the most widely used techniques for resection of these lesions. In such cases reconstruction of the parotid bed is not feasible, and, as largely reported in the international literature, the use of local flaps as SMAS or SCM is indicated [4].

SMAS is probably the most used technique worldwide because it is easy to harvest; usually spared during resection; provides a good separation between the parotid bed and skin, thus helping to prevent Frey's syndrome; and ensures good cosmetic results because it gives support to the overlying skin by avoiding its depression during healing. As an alternative, or sometimes in addition, the SCM can be used as a donor site for harvesting of a muscular flap that can be used with the inferior or superior base (even a bi-pedicled flap is reported in the literature), and provides well-vascularised muscular tissue for filling the defect. Despite no differences in results when one or the other flaps are used as reported in literature, in general it can be useful to propose the SCM flap, especially for reconstruction of the inferior area of the parotid, which is closer to the SCM, while the SMAS is more easily applied for the superior portion of the area.

Nonetheless, when "pure" parotid gland defects are approached, the cosmetic results are usually good, especially because the skin is preserved, but even if SMAS and SCM flaps are properly used, they can be certainly improved upon. However, if some focal contour impairment still persists after healing, ancillary procedures, mainly represented by fat injection, can easily be associated to further improve patient satisfaction [5].

9.2 Reconstruction of Defects Extending to the Skin

Composite defects involving the whole gland and skin are often encountered in this area, especially when recurrences are treated. As already explained at the beginning of this chapter, skin replacement with tissue that has similar features in terms of colour, texture, hair-bearing and thickness is a key point of the reconstructive procedure because of the critical aesthetic relevance of this area in the frontal and lateral appearance of the patient. While a free flap is certainly an option in such cases, if a fasciocutaneous regional flap is used, the skin features will better match the native one, with superior aesthetic results [6]. Among the different options available, cervicofacial/cervicopectoral, supraclavicular and submental flaps are the most indicated [7].

9.2.1 Cervicofacial/Cervicopectoral Flap

Cervicofacial and cervicopectoral flaps are two very similar flaps that are harvested as random flaps from the facial area (cervicofacial) or designed to include anterior thoracic perforators from mammary artery (cervicopectoral), especially if associated with neck dissection. A wide range of skin defects can be managed with these flaps, especially when thin skin is required. The greatest advantage is that the skin of the face is merely advanced or rotated with perfect match in terms of skin features (Fig. 9.1a, b). Unfortunately, with these techniques only small defects can be properly reconstructed because of the relatively small arch of rotation of the flap. As already mentioned, if neck dissection is indicated, the cervicopectoral flap can be elevated during neck treatment and provides more tissue than a cervicofacial flap [8].

9.2.2 Supraclavicular Flap

Supraclavicular flap is an "old" flap that has again gained popularity after the year 2000, thanks to its great versatility in head and neck defects. In the parotid area, it is especially useful in cases with skin defects that cannot be managed with a

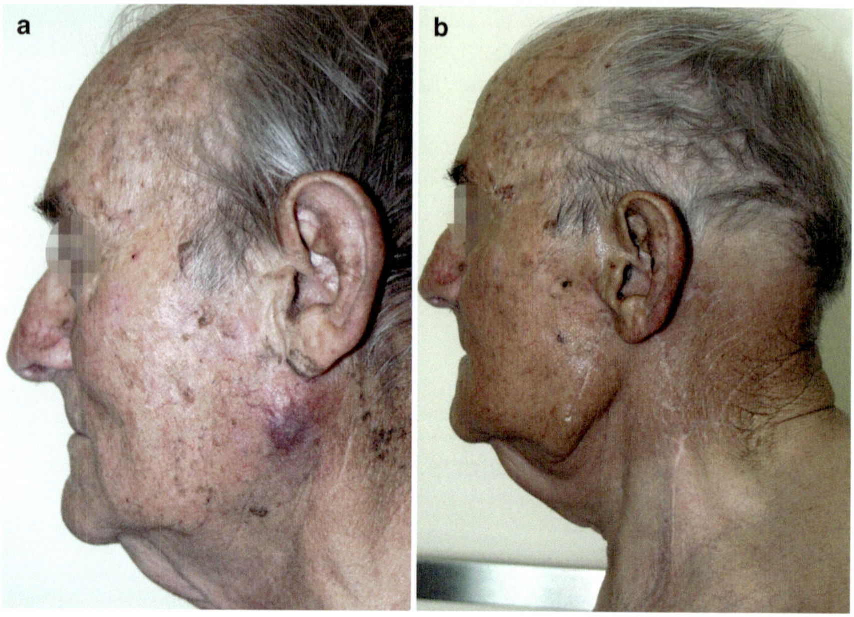

Fig. 9.1 Adenocarcinoma of the left parotid gland extended to pre-auricular skin (**a**) and results of reconstruction with cervicopectoral flap (**b**)

cervicofacial/cervicopectoral flap, and today it represents the first choice in the vast majority of patients. The tissue provided is thin, pliable and reliable and can reach easily the parotid area, even in its most superior part. The skin of the shoulder is very similar to that of the face and is often without hair, thus offering a good solution from a cosmetic point of view [9]. Furthermore, the whole flap or only a part of it can be de-epithelised to provide vascularised tissue for filling the defect and to restore adequate volume and facial contour, even when facial skin is not resected. The greatest disadvantage of the flap is donor site morbidity and scars that can be increased in cases of harvesting large flaps when donor site closure, which is usually performed primarily, requires skin grafts that reduce cosmetic outcome. Finally, the pedicle may necessitate sectioning after healing if it interferes with the patient's daily function but in most cases is not required [10].

9.2.3 Submental Flap

Submental flap is a well-known flap that has several indications in oral cavity and face reconstruction. Its use in the parotid area is not so popular, but this flap has some advantages that can improve cosmetic results. It is thin and pliable and provides hair-bearing skin that can be used for reconstruction of the pre-auricular hair-bearing area overlying the parotid, especially in males (Fig. 9.2a–c). Furthermore, colour and texture are very similar to native skin, which further

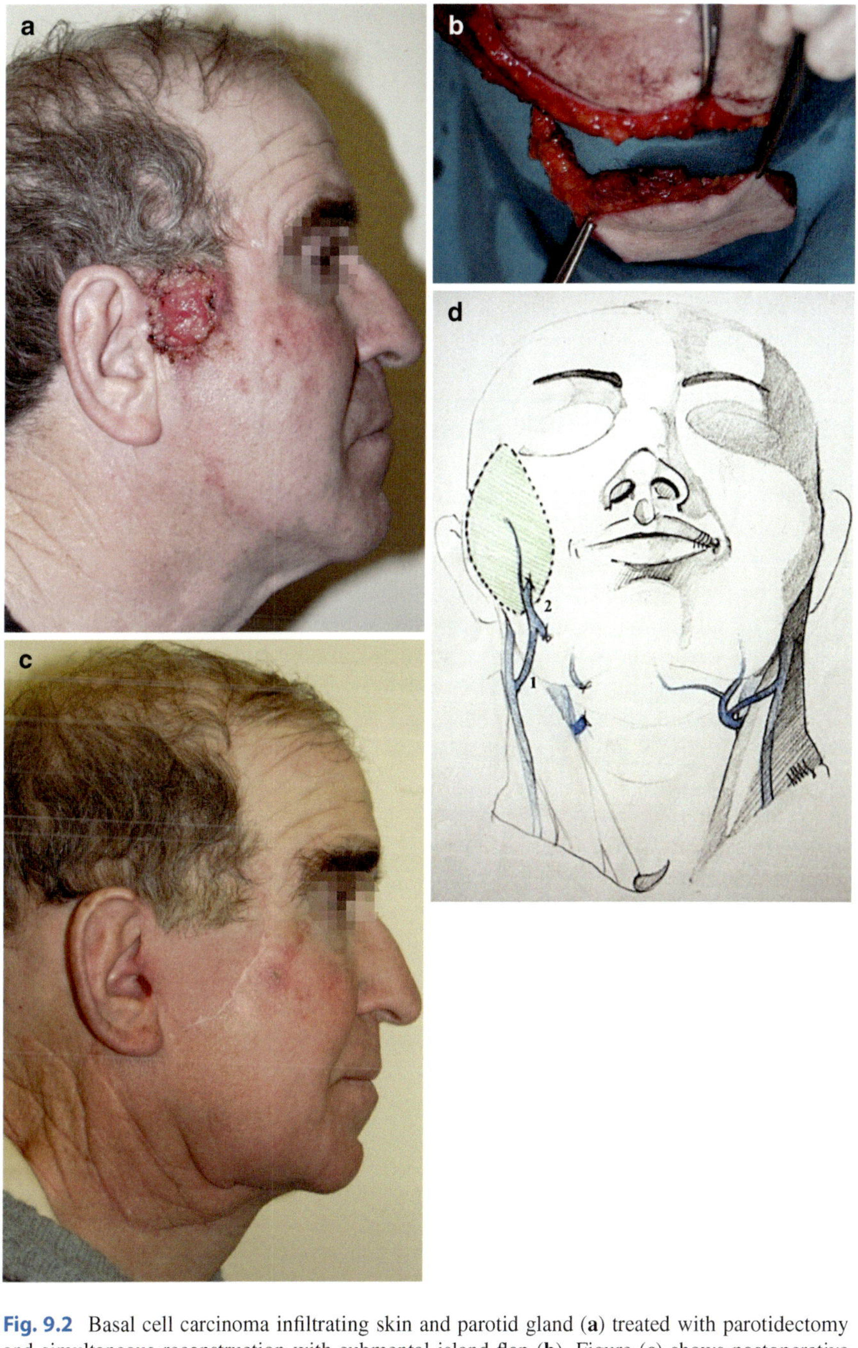

Fig. 9.2 Basal cell carcinoma infiltrating skin and parotid gland (**a**) treated with parotidectomy and simultaneous reconstruction with submental island flap (**b**). Figure (**c**) shows postoperative results, especially concerning hairy skin replacement. Figure (**d**) represents the V-Y technique used for pedicle elongation

improves the results. Finally, donor site morbidity is very low, and its harvest may even be ameliorative in overweight patients when a more pronounced double chin is removed as a consequence of flap harvest [11]. However, this flap also has some disadvantages, mainly represented by the technical difficulty of its harvesting: pedicle dissection is difficult and requires skills in microvascular management and magnification that is mandatory for safe harvesting. The pedicle is short and the V-Y technique used for its elongation is often required to reach the upper portion of parotid area and can be difficult if not performed by experienced hands (Fig. 9.2d). Finally, oncological safety can be reduced in case of positive neck lymph nodes, when preservation of facial and submental artery and veins can invalidate the efficacy of neck clearance [12].

9.3 Extensive Composite Defects

Management of defects involving not only the parotid and the overlying skin but also adjacent structures, such as the masseter or other masticatory muscles, wider skin areas, temporal region, mastoid or skull base and SCM muscle or others, requires more tissue to be properly reconstructed. In this regard, musculocutaneous flaps are usually preferred over fasciocutaneous ones because of the possibility to provide the needed bulk. As mentioned in the introduction of this chapter, the parotid area is quite easily reached by pedicled musculocutaneous flaps harvested either from the thorax or from the back, and therefore pectoralis major, trapezius island and latissimus dorsi flaps are some of the most used techniques [13]. Free flaps, especially musculocutaneous as ALT or latissimus dorsi, are certainly another option and sometimes, especially in microvascular expert centres, can be easier than pedicled ones [14]. However, the distant skin is often worse than that provided by a pedicled flap, and they are therefore mainly indicated in extremely extensive defects (when the possibility to harvest large amount of tissue is required) or in patients with a compromised healing process, mainly in those with previous radiation therapy or with diabetes, when well-vascularised tissue helps prevent marginal necrosis and decrease the healing time (especially when heavy flaps are harvested and gravity works against healing in the upper portion of the suture).

9.3.1 Pectoralis Major Flap

Pectoralis major is one of the most popular pedicled flaps for head and neck reconstruction, and almost all reconstructive surgeons are very familiar with it. It is very easy and fast to harvest, and donor site morbidity is negligible, with the exception of the aesthetic impact of the cutaneous scar on the chest. When the flap needs to reach the auricular-parotid area, pedicle elongation should be maximised, with harvesting of the cutaneous paddle in its more lower portion, island dissection of the pedicle and careful resection of all the muscular branches surrounding the vessels, in order to increase as much as possible its arch of rotation. Another important trick

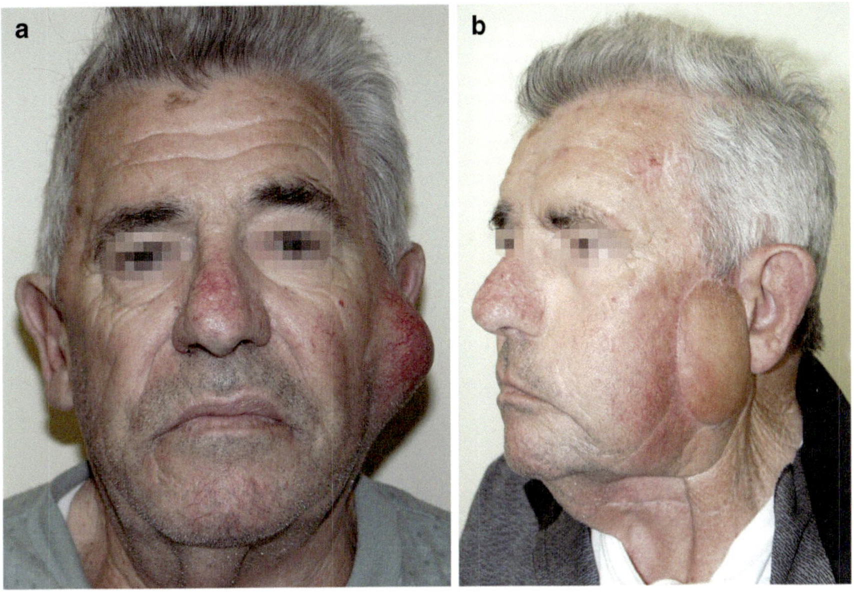

Fig. 9.3 Adenoid cystic carcinoma of the left parotid gland extending to the skin (**a**) and results of reconstruction using pectoralis major pedicled flap (**b**)

is to properly manage the patient's head positioning: a downward and medially rotated position is often ideal to prevent pedicle stretching and other vascular complications. Pectoralis flap is therefore indicated in the reconstruction of lower parotidectomy defects, not extending to the temporal area, especially when bulk is required, as in cases of wide soft-tissue resections (Fig. 9.3a, b).

9.3.2 Trapezius Island Flap

Trapezius island flap is rarely used in head and neck reconstruction, mainly because of the need to change the patient's position during surgery. Therefore, other techniques that allow a supine position and possibly a double team approach are usually preferred. The auricular-parotid area is probably the main indication in head and neck surgery for this flap because of its unique advantages. First of all, being parotid lateral in the head, the patient can be positioned from the beginning in lateral decubitus to allow tumour resection and flap harvest without the need to change the patient's position (this could be uncomfortable in case of neck dissection). Furthermore the trapezius flap has a long pedicle that can reach easily the parotid area with a low rate of vascular complication. The tissue harvested has an ideal thickness for the parotid area, because it is usually a compromise between the bulk of the pectoralis major flap and the thinness of fasciocutaneous flaps, which is a major advantage when facial contour needs to be restored (Fig. 9.4a–d). Donor

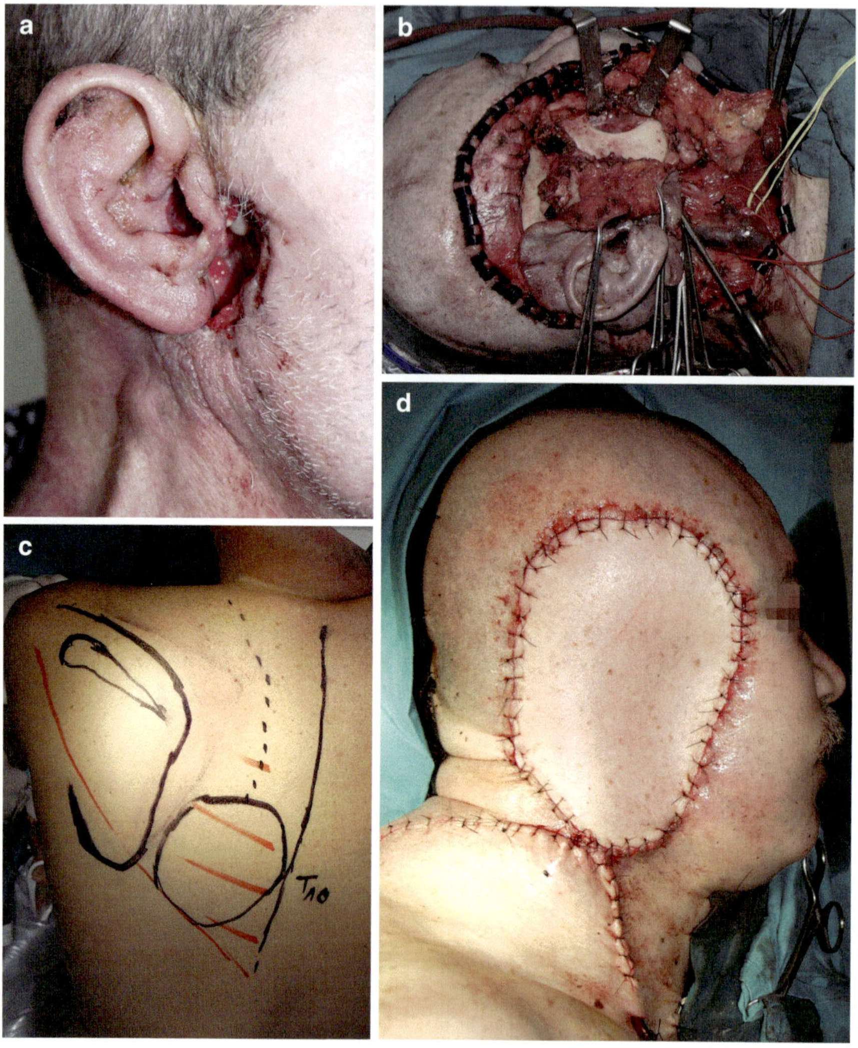

Fig. 9.4 Adenoid cystic carcinoma of the right parotid gland with invasion of the skin and of the lateral skull base (**a**, **b**). Trapezius island flap design (**c**) and its rotation to reconstruct the wide parotid defect (**d**)

site morbidity is low, but its postoperative management can be complicated by the position of the patient in bed [15]. Furthermore, the skin of the back is not as mobile as the lateral thoracic wall, and donor site closure can be difficult in cases of large skin paddle harvesting. In conclusion, this flap is optimal for reconstruction of the parotid area, but difficulty in donor site management, the surgeon's discomfort during the operation and, last but not least, the scarce familiarity of many head and neck surgeons with this technique often limit its use even in reconstruction of parotid defects [16].

9.3.3 Latissimus Dorsi Free Flap

The lateral thoracic wall and, in particular, free flaps harvested from the thoracodorsal arterial system gained great popularity starting from 2010, especially after the description of the scapular tip free flap with its chimeric variations. In the parotid area, bone reconstruction is usually not required, with the exception of rare, extremely advanced tumours involving the mandibular ramus. Therefore, the most widely used flap harvested from the thoracodorsal system is the latissimus dorsi free flap. It can be also harvested on the same pedicle as a pedicled flap, as routinely done in the 1980s, but in this case pedicle transposition to the parotid area can be difficult, and today its free version is usually preferred. Latissimus dorsi free flap has the great advantage of providing an extremely wide amount of tissue, especially in the presence of very large skin defects. Muscle and the subcutaneous fat layer are often thinner than other areas (such as the thigh), which can improve cosmetic outcomes. The pedicle is long and usually spared by vascular sclerosis, even in the elderly, and this can be of help during microvascular anastomosis, even though a long pedicle is usually not mandatory in the parotid area because of the proximity of temporal and facial vessels. One of its greatest advantages is the very low donor site morbidity: the lateral thoracic wall is usually easily closed primarily, and impairment of the patient's functions is also low in the long term. Furthermore, there is no impairment of limbs, and mobilisation is possible starting from day 2 to day 3 after surgery. The main drawback of this technique is the difficulty of simultaneously harvesting the flap with tumour resection, but if the contralateral side is chosen and the patient is carefully positioned before surgery, this problem can be easily overcome.

9.3.4 Anterolateral Thigh Free Flap

Anterolateral thigh free flap is one of the most used soft-tissue free flaps worldwide. In particular its perforator harvesting has many indications in head and neck defects, especially when the oral cavity needs to be reconstructed. The pedicle is long and of good calibre, and chimeric variations of the flap can also be harvested. Therefore, many surgeons are familiar with this donor site, and this flap is often used even in the parotid area. However, in this particular region, a useful modification of this flap includes the vastus lateralis muscle, harvesting a musculocutaneous free flap rather than a perforator or a chimeric one. This is very useful especially when extensive defects are approached, and restoration of adequate bulk is one of the goals of treatment (Fig. 9.5a–c). In this variation ALT is even easier, safe and fast to harvest, because there is no need for musculocutaneous perforators dissection, even if a septocutaneous perforator is not found. The pedicle is elevated without separating it from the vastus lateralis, including all the perforator branches to the skin. The amount of muscle harvested depends on the need of the defect and the thickness of the subcutaneous fat layer of the thigh [17]. This possibility to "modulate" the amount of muscle is a precious advantage for

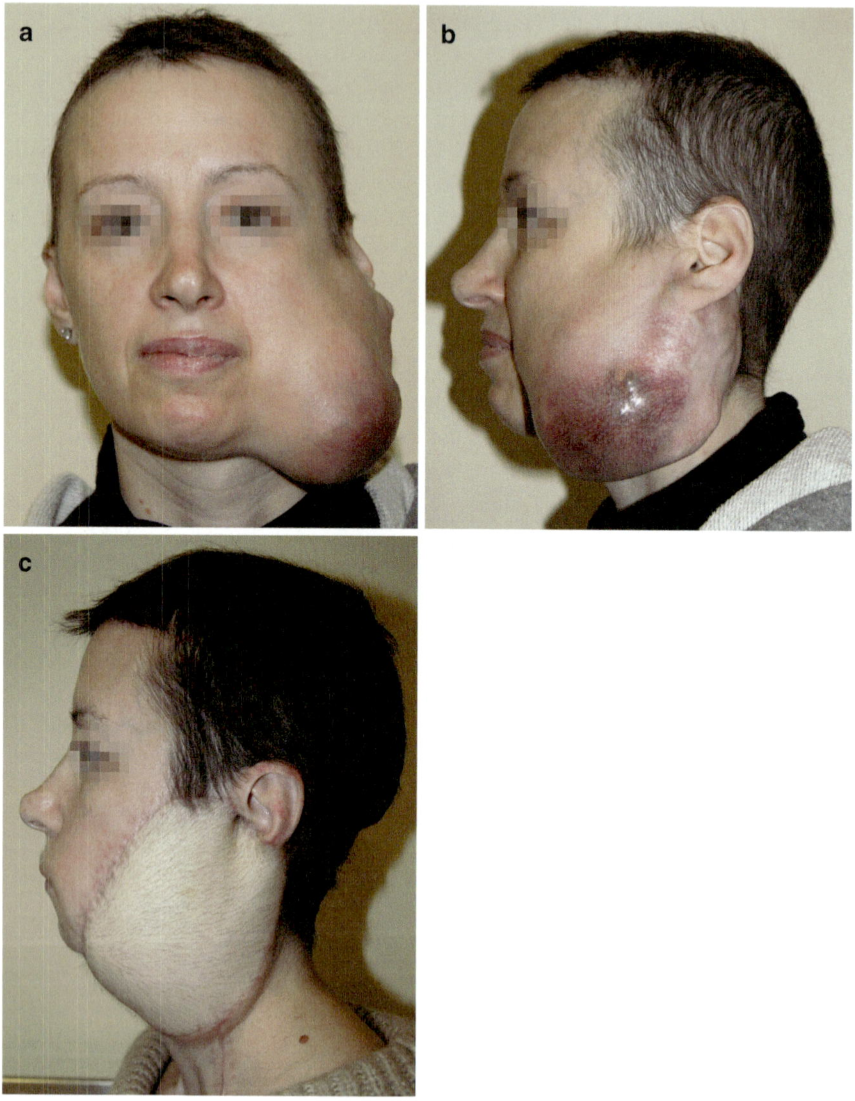

Fig. 9.5 Huge adenoid cystic carcinoma of the left parotid gland with extensive skin invasion (**a**, **b**) and results after reconstruction with a musculocutaneous anterolateral thigh free flap (**c**)

the parotid area, helping to prevent excesses or defects of bulkiness. Moreover, morbidity associated with muscle harvesting is paltry and does not interfere with the patient's normal activity. However, around 1 week is usually required before the patient returns to walking in a satisfactory way, and crutches are often used during the first weeks after surgery [18, 19].

9.4 Management of Facial Nerve

The facial nerve is certainly the most difficult issue to address in management of parotid malignancies. Principles of preservation or sacrifice of the nerve have already been analysed in previous chapters, and the purpose of this section is to provide a guide for facial nerve reconstruction after its resection. The techniques for immediate facial nerve repair include simple neurorraphy and nerve grafting and can be used within 30 days after nerve damage. After this time treatment consists in facial reanimation with different procedures based mainly on the time elapsed from palsy: in recent forms (before 18–20 months), the facial nerve can be recovered with facial cooptation procedures (cross-facial nerve grafting, masseteric-facial, hypoglossal-facial), while in established forms neuromuscular transplants are currently the gold standard [18–20]. However, this is not the topic of this chapter.

When the facial nerve is damaged during parotid surgery for salivary gland malignancies, the first and most important paradigm is that immediate reconstruction is always the best solution. In fact, it is widely reported in the literature that delays in reconstruction are related to poorer outcomes because of scars and difficulties in isolation of facial nerve branches. Furthermore identification of facial nerve branches during tumour resection is usually easier, and it is possible to identify and isolate the main branches (a neurostimulation device is mandatory) that will be grafted during reconstruction.

The second key point is the use of tension-free sutures, meaning that reparative techniques for facial nerve damage, being sutures or reconstruction, must be performed without tension that could interfere with the axonal regeneration process. In order to prevent tension, it is very useful to proceed in dissection of the branches or the main trunk to increase their mobility and to facilitate neurorraphy.

Finally, in case of nerve grafting, an adequate match of diameter between the facial nerve and the graft is an important element to ensure good neural regeneration through the graft [21].

From a technical point of view, neural suture must always be done under magnification, to improve precision, and care must be taken to provide good closure of the perineural sheath, in order to prevent scarring that will interfere with regeneration of the nerve. At the end of the procedure, fibrin glue can be used to further isolate the neurorraphy from scarring processes. Other procedures such as vein grafts or synthetic materials can be also used for this purpose, although clear evidence of their benefit is not well documented in literature.

A key point of the procedure is selection of the donor nerve that will be used for grafting: the great auricular, the sural and the thoracodorsal nerves are the most widely used worldwide. The great auricular nerve has the advantage that is located very close to the parotid bed and is usually already dissected during parotidectomy. Therefore, its use is morbidity-free (with the exception of numbness in the ear lobe) and very fast and comfortable for surgeon. However, only a limited length of nerve is available, and the diameter provided is usually small. Therefore, its use is indicated mainly in small reconstruction of single branches.

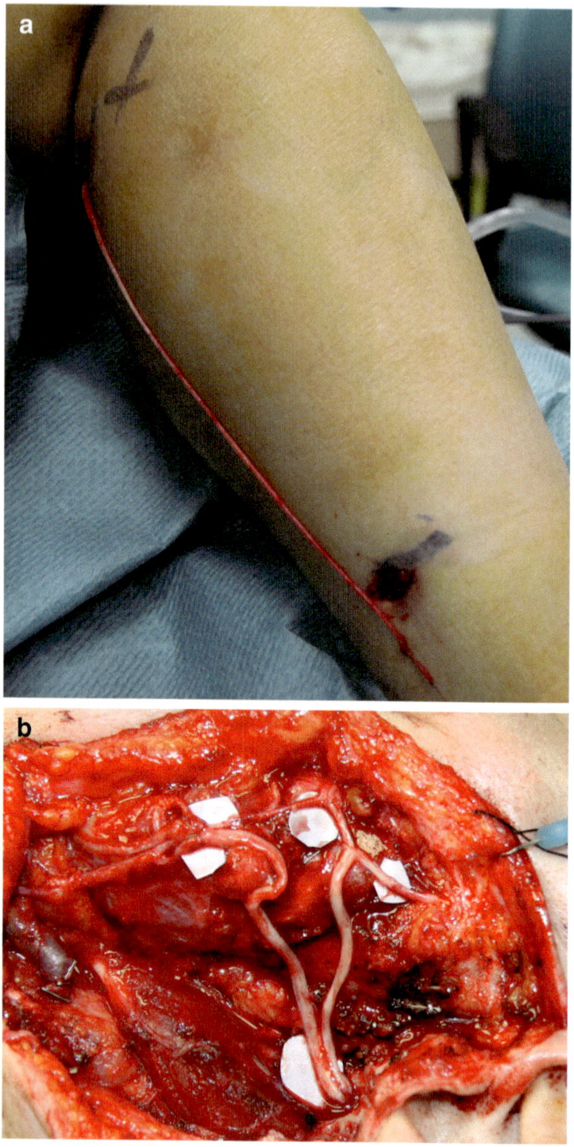

Fig. 9.6 Harvesting of the sural nerve from the leg (**a**) and its grafting to reconstruct multiple branches of the resected facial nerve (**b**)

The sural nerve (Fig. 9.6a) is probably the most used for facial nerve grafting, probably because it is also used in more complex facial reanimation procedures and surgeons are familiar with it. The main advantages are the possibility of harvesting the nerve with a second team during tumour resection (thus reducing surgical time), its low morbidity (just stripping the nerve through two small incisions in the posterior calf and a small area of numbness in the lateral malleolus), the possibility of endoscopic harvesting (with only one incision) and the availability of a long nerve (such as the leg, if required), with a large diameter, which

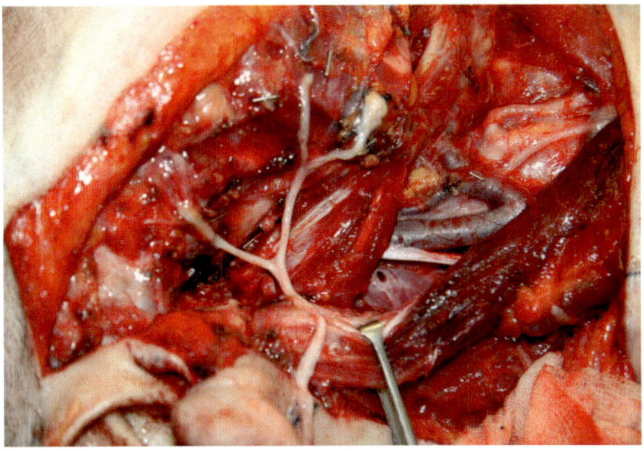

Fig. 9.7 The thoracodorsal nerve can also be used for facial nerve reconstruction thanks to its multiple branches that reproduce facial nerve anatomy

can also be split to provide an ideal match with the facial nerve. In case of resection of the main trunk, the whole diameter of the sural nerve can be used to better match the trunk size, and the other end can be split to match with two terminal facial nerve branches. In case of complex or complete reconstruction, multiple grafts should be used to restore the physiologic anatomy of the VII nerve as much as possible (Fig. 9.6b). In these cases, accurate identification of the branches that actually need reconstruction should be done by mapping all the branches with a neurostimulator and selecting those to reconstruct based mainly on facial movements rather than dimension or position: this is very important to reduce synkineses, which are the main complications of such reconstructions.

The thoracodorsal nerve is less well described in the international literature but certainly represents a good alternative to the sural nerve. The main advantage is that it is composed of a main trunk and multiple branches and presents an anatomy that is very similar to the facial nerve (Fig. 9.7). This means that splitting or multiple neurorraphies with the main trunk are not required. Concerning its harvesting, the scar is placed on the lateral thoracic wall, is well hidden and can be obtained simultaneously with tumour resection, even if with less comfort than with the sural nerve. In this case, the dissection is open and stripping is not possible. Unfortunately, while limited data concerning functional impairment (being a motor nerve) are available, it can be inferred that it has minimal impact on the patient's shoulder and arm movements.

References

1. Ch'ng S, Ashford BG, Gao K, McGuinness J, Clark JR. Reconstruction of post-radical parotidectomy defects. Plast Reconstr Surg. 2012;129:275e–87e.
2. Bianchi B, Ferri A, Ferrari S, Copelli C, Poli T, Sesenna E. Free and locoregional flap associations in the reconstruction of extensive head and neck defects. Int J Oral Maxillofac Surg. 2008;37(8):723–9.
3. Irvine LE, Larian B, Azizzadeh B. Locoregional parotid reconstruction. Otolaryngol Clin N Am. 2016;49:435–46.

4. Bianchi B, Ferri A, Ferrari S, Copelli C, Sesenna E. Improving aesthetic results in benign parotid surgery: statistical evaluation of the facelift approach, sternocleidomastoid flap, and SMAS flap application. J Oral Maxillofac Surg. 2011;69:1235–41.
5. Pham M, Eviston TJ, Clark JR. Reconstruction of limited parotidectomy defects using the dermofat graft. ANZ J Surg. 2017;87:E256.
6. Behan FC, Lo CH, Sizeland A, Pham T, Findlay M. Keystone island flap reconstruction of parotid defects. Plast Reconstr Surg. 2012;130:36e–41e.
7. Shestak KC, Roth AG, Jones NF, Myers EN. The cervicopectoral rotation flap—a valuable technique for facial reconstruction. Br J Plast Surg. 1993;46:375–7.
8. Liu FY, Xu ZF, Li P, Sun CF, Li RW, Ge SF, Li JL, Huang SH, Tan X. The versatile application of cervicofacial and cervicothoracic rotation flaps in head and neck surgery. World J Surg Oncol. 2011;23:135–8.
9. Emerick KS, Herr MW, Lin DT, Santos F, Deschler DG. Supraclavicular artery island flap for reconstruction of complex parotidectomy, lateral skull base, and total auriculectomy defects. JAMA Otolaryngol Head Neck Surg. 2014;140:861–6.
10. Ramirez CA, Fernandes RP. The supraclavicular artery island and trapezius myocutaneous flaps in head and neck reconstruction. Oral Maxillofac Surg Clin North Am. 2014;26:411–20.
11. Multinu A, Ferrari S, Bianchi B, Balestreri A, Scozzafava E, Ferri A, Sesenna E. The submental island flap in head and neck reconstruction. Int J Oral Maxillofac Surg. 2007;36(8):716–20.
12. Ferrari S, Copelli C, Bianchi B, Magri AS, Ferri A, Varazzani A, Poli T, Ferri T, Sesenna E. The submental island flap: pedicle elongation and indications in head and neck reconstruction. J Craniomaxillofac Surg. 2014;42(6):1005–9.
13. Ioannides C, Fossion E. Reconstruction of extensive defects of the parotid region: experience with the pectoralis major and free latissimus dorsi flaps. J Craniomaxillofac Surg. 1997;25:57–62.
14. Fritz MA, Rolfes BN. Microvascular reconstruction of the parotidectomy defect. Otolaryngol Clin N Am. 2016;49:447–57.
15. Dinner MI, Guyuron B, Labandter HP. The lower trapezius myocutaneous flap for head and neck reconstruction. Head Neck Surg. 1983;6:613–7.
16. Ou KL, Dai YH, Wang HJ, Chen TM, Dai NT, Chang SC, Deng SC, Tzeng YS, Wang CH, Chen SG. The lower trapezius musculocutaneous flap for head and neck reconstruction: two decades of clinical experience. Ann Plast Surg. 2013;71(Suppl 1):S48–54.
17. Elliott RM, Weinstein GS, Low DW, Wu LC. Reconstruction of complex total parotidectomy defects using the free anterolateral thigh flap: a classification system and algorithm. Ann Plast Surg. 2011;66:429–37.
18. Bianchi B, Ferri A, Ferrari S, Copelli C, Boni P, Ferri T, Sesenna E. The free musculocutaneous anterolateral thigh free flap for head and neck reconstruction: one surgeon's experience in 92 cases. Microsurgery. 2012a;32(2):87–95.
19. Bianchi B, Ferri A, Sesenna E. Facial animation after nerve sacrifice in the treatment of head and neck cancers. Curr Opin Otolaryngol Head Neck Surg. 2012b;20:114–9.
20. Renkonen S, Sayed F, Keski-Säntti H, Ylä-Kotola T, Bäck L, Suominen S, Kanerva M, Mäkitie AA. Reconstruction of facial nerve after radical parotidectomy. Acta Otolaryngol. 2015;135:1065–9.
21. Biglioli F, Colombo V, Pedrazzoli M, Frigerio A, Tarabbia F, Autelitano L, Rabbiosi D. Thoracodorsal nerve graft for reconstruction of facial nerve branching. J Craniomaxillofac Surg. 2014;42:e8–14.

Principles of Reconstruction: Palatomaxillary Reconstruction

10

Cesare Piazza, Alberto Paderno, and Piero Nicolai

The hard palate and maxillary sinus are among the most frequently involved sites by minor salivary gland tumours, and reconstruction of these structures is particularly challenging in consideration of their essential aesthetic and functional roles. The maxillary bone (together with the zygomatic) contributes to the anterior projection of the midface and constitutes the bony scaffold of the hard palate and superior alveolus. Consequently, its role is essential in mastication, deglutition and speech, and it determines the shape of the midfacial region. In this view, reconstruction should be primarily focused on reconstituting this structural framework, withstanding the forces applied during mastication, giving adequate separation between the oral cavity and nasal fossa/residual maxillary sinus and granting a symmetric facial appearance. This is even more complex when adjunctive structures are involved by resection, such as the orbital floor, orbital content, contralateral portion of the hard palate, facial skin and (less frequently) the skull base.

A number of reconstructive approaches may be applied to such a diverse group of defects, ranging from obturator prostheses and local flaps to more complex techniques such as free flaps. For these reasons, an adequate classification system precisely addressing the defect extension and its characteristics is particularly useful for surgical planning of the reconstructive approach.

C. Piazza (✉)
Department of Otorhinolaryngology, Maxillofacial and Thyroid Surgery, Fondazione IRCCS Istituto Nazionale dei Tumori, Milan, Italy
e-mail: cesare.piazza@istitutotumori.mi.it

A. Paderno · P. Nicolai
Department of Otorhinolaryngology—Head and Neck Surgery, Spedali Civili of Brescia, University of Brescia, Brescia, Italy
e-mail: piero.nicolai@unibs.it

© Springer Nature Switzerland AG 2019

L. Licitra, L. D. Locati (eds.), *Salivary Gland Cancer*,
https://doi.org/10.1007/978-3-030-02958-6_10

10.1 Classification of the Surgical Defect

A number of classifications have been proposed in the international literature [1–5], mostly aimed at precisely describing the horizontal and vertical extension of the resection. In particular, Okay's classification [1] has proven to be simple, easy to use and applicable to most of the defects. Its rationale is to define the structural properties of the defect in relation to the biomechanics that determine the stability of an obturator prosthesis or that of any other type of reconstruction. The horizontal extension is defined by the following:

- *Class Ia*: defect involving any portion of the hard palate not extending to the tooth-bearing maxillary alveolus.
- *Class Ib*: defect involving the premaxilla or any portion of the maxillary alveolus and dentition posterior to the canines.
- *Class II*: defect involving any portion of the hard palate and tooth-bearing maxillary alveolus and only one canine. The anterior margin of defect lies within the premaxilla. This class includes transverse palatectomy defects involving less than 50% of the hard palate.
- *Class III*: defect involving any portion of the hard palate and tooth-bearing maxillary alveolus, including both canines. This class includes total and transverse palatectomy defects extending to more than 50% of the hard palate.

On the other hand, the vertical extension is defined by these suffixes:

- *z*: defect involving any portion of the zygomatic bone
- *f*: defect involving the floor of the orbit
- *o*: defect extending to the orbital content
- *s*: concomitant resection of the facial skin

The conjunction of these two components (horizontal and vertical) leads to a three-dimensional definition of the surgical defect and, consequently, can orientate the choice of the ideal reconstructive approach.

10.2 Reconstruction of Partial Palatal Defects (Class I)

Defects involving the hard palate, but not extending to the tooth-bearing maxillary alveolus, and those involving the maxillary alveolus and dentition posterior to the canines may be easily rehabilitated by an obturator prosthesis, local flaps or (in larger defects and according to the patient's preference) fascio-cutaneous free flaps, in particular the radial forearm (RF). In fact, in these defects the structural stability of the hard palate and maxilla is maintained, and residual structures are able to sustain the cantilever forces applied to an obturator prosthesis by mastication. Similarly, soft tissue flaps can fill the palatal gap, avoiding oronasal/oro-antral fistula and allowing mastication and deglutition with the residual dentition or dental fittings. Considering local flaps, the most frequently employed in this scenario are:

- Buccal fat pad flap
- Palatal island flap
- Facial artery musculo-mucosal (FAMM) flap

Among regional flaps, the temporalis myofascial pedicled flap, even though less popular than some decades ago, can still be used for closure of limited palatal gaps even though at a relatively high functional cost, mainly related to the loss of a potent masticatory muscle with ensuing risk of postoperative trismus.

When a free flap is considered, the radial forearm (RF) is frequently the most suitable choice thanks to its long pedicle and favourable surface-to-volume ratio, with the anterolateral thigh (ALT) being the second choice for thin patients.

10.2.1 Obturator Prosthesis

Historically, this is one of the first techniques employed for palatal reconstruction, in particular for congenital defects. It is a prosthetic device aimed at separating the oral cavity from the nasal fossa and maxillary sinus while restoring complete dentition (when necessary) by means of dental fittings. This is fixed to the residual palate and alveolus and depends on these structures to obtain sufficient stability to sustain the forces implied in mastication and to avoid oronasal regurgitation of food or liquids [6] (Fig. 10.1). Therefore, its effectiveness is directly related to the structural characteristics of each defect:

- Class Ia and b defects are easily rehabilitated by an obturator.
- Class II defects may be effectively covered by such a device, but residual functional problems may be encountered especially due to the overall bulkiness of the obturator required, usually needing optimal mouth opening for its positioning and careful hygiene/maintenance [7].
- Class III defects rarely (if ever) give sufficient stability to the prosthesis, leading to malposition and functional issues such as liquid leakage into the nasal cavities.

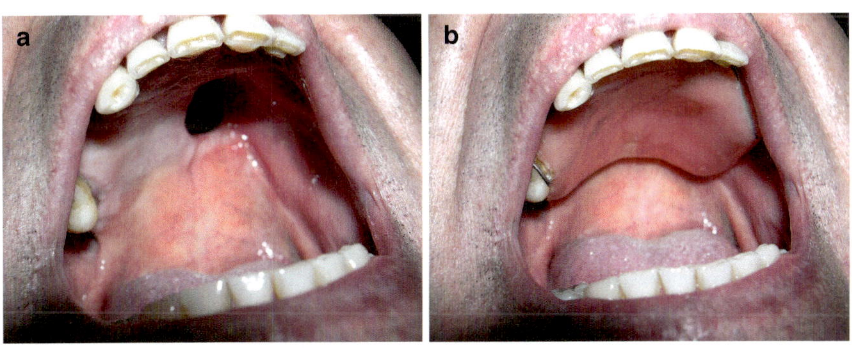

Fig. 10.1 (**a**) Okay Class Ib defect with limited involvement of the superior alveolar crest and hard palate; (**b**) obturator prosthesis fixed on the contralateral teeth filling the palatal defect

In fact, obturator stability may be determined by the so-called prosthodontist's triangle [1], a figure defined by the fulcrum line connecting the two teeth that distally delimit residual dentition and the most distant point from this line at the level of the alveolus. The surface of this triangle may be employed as a "prognosticator" of prosthesis stability: a low surface determines a poor result and vice versa. Furthermore, residual canines and molars are particularly important because they serve as attachment points for retaining clasps.

The process for producing an adequate obturator prosthesis starts in the preoperative setting and ends at approximately 6 months from surgery, when wound healing is complete. For this reason, obturators may be distinguished in three types:

- Surgical obturator
- Temporary obturator
- Definitive obturator

The process starts by taking an impression cast of the patient's dentition and hard palate before surgery. This is used to produce a surgical obturator that is inserted at the level of the defect immediately after resection, allowing initial separation between the oral cavity and the nasal fossa/maxillary sinus, giving support to postoperative wound dressings and allowing early rehabilitation of deglutition (with ensuing early removal of the nasogastric feeding tube).

After this phase, a temporary obturator is produced based on the patient's postoperative impression cast. This is composed of a horizontal portion covering the palatal defect and fixed to the residual teeth and palate and a vertical portion formed by a hollow bulb extending in the nasal fossa through the palatal defect. In case of resections extending to the teeth, it is possible to add dental fittings to the structure. This prosthesis is progressively adapted according to the wound modifications (scarring and remucosalisation) and patient needs.

When the healing process is complete and the structure of the obturator does not need further modifications, a permanent obturator is fabricated. This is composed of a false palate, a false alveolus with its attached dentition and a hollow bulb that avoids passage of liquids and food in the nasal cavity.

10.2.2 Palatal Island Flap

Small defects involving only a small portion of the palate may be easily reconstructed with the rotation of a palatal island flap if sufficient residual mucosa is present. Clearly, flap design is limited by the fact that the resection itself reduces the amount of tissue available for closure. However, the transfer of well-vascularised, sensate mucosa is particularly appealing [8, 9].

After incision and dissection of the palatal mucoperiosteum pedicled on the greater palatine artery and vein, the flap can be rotated to cover a defect at the level of the contralateral palate. The secondary defect of exposed bone can heal by secondary intention, with no functional morbidity or risk of wound contraction thanks to the underlying bone. However, as mentioned before, the main limits of this flap are the lack of healthy tissue after resection, as well as the limited elasticity of the palatal mucoperiosteum and its pedicle.

10.2.3 Buccal Fat Pad Flap

This intraoral flap may be useful in reconstruction of small defects of the hard palate and alveolus thanks to its close proximity to these sites [10–12] (Fig. 10.2). It is represented by the buccal fat pad, an encapsulated fat mass of the cheek located on either side of the face between the buccinator muscle and several more superficial muscles (including the masseter, zygomaticus major and zygomaticus minor). It may be divided into three lobes according to the structure of lobar envelopes, ligaments and feeding vessels: anterior, intermediate and posterior. The posterior lobe gives origin to the buccal, pterygoid, pterygopalatine and temporal extensions. The facial artery, transverse facial vessel and internal maxillary artery (together with their anastomosing branches) enter the fat tissue and form a lobar subcapsular vascular plexus by anastomosing with each other.

The approach for buccal fat pad in case of reconstruction of the hard palate or superior alveolus is through an incision along the superior vestibular sulcus at about the level of the upper second molar and backwards. The incision through the mucosa and buccinator exposes the maxillary periosteum and buccal fat pad, allowing blunt dissection and fat herniation without tearing its capsule or surrounding vessels. The flap is then positioned at the level of the defect maintaining minimal tension in order to avoid compromise of its vascularisation.

This flap may be effectively employed for reconstruction of maxillary defects of approximately 4 cm not requiring significant structural stability.

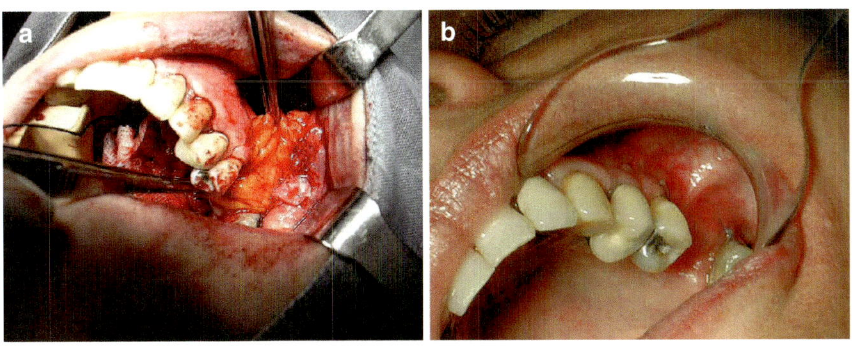

Fig. 10.2 (**a**) Bichat fat pad covering a maxillary tuberosity defect; (**b**) postoperative view after complete healing and flap remucosalisation

10.2.4 FAMM Flap

This is a local flap suitable for small-to-moderate palatal defects that do not need rigid structural support but which only require adequate separation between the oral cavity and the nasal fossa or maxillary sinus. It is based on the facial artery (and its venous plexus), which allows isolating a flap composed of the buccal mucosa, underlying submucosa, a portion of the buccinator muscle and deeper fibres of the orbicularis oris [13–15]. In palatal reconstruction, the flap is based superiorly, with retrograde flow coming from the angular artery. This leads to a wide arc of rotation that allows reconstruction of defects of the hard palate, alveolus and nasal lining.

In flap harvesting, the facial artery is identified at the level of the buccal mucosa by means of palpation or a Doppler ultrasound probe. The vessel is then isolated and ligated at the antero-inferior edge of the flap after incision of the mucosa, submucosa and buccinator muscle. The remaining edges of the flap are then incised along the course of the facial artery, maintaining the vessel at the centre of the mucosal paddle. The flap is then elevated from inferior to superior including the artery itself and all three soft tissue layers (mucosa, submucosa and buccinator). With this design, it is possible to harvest a long (7–8 cm) and narrow axially perfused flap with a thickness of approximately 8–10 mm.

10.3 Reconstruction of Unilateral Inferior Maxillectomy (Okay Class II)

Inferior maxillectomy consists of total or subtotal removal of the inferior portion of the maxilla (i.e. ipsilateral hard palate and alveolus) without involvement of its suprastructure. Consequently, the ipsilateral alveolar ridge is removed up to the midline or at least the canine teeth. As in smaller defects, the aim of reconstruction is to restore the physiologic separation between the oral cavity and nasal fossa/maxillary sinus, since there are generally no issues concerning the anterior projection of the maxilla or the orbital floor.

Obturator prostheses remain a useful tool in this kind of defect even if cantilever forces generated during mastication are applied to a smaller "prosthodontist's triangle", thus leading to inferior stability, more frequent malposition and a higher risk of nasal regurgitation (Fig. 10.3). In this view, patient preference also plays an important role in the choice of treatment, since younger subjects may prefer a more definitive type of reconstruction without the above-mentioned downsides and constant maintenance needed by an obturator. In these cases, fascio-cutaneous free flaps (in particular the RF) represent an ideal choice for closure of such gaps. In most cases, sufficient mastication is maintained by the contralateral dentition, and the anterior teeth may be replaced by dental fittings for aesthetic purposes. In selected cases and highly motivated patients, a bony free flap (i.e. scapula, fibula or iliac crest) could be considered in view of a subsequent insertion of osteo-integrated implants for complete dental rehabilitation. However, this is not the main indication for this kind of flap.

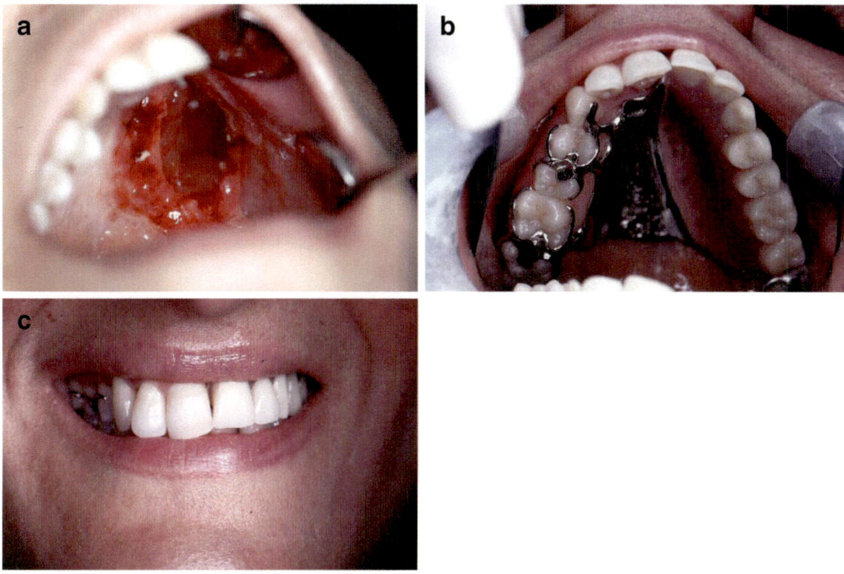

Fig. 10.3 (a) Okay Class II defect (involvement of the entire hemi-palate and alveolar crest); (b) rehabilitation of the Okay Class II defect by means of an obturator prosthesis; (c) post-rehabilitative appearance with the obturator in place

10.3.1 Radial Forearm Free Flap

The RF is a highly versatile free flap, widely employed in head and neck reconstruction in a variety of clinical scenarios. It almost invariably consists of a fasciocutaneous free flap based on the radial artery and the cephalic vein (or the comitant veins of the radial artery), while portions of the bone, muscle or tendon may also be transferred concomitantly. Typically, it allows harvesting of a wide surface of thin and pliable cutaneous tissue that can effectively reconstruct partial defects of the palate [16, 17]. Its long vascular pedicle is particularly suitable to reach the maxillofacial region without the need for vein grafts. The anatomical separation between artery (in a deeper plain) and vein (in the subcutaneous layer of fat more superficially located in the forearm) also allows for a significant degree of freedom in the choice of recipient vessels. A further advantage is represented by the fact that the donor site is relatively distant from the head and neck area, thus allowing concomitant flap harvesting and surgical resection.

On the other hand, the main drawbacks are related to donor site morbidity, since there may be negative outcomes both in terms of aesthetic appearance and subtle loss of functionality of the forearm and hand [18]. In particular, local flaps or a skin graft is almost invariably needed for wound closure, sometimes leading to diffuse scarring or a different type of skin texture at the level of the donor site. In addition, patients may experience mild functional sequelae that rarely influence their overall quality of life: altered skin sensibility, reduced tolerance to low temperatures (especially concerning the hand) and impaired accuracy of the hand fine motor control (mainly due to the potentially reduced sensitivity of the first two fingers).

10.4 Reconstruction of Subtotal and Total Maxillectomies (Okay Class II z, II f and II z, f)

Total maxillectomy is defined as the complete resection of the maxillary infra- and suprastructures and may involve the floor of the orbit (f), the zygomatic process (z) or both structures. Resection of these elements should be always precisely specified due to its significant impact on the reconstructive approach chosen for the patient. In fact, the anterior projection of the maxilla (defined by the zygomatic process and the zygomatic bone), as well as the orbital floor, often needs to be reconstructed by means of rigid structures (such as a bony free flap) to obtain an optimal result in terms of aesthetic appearance and stereoscopic visual function. While metallic meshes and bone grafts may also be employed, they generally do not represent a first choice in malignant salivary neoplasms because of the frequent need for adjuvant radiotherapy and the consequent risk of infection, exposure or necrosis.

In particular, reconstruction of the orbital floor should be carefully planned to symmetrically reposition the eye, avoid enophthalmos or proptosis and allow a complete degree of movement of the extraocular muscles.

The main free flaps containing a bone component that have been proposed for these defects are:

- Tip of the scapula
- Iliac crest
- Fibula

Each of these flaps is characterised by distinct advantages and drawbacks that should be considered in relation to the defect and characteristics of the patient.

10.4.1 Tip of the Scapula Free Flap

The tip of the scapula osteo-muscular free flap is the latest acquisition in the field of palatomaxillary reconstruction [19–21]. It is based on the angular branch of the thoracodorsal artery and includes the tip of the scapula together with the teres major and/or the serratus anterior and/or part of the latissimus dorsi muscles. The vascular pedicle is the longest available for osseous donor sites (up to 15–20 cm) and is rarely involved by atherosclerosis, even in elderly patients with impending peripheral vascular disease.

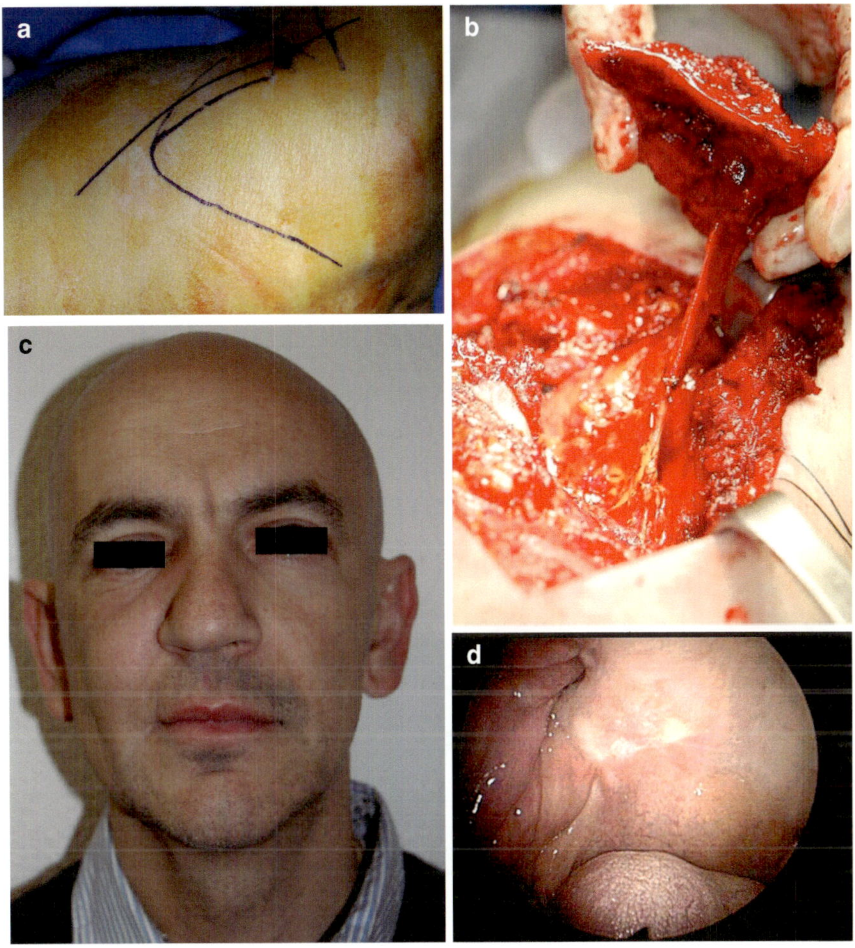

Fig. 10.4 (**a**) Preoperative drawing showing the planned incision for tip of the scapula free flap harvesting; (**b**) intraoperative view of the left tip of the scapula harvested with its vascular pedicle (angular branch of the thoracodorsal artery and vein); (**c**) postoperative result after 3 months following total maxillectomy (Okay Class II z, f); (**d**) intraoral view showing complete muscle remucosalisation (at 3 months)

Vascularised bone provides an effective support for palatal and midfacial structures and allows subsequent dental rehabilitation with osteo-integrated implants. Its main application is in Class II z, f defects with involvement of the zygomatic-maxillary buttress and orbital floor (Fig. 10.4). In these defects, the tip of the scapula is positioned vertically to restore the alveolar bone with its lateral border and the naso-maxillary buttress with its medial part. In this case, the hard palate is restored using the teres major muscle, sutured posteriorly to the soft palate. Reconstruction of the orbital floor can be provided by contouring the scapular bone with a greenstick osteotomy on its superior portion, obtaining a perpendicular surface oriented in the horizontal plane to support the orbital content. Postoperative positioning of osteo-integrated implants has been described by different authors, even though the quality of bone is usually inferior to that obtained from the fibula or iliac crest, with the only exception of young males in which the lateral edge of the scapula closely resembles the thickness of a fibular bone. Moreover, the tip of the scapula free flap is unique in the possibility to harvest generous chimeric flaps composed of multiple skin paddles (based on perforators coming from the circumflex scapular artery) and muscles (teres major, latissimus dorsi, serratus anterior with/without costal cartilages) which are rarely needed for reconstruction of extended resections involving the entire maxilla, mandibular ramus and condyle, orbital content and facial skin (Okay Class II z, f, o, s) [22] (Fig. 10.5).

Donor-site complications after tip of scapula harvesting are rarely described, and postoperative upper limb function has been evaluated by different authors, which shows mild dysfunction with little influence on patients' quality of life.

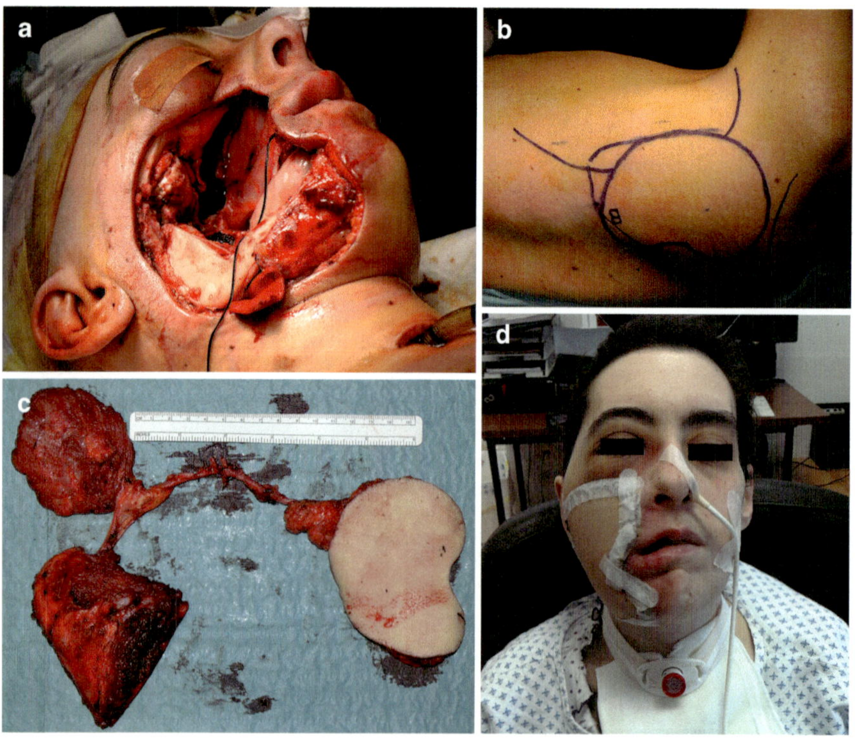

Fig. 10.5 (**a**) Complex surgical defect following right maxillectomy (Class II z, f) extended to the pterygopalatine fossa and the masticatory space, marginal mandibulectomy and wide skin paddle; (**b**) preoperative planning for flap harvesting; (**c**) chimeric flap including the tip of the scapula, latissimus dorsi muscle and parascapular skin; (**d**) postoperative result 1 week after surgery

10.4.2 The Iliac Crest Free Flap

This is an osteo-cutaneous, osteo-muscular or osteo-myocutaneous free flap based on the deep iliac circumflex artery and vein. It allows harvesting of a significant amount of uni- or bi-cortical bone from the iliac crest together with the overlying skin and/or the internal oblique muscle [23]. While it has been more frequently employed in mandibular reconstruction, several authors have described its potential in restoring both the superior alveolus and anterior maxillary projection without the need for multiple osteotomies (Fig. 10.6). Furthermore, the thick bone-stock is always suitable for implantation, even when harvested in a uni-cortical fashion. However, its main drawbacks are represented by the relatively short pedicle, the reduced degree of freedom in the orientation of each of its component (bone, skin and muscle) and the non-negligible donor site morbidity and sequelae [24, 25]. In fact, abdominal wall integrity is the first concern after reconstruction with this flap, since in approximately 10% of cases, subsequent development of abdominal hernias is observed, while another significant problem is related to the occasional development of chronic pain or gait disturbances.

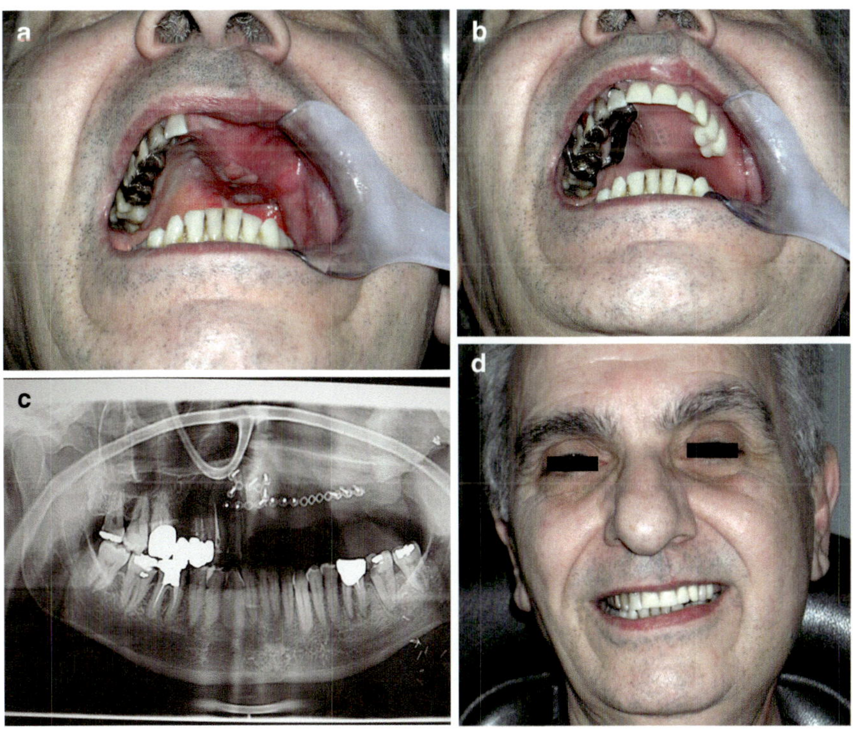

Fig. 10.6 (**a**) Intraoral view after total maxillectomy (Class II z, f) and reconstruction with iliac crest free flap; (**b**) intraoral view after customised obturator prosthesis positioning; (**c**) dental panoramic radiograph showing the iliac bone matching the contralateral maxilla; (**d**) patient's appearance after complete healing

10.4.3 The Fibula Free Flap

The fibula free flap offers a large amount of cortical bone (up to 25 cm if the entire fibula is taken) that may be associated with a skin paddle perfused by perforator vessels (Fig. 10.7). The pedicle is represented by the peroneal artery and its comitant veins, thus obtaining a moderately long pedicle with high-calibre vessels [26]. As mentioned before, it may be employed in the reconstruction of the superior alveolar crest in very selected Class II defects where resection does not involve the maxillary suprastructure [27]. When dealing with total maxillectomy defects (Class II z, II f and II z, f), complex tridimensional flap contouring is essential to restore all the main components of the maxilla [28] with an ensuing risk of pedicle kinking and compression. This is described as particularly cumbersome and may lead to a higher risk of bone devascularisation due to the numerous osteotomies needed. On the other hand, this flap offers a high-quality bone stock that effectively withstands the forces applied by mastication and which is ideal for intra- or postoperative implantation.

Concerning donor site complications, delayed wound healing (especially in case of skin grafting), wound necrosis and dehiscence are not infrequent. Additionally, a moderate number of functional issues have been reported, including limited range

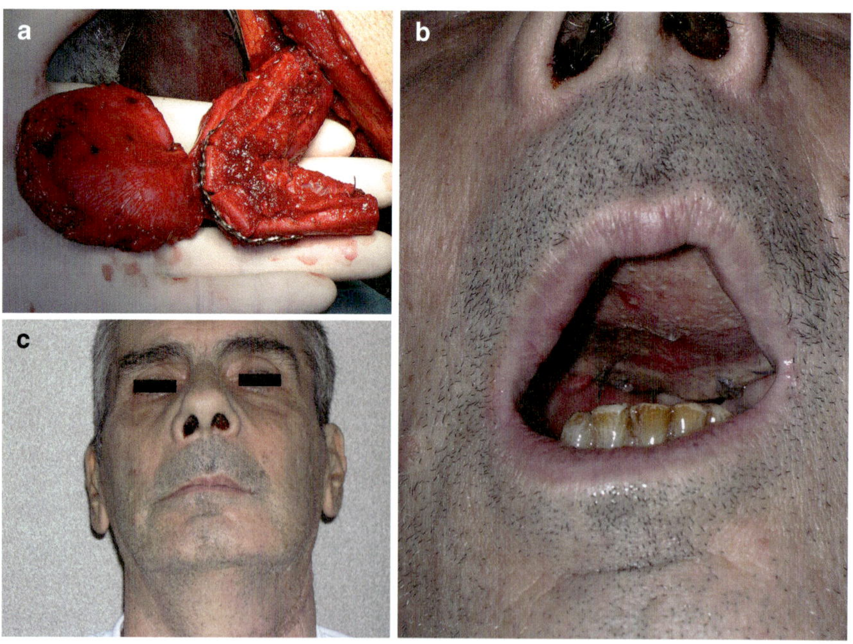

Fig. 10.7 (**a**) Right fibula free flap after complete harvesting and contouring; (**b**) intraoral postoperative view 3 weeks after surgery: the skin paddle has been positioned in order to restore the subtotal palatal defect; (**c**) postoperative result 3 weeks after surgery

of motion of the ankle, sensory deficit, chronic pain, ankle instability and reduced muscle strength [29]. Finally, arterial anomalies (as well as venous insufficiency) may put residual foot vascularisation at risk, necessitating adequate preoperative clinical and radiological assessment.

10.5 Reconstruction of Total Maxillectomy with Orbital Exenteration (Okay Class II z, f, o)

Total maxillectomy with orbital exenteration requires reconstruction with a high volume of tissue in order to completely fill the defect. In this view, the aim of reconstruction is to fill the orbital cavity while simultaneously restoring the resected hard palate. This is essential to avoid aesthetically and functionally disabling defects with direct communication between the oral cavity, nasal fossa and orbital cavity. In addition, when the orbital cavity is left healing by secondary intention, remucosalisation and frequent occurrence of orbito-nasal fistulae lead to accumulation of secretions needing frequent medications. For these reasons, soft tissue free flaps with a low surface-to-volume ratio such as the rectus abdominis, anterolateral thigh (see Sect. 8.3.4) and latissimus dorsi (see Sect. 8.3.3) are ideal candidates for reconstruction of these types of defects. As already mentioned above, the use of the angular branch-based tip of the scapula free flap after total maxillectomy with orbital clearance (Class II z, f, o) has been implemented to obtain better functional and aesthetic results while granting the possibility of dental rehabilitation by secondary osteo-integration. However, this should be only considered as an alternative in young, highly motivated patients with no significant comorbidities.

10.5.1 The Rectus Abdominis Free Flap

This is a myocutaneous, muscular or fascio-cutaneous free flap based on the deep inferior epigastric artery and vein, which has been widely popularised by its application in breast reconstruction. When both the abdominal skin and the underlying rectus abdominis muscle are harvested (myocutaneous flap), it offers one of the largest volumes of soft tissues available for head and neck reconstruction. Neck recipient vessels can be easily reached thanks to the long- and high-calibre pedicle, and the skin paddle can be placed in different orientations according to each specific defect. The hard palate is often reconstructed using the abdominal skin, which may also be extended to cover midfacial cutaneous defects and the orbital cavity [30, 31] (Fig. 10.8). The main drawbacks of this flap are related to removal of the rectus abdominis muscle, an important structure of the abdominal wall. In fact, the most frequent sequelae are development of postsurgical hernias (which may be reduced by careful reconstruction of the abdominal wall using synthetic meshes) and a mild functional deficit in the flexion of the trunk (due to removal and denervation of the rectus abdominis).

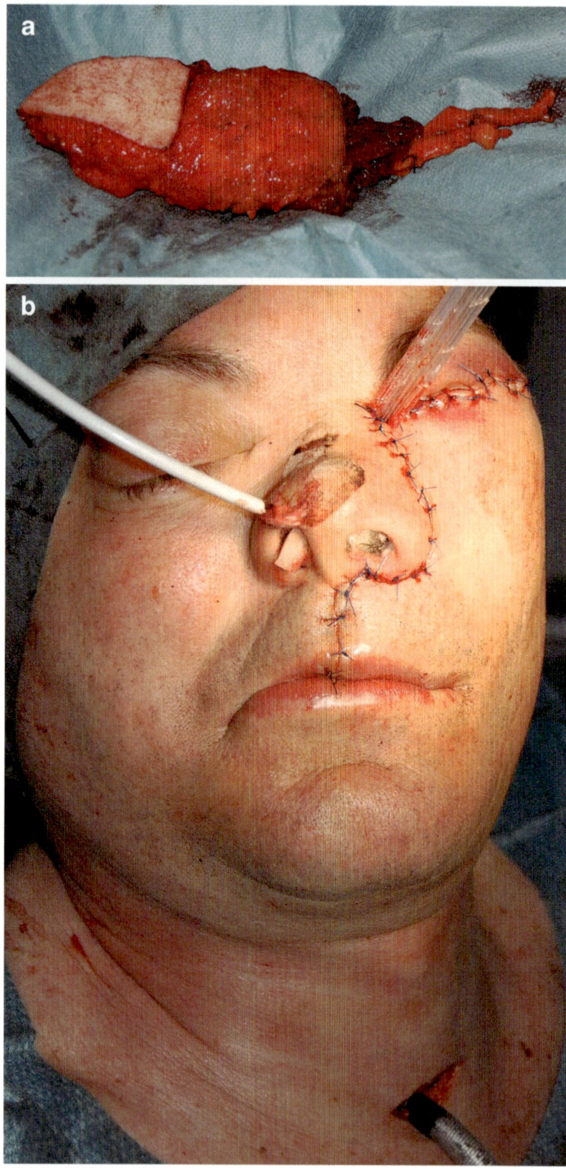

Fig. 10.8 (**a**) Rectus abdominis myocutaneous free flap after harvesting; (**b**) intraoperative view after total maxillectomy with orbital exenteration (Class II z, f, o) and reconstruction with rectus abdominis myocutaneous free flap

10.6 Reconstruction of Bilateral Inferior Maxillectomy (Okay Class III)

Class III defects (total or subtotal palatectomies) are extensive resections that may be needed in case of tumours arising from the hard palate and the superior alveolar crest with significant infiltration of these structures crossing the midline. In such advanced cases, there is no sufficient structural support to adequately sustain an obturator prosthesis due to the lack of a significant portion of the alveolar crest. For

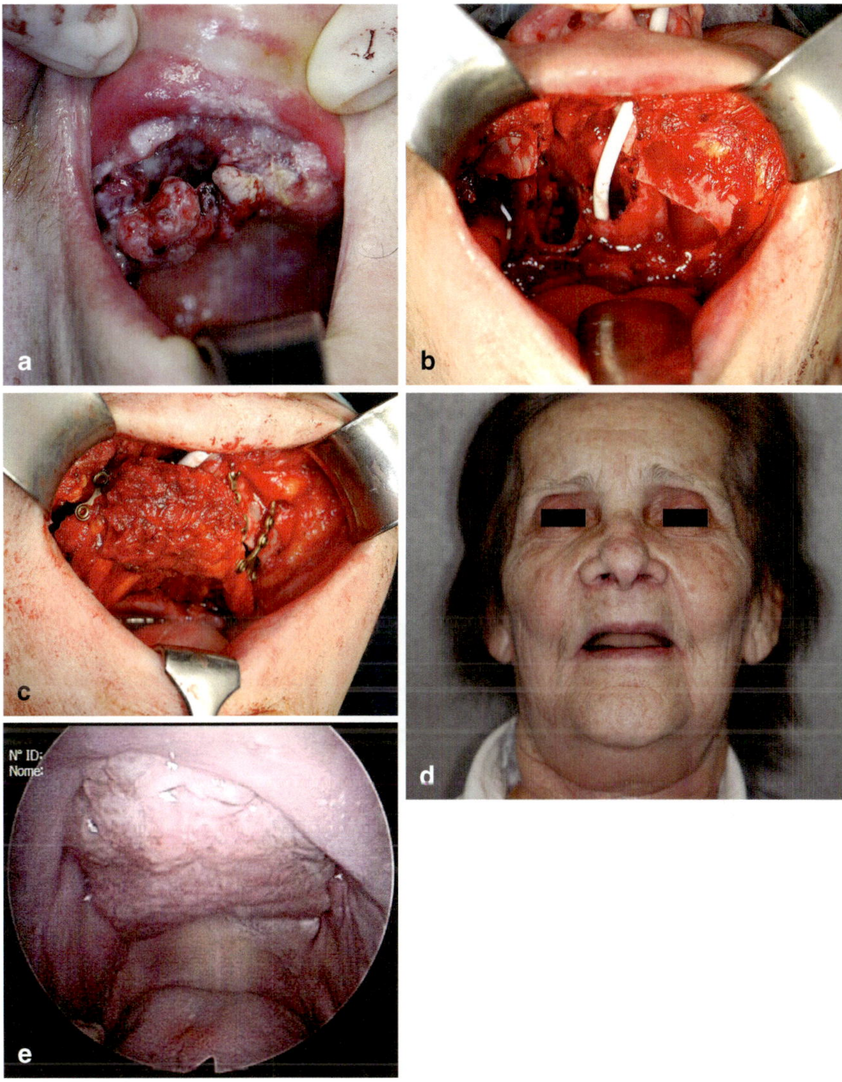

Fig. 10.9 (**a**) Squamous cell carcinoma involving the entire hard palate; (**b**) intraoperative view after complete tumour resection (Class III defect); (**c**) intraoperative view after right tip of the scapula free flap insetting; (**d**) external postoperative appearance 2 months after surgery; (**e**) intra-oral postoperative view 2 months after surgery with complete remucosalisation

this reason, a complex reconstruction by means of bone-containing flaps is essential to obtain an optimal functional result. The aim of this reconstruction is to separate the oral cavity from the paranasal sinuses while providing a stable structure for dental fittings or postoperative implantation. In this view, the tip of the scapula is an ideal donor site thanks to its remarkable tridimensional structural homology with the hard palate, as also demonstrated by radiological comparisons [32]. The scapula can be positioned horizontally at the level of the resected palate, with its bony tip oriented anteriorly, the ventral portion intraorally, the dorsal surface endonasally and the donor vessels on the side of the selected recipient vessels (considering that harvesting a right-sided tip of the scapula will bring the vessels to be anastomosed on the left side of the neck and vice versa). The bare muscles covering the ventral surface of the scapula (thus becoming the endo-oral part of the flap) undergo a quick process of shrinkage and remucosalisation that closely resembles the native palatal mucosa (Fig. 10.9).

Another option is represented by the fibula free flap, in which the bone can be used to replace the entire alveolar crest and the skin paddle used for closure of the palatal gap. However, the need for a significant length of bone results in a shorter pedicle that may frequently need vein grafts to reach the neck vessels. Moreover, the skin paddle used to reconstitute the palatal mucosal lining is suboptimal in terms of intraoral feeling and bolus processing.

References

1. Okay DJ, Genden E, Buchbinder D, Urken M. Prosthodontic guidelines for surgical reconstruction of the maxilla: a classification system of defects. J Prosthet Dent. 2001;86:352–63.
2. Brown JS, Shaw RJ. Reconstruction of the maxilla and midface: introducing a new classification. Lancet Oncol. 2010;11:1001–8.
3. Cordeiro PG, Santamaria E. A classification system and algorithm for reconstruction of maxillectomy and midfacial defects. Plast Reconstr Surg. 2000;105:2331–46.
4. Cordeiro PG, Chen CM. A 15-year review of midface reconstruction after total and subtotal maxillectomy: part I. Algorithm and outcomes. Plast Reconstr Surg. 2012;129:124–36.
5. Yamamoto Y, Kawashima K, Sugihara T, et al. Surgical management of maxillectomy defects based on the concept of buttress reconstruction. Head Neck. 2004;26:247–56.
6. Sharma AB, Beumer J. Reconstruction of maxillary defects: the case for prosthetic rehabilitation. J Oral Maxillofac Surg. 2005;63:1770–3.
7. Keyf F. Obturator prostheses for hemimaxillectomy patients. J Oral Rehabil. 2001;28:821–9.
8. Gullane PJ, Arena S. Palatal island flap for reconstruction of oral defects. Arch Otolaryngol. 1977;103:598–9.
9. Ducic Y, Herford AS. The use of palatal island flaps as an adjunct to microvascular free tissue transfer for reconstruction of complex oromandibular defects. Laryngoscope. 2001;111:1666–9.
10. Hao SP. Reconstruction of oral defects with the pedicled buccal fat pad flap. Otolaryngol Head Neck Surg. 2000;122:863–7.
11. Meyer E, Liebenberg SJ, Fagan JJ. Buccal fat pad – a simple, underutilised flap. S Afr J Surg. 2012;50:47–9.
12. Kim MK, Han W, Kim SG. The use of the buccal fat pad flap for oral reconstruction. Maxillofac Plast Reconstr Surg. 2017;39:5.
13. Pribaz J, Stephens W, Crespo L, Gifford G. A new intraoral flap: facial artery musculomucosal (FAMM) flap. Plast Reconstr Surg. 1992;90:421–9.
14. Dupoirieux L, Plane L, Gard C, Penneau M. Anatomical basis and results of the facial artery musculomucosal flap for oral reconstruction. Br J Oral Maxillofac Surg. 1999;37:25–8.
15. Ashtiani AK, Emami SA, Rasti M. Closure of complicated palatal fistula with facial artery musculomucosal flap. Plast Reconstr Surg. 2005;116:381–6.
16. Duflo S, Lief F, Paris J, et al. Microvascular radial forearm fasciocutaneous free flap in hard palate reconstruction. Eur J Surg Oncol. 2005;31:784–91.
17. Ciuman R, Mohr C, Kroger K, Dost P. The forearm flap: assessment of functional and aesthetic outcomes and quality of life. Am J Otolaryngol. 2007;28:367–74.

18. Toschka H, Feifel H, Erli HJ, et al. Aesthetic and functional results of harvesting radial forearm flap, especially with regard to hand function. Int J Oral Maxillofac Surg. 2001;30:42–8.
19. Clark JR, Vesely M, Gilbert R. Scapular angle osteomyogenous flap in postmaxillectomy reconstruction: defect, reconstruction, shoulder function, and harvest technique. Head Neck. 2008;30:10–20.
20. Miles BA, Gilbert RW. Maxillary reconstruction with the scapular angle osteomyogenous free flap. Arch Otolaryngol Head Neck Surg. 2011;137:1130–5.
21. Piazza C, Paderno A, Del Bon F, et al. Palato-maxillary reconstruction by the angular branch-based tip of scapula free flap. Eur Arch Otorhinolaryngol. 2017;274:939–45.
22. Janus JR, Carlson ML, Moore EJ. The scapular, parascapular, and latissimus dorsi flap as a single osteomyocutaneous flap for repair of complex oral defects. Clin Anat. 2012;25:120–8.
23. Brown JS. Deep circumflex iliac artery free flap with internal oblique muscle as a new method of immediate reconstruction of maxillectomy defect. Head Neck. 1996;18:412–21.
24. Rogers SN, Lakshmiah SR, Narayan B, et al. A comparison of the long-term morbidity following deep circumflex iliac and fibula free flaps for reconstruction following head and neck cancer. Plast Reconstr Surg. 2003;112:1517–25.
25. Valentini V, Gennaro P, Aboh IV, et al. Iliac crest flap: donor site morbidity. J Craniofac Surg. 2009;20:1052–5.
26. Baj A, Youssef DA, Monteverdi R, et al. Reconstruction of partial maxillary defects with the double-barrel fibula free flap. Acta Otorhinolaryngol Ital. 2010;30:299–302.
27. Peng X, Mao C, Yu GY, et al. Maxillary reconstruction with the free fibula flap. Plast Reconstr Surg. 2005;115:1562–9.
28. Zhang WB, Wang Y, Liu XJ, et al. Reconstruction of maxillary defects with free fibula flap assisted by computer techniques. J Craniomaxillofac Surg. 2015;43:630–6.
29. Ling XF, Peng X. What is the price to pay for a free fibula flap? A systematic review of donor-site morbidity following free fibula flap surgery. Plast Reconstr Surg. 2012;129:657–74.
30. Browne JD, Burke AJ. Benefits of routine maxillectomy and orbital reconstruction with the rectus abdominis free flap. Otolaryngol Head Neck Surg. 1999;121:203–9.
31. Bianchi B, Bertolini F, Ferrari S, Sesenna E. Maxillary reconstruction using rectus abdominis free flap and bone grafts. Br J Oral Maxillofac Surg. 2006;44:526–30.
32. Pagedar NA, Gilbert RW, Chan H, et al. Maxillary reconstruction using the scapular tip free flap: a radiologic comparison of 3D morphology. Head Neck. 2012;34:1377–82.

Salivary Gland Tumors: Radiotherapy

11

Ester Orlandi, Giuseppe Sanguineti, and Carlo Fallai

Abbreviations

3DRT	3-dimensional conformal radiation therapy
ACC	Adenoid cystic carcinoma
AciCC	Acinic cell carcinoma
CRT	Chemoradiotherapy
CT	Chemotherapy
CXPA	Ex pleomorphic adenoma
DFS	Disease-free survival
DSS	Disease-specific survival
ECE	Extracapsular extension
END	Elective neck dissection
ENI	Elective neck irradiation
HG	High grade
IG	Intermediate grade
IMRT	Intensity-modulated radiation therapy
LC	Local control
LF	Local failure
LG	Low grade
LGSGTs	Low-grade salivary glands cancers
LRC	Locoregional control
MEC	Mucoepidermoid carcinoma

E. Orlandi (✉) · C. Fallai
SC Radioterapia 2, Fondazione IRCCC, Istituto Nazionale dei Tumori, Milano, Italy
e-mail: ester.orlandi@istitutotumori.mi.it; carlo.fallai@istitutotumori.mi.it

G. Sanguineti
UOC Radioterapia, Istituto Nazionale Tumori Regina Elena, Roma, Italy
e-mail: giuseppe.sanguineti@ifo.gov.it

© Springer Nature Switzerland AG 2019

L. Licitra, L. D. Locati (eds.), *Salivary Gland Cancer*,
https://doi.org/10.1007/978-3-030-02958-6_11

OS	Overall survival
PLGA	Polymorphous low-grade adenocarcinoma
PNI	Perineural involvement
PORT	Postoperative radiation therapy
RFS	Recurrence-free survival
RT	Radiotherapy
SBRT	Stereotactic radiotherapy
SEER	Surveillance, epidemiology, and end results
SGTs	Salivary gland tumors
SOR	Standards, options, and recommendations
VMAT	Volumetric modulated arc therapy

11.1 Introduction

SGTs are rare diseases, accounting for 2–6.5% of all head and neck cancers, and characterized by considerable heterogeneity in their histology, biology, and clinical behavior [1]. Mucoepidermoid carcinoma (MEC), ACC, and adenocarcinoma, NOS, are the most frequent diagnoses, representing >70% of all SGTs, although their frequency varies depending on the site of origin (major vs minor salivary glands) [2]. Among benign lesions, the most common tumor is the pleomorphic adenoma, although it shows great histopathological diversity with a relative proportion of malignancy increasing in smaller glands [3].

Prognosis depends on histology and grading: among non-ACC, high-grade carcinomas are associated with a poorer prognosis compared with low-grade carcinomas [4, 5]. ACC frequently displays an indolent course with a propensity for local or distant recurrence, in particular up to 10–15 years after initial treatment, and it is often highly fatal. Histology, involved gland, and location within the gland have a pivotal role in choosing the best therapeutic management. Complete surgical resection with adequate free margins is the mainstay of treatment for resectable cases. Small, well-localized, low-grade carcinomas excised with clear margins are best treated with surgery alone [2]. PORT is recommended in high-risk patients when adverse prognostic factors based on pathology (T3–T4, lymph node involvement, close/microscopically positive margins, vascular/perineural invasion, and high-grade) can be identified [2]. Unresectable or inoperable SGTs can be managed with RT alone, even though curative purposes are hardly achievable [2].

Overall, SGTs represent a major challenge for the radiation oncologists' community not only for their historically known radioresistance but also for frequently horseshoe-shaped target volume (e.g., in case of perineural invasion) and their proximity to radiosensitive normal structures (e.g., tumors arising from minor salivary glands in paranasal sinuses).

The last two decades has seen significant technological advances for photon radiation delivery in terms of precision by using IMRT, VMAT, and SBRT. These approaches can generate extremely conformal dose distributions including concave isodose volumes that provide conformal target volume coverage and avoidance of specific sensitive normal structures [6, 7]. Further improvements in therapeutic ratio could be achieved by using particle beam RT, in particular proton and carbon ion therapy (see Chap. 11). This can lead to several advantages in terms of normal tissue sparing, better dose homogeneity, and a reduced dose bath effect (low radiation dose to normal tissue). However, both modern photon- and hadron-based treatments have been shown to be effective and are characterized by a favorable toxicity profile [8]. Dosimetric and/or clinical comparison studies between photon and hadron therapy for SGTs are very scant [8, 9]. Besides, due to the high cost of particle therapy and the very low number of equipped facilities, a careful selection of patients is absolutely critical.

In this chapter, we will focus on the role and the impact of photon RT for SGTs both in malignant and benign lesions. The majority of published retrospective papers includes heterogeneous series taking into account number of patients, histology, tumor sites (major vs minor salivary glands), stages, and RT settings (i.e., definitive, postoperative, or reirradiation); for this reason we have dedicated different paragraphs to detail curative RT treatment based on the following histopathologies: ACC, non-ACC high-grade, non-ACC low-grade, and non-malignant neoplasms.

11.2 Adenoid Cystic Carcinoma (ACC)

11.2.1 Indications and Role of Postoperative Radiotherapy (PORT)

The "gold-standard" treatment for potentially resectable ACCs consists in radical surgery providing free margins followed by PORT, although the role of RT has been debatable in the absence of randomized trials or prospective studies. The addition of RT with surgery has been reported to improve local control (LC) rates compared with surgical resection alone in all ACC sites. Five- and 10-year LC rates for combined modality treatment were 88–95% and 84–91%, respectively [10–13]. Garden et al. studied 198 patients with ACC of the head and neck treated with surgery followed by radiation. They demonstrated LC rates of 95%, 86%, and 79% at 5, 10, and 15 years, respectively. Improved treatment outcome led the investigators to recommend PORT as the routine treatment approach for most patients with ACC. In addition, Mendenhall et al. also stated that the optimal treatment for these patients is surgery followed by adjuvant radiotherapy [11]. The omission of adjuvant radiation was found to be an independent predictor of local recurrence in the study by the University of California at San Francisco (UCSF), including 140 patients [14]. Furthermore, the experience of Memorial Sloan Kettering Cancer Center published in 2008 showed improved LC for patients treated with PORT and supported the routine use of combined treatment in ACC [15]. However, some authors do not find a statistically significant effect of PORT on LC [16, 17]; others postulated that PORT may delay rather than prevent recurrence instead [18, 19].

The effectiveness of RT has been questioned by some other studies because of its lack of advantage in overall survival (OS) for the high rate of distant metastases and a relatively high probability of long-term survival after salvage therapy [14, 16, 20].

A recent study from the SEER database on 3026 patients reported by Ellington et al. suggested that PORT confers no survival benefit [21]; this was also confirmed by Lloyd et al. [22]. Some papers with opposed conclusions have been published. A retrospective series by Shen, on 101 patients diagnosed with ACC arising from all head and neck sites, showed at multivariate analysis that the addition of RT was a favorite predictor for LC and survival rates [23].

Several authors have retrospectively studied clinical and pathological features, attempting to identify significant prognostic factors in the presence of which PORT was highly suggested, but these factors still remain controversial. Various adverse parameters such as advanced tumor lesions, positive surgical margins, perineural invasion, and major nerve involvement have been suggested as the indication for PORT in ACC [11, 12, 14, 15, 24, 25].

In a recent paper by Ali at al. [26], pathological T4 stage without PORT was an independent predictor of local failure. However, after adjusting for T stage, patients who do not get PORT were more likely to have local recurrence: they had a 13-fold increased risk of local failure compared to patients treated with PORT. Vikram et al. recommended that patients with high-grade tumors and/or high-stage tumors benefited from PORT [27]. Histological grade was also considered in the paper by da Cruz Perez et al. They affirmed that grade 3 ACC should be considered as a specific entity within the ACC group, due to its typical aggressive biological behavior and relatively poor outcome; therefore it is needed an improved adjuvant treatment [28].

As for perineural involvement (PNI), it is not currently clear if microscopic evidence of perineural invasion has true prognostic significance in ACC and also available data are conflicting. Nevertheless, when the nerve involved is above a certain size, or "named," a prognostic factor can be established [29].

It is known that PNI occurs via contiguous spread along perineural spaces or within the nerve itself, and it is a microscopic feature of malignancy often confined to the main tumor mass. The PNI, even microscopic, may be an indication for PORT. In fact, it is sometimes associated with skip lesions along the nerve that significantly increase the risk of recurrence after resection even if negative margins are obtained [29]; besides, Chen et al. at the UCSF found that PNI was associated with local recurrence in patients treated with surgery alone but not in those who received postoperative radiation [14]. The authors regarded PNI invasion as a marker for subclinical extension of disease that may not be adequately addressed by surgery alone, even in the setting of an apparently complete surgical resection [14]. Besides, there is an association between PNI and margin status. In a paper by Khan, 15 out of 20 patients with positive margins displayed PNI as well, while only 5 of 17 with negative margins showed nerve invasion ($P = 0.02$) [20].

Bone invasion from ACC can be identified in advanced tumor arising from sublingual and submandibular gland, paranasal sinuses, nasopharynx, and lacrimal gland. Thompson et al. stated that an increased incidence of either recurrence or dying with disease in patients with both skull base involvement and bone invasion suggests an adjuvant treatment [30]. Williams et al. found radiologically and histologically documented bony invasion of the lacrimal gland fossa by ACC very high, up to 76%. In this case, PORT could be hardly recommended, due to its poorly prognostic role [31].

Some reports have been shown that nodal involvement, with or without extracapsular extension (ECE), is independently associated with decreased overall and cause-specific survival, probably because it is a risk factor for subsequent distant metastasis [32]. The role of adjuvant RT after therapeutic neck dissection has been highly debated. Generally, patients treated with surgery and adjuvant RT showed comparable outcome with those treated by surgery alone [33]. Furthermore, regional recurrences are not usually identified in clinically positive node patients who undergo therapeutic neck dissection, whether or not adjuvant RT is administered [34].

The overall rate, from 15% to 44%, of occult neck metastasis for all ACC head and neck sites seems to be higher in oral cavity and oropharynx (22–31%) than those in the sinonasal tract (17%) or in the major glands (11–23%) [32–35]. Level II was the most frequently involved, with a reported incidence of 59.6%. Level III and IV regions were affected only in 22.5% of cases [32]. Besides, Lee et al. noted that the primary tumor site and peri-tumoral lymphovascular invasion were significantly associated with cervical lymph node metastasis [35]. On this basis, selective neck dissection should be considered for tumors of those sites showing lymphovascular invasion, in high-risk oral and oropharyngeal ACC [23, 32].

Lee et al. observed that regional recurrence was not identified in cN+ patients who underwent therapeutic neck dissection or in cN0 patients who had elective neck treatment, whereas regional recurrence was identified in four patients staged cN0 who did not have elective treatment of the neck [34, 35]. Although there was no significant difference in distant metastases or survival rates when END was performed in N0 necks, END could remove occult regional disease and provide patients with a regional recurrence-free life [34, 35]. However, elective neck irradiation (ENI) remains controversial. Balamucki et al. employed ENI in 64 out of 101 patients with undissected cN0; the remaining 37 were observed. Multivariate analysis of neck control revealed that ENI significantly influenced rates of neck control at 5 and 10 years [10]. On this basis, the authors advised to electively treat the first echelon nodes, particularly in patients with primary tumors at sites that are rich in lymphatics. However, contrary results have been published. Chen et al. [36] compared outcomes in a group of patients receiving neck irradiation and another group submitted to observation. There were no relapses in either group. In accordance with these results, their current policy is not recommending elective neck irradiation routinely.

Overall, PORT is suggested in all patients or at least in the presence of various adverse parameters such as advanced tumor stages (e.g., T3–4), positive or close surgical margins, PNI, and bone involvement [37]. Patients with T1/T2 tumors, negative margins, and negative neck disease did not have any benefit [38]. Radiotherapy treatment of the neck should be made on a case-by-case basis. However, ENI could be considered for tumors of those sites showing lymphovascular invasion and in high-risk oral and oropharyngeal ACC, when END is not performed [34, 35].

11.2.2 Definitive Radiotherapy

RT alone can be given to a subset of patients with early-stage resectable cancers depending on the location of the tumor, patients' wishes, and philosophy of the attending physician [10].

Patients with unresectable ACCs or gross residual diseases receiving conventional RT alone showed the poorest results in terms of LC ranging from 10% to 48% [27, 39, 40]. ACCs from paranasal sinuses can receive advanced photon beam techniques (IMRT and VMAT) allowing for a higher therapeutic ratio when a complete surgery cannot be performed because of invasion of the dura, brain, orbit, or nasopharynx. Spratt DE et al. stated that IMRT techniques with doses ≥70 Gy are a reasonable alternative to neutron radiotherapy in patients who present unresectable SGTs showing comparable disease control with fewer late complications [41]. Today, a more state-of-the-art radiotherapeutic approach is applied: instead of photon external beam treatment, a proton- or carbon ion-based irradiation is currently used. Exclusive modern particle therapy is not the object of the present chapter, but we want just to make a brief reference to mixed beam RT, based on photon and heavy particle. Pommier et al. studied 23 patients with nonmetastatic ACCs with skull base extension treated with both proton and photon RT to a total dose of 75.9 cobalt-Gy equivalent. The DFS and OS rates at 5 years were 56% and 77%, respectively [42]. Huber et al. compared RT with neutrons, photons, and a photon/neutron mixed beam in 75 patients with locally advanced, recurrent, or incompletely resected disease. They found the 5-year LC rate to be 75% for neutrons and 32% for the other two groups [43].

The advantage of neutrons over photons has also been shown in a prospective phase III trial conducted by RTOG and MRC [44]. However, the study was prematurely interrupted, but data from the 32 enrolled patients showed a 10-year LC of 56% in the neutron arm vs 17% in the photon arm. Long-term, treatment-related severe morbidity was greater in the neutron arm even if there was no significant difference in "life-threatening" complications. Neutrons were responsible for the increase in LC and toxicity [44].

More recently, carbon ion RT has been used in ACC, in the attempt to reproduce the high LC of neutron therapy without its toxicity. In the Heidelberg experience, a phase II trial (COSMIC) was designed to investigate the effects of dose escalation in the established mixed-beam regimen (photons+ carbon ions) with a total biologically effective dose of 80 Gy [45]. This study included patients with either inoperable disease or R2 or R1 resection (N = 53 patients), and most of them had ACC (89%). Three-year LC was 82%, and there was no significant difference between R1, R2, and inoperable patients. In the COSMIC trial, there were two patients with late osteoradionecrosis and one case of late internal carotid aneurysm [45].

Main characteristics and relative reported outcomes of ACC selected studies are reported in Table 11.1.

Table 11.1 Main characteristics and relative reported outcomes of ACC studies included in this chapter

Author	Observation period	No. of patients	Site	Histology	Type of treatment (pts)	RT technique (pts)	Dose/fractionation	Local control	Overall survival
van Weert et al. [13]	1979–2009	105	All sites	ACC	Surgery alone (6) PORT (81) RT alone (13) Not treated (5)	n.s.	50 Gy (2 Gy/fr) + 10–20 Gy (2–2.5 Gy/fr)	58% at 10 years	52% at 10 years
Balamucki et al. [10]	1966–2008	120	All sites	ACC	RT alone (44) PORT (76)	n.s.	72.4 Gy (range 60–79.2) 69.6 Gy (range 10.5–75.6) Conventional fractionation, hyperfractionation, or concomitant-boost	36% at 10 years 84% at 10 years	37% at 10 years 57% at 10 years
Gomez et al. [15]	1990–2004	59	All sites	ACC	PORT (54) RT alone (5)	IMRT (17) 3D-CRT (15) Conventional (27)	63 Gy (range 52.2–70.2)	81% at 10 years	65% at 10 years
Chen et al. [46]	1960–2004	140	All sites	ACC	Surgery alone (50) PORT (90)	Wedged pairs (21) Mixed beams (24) 2-field (11) 3-field (12) IMRT (22)	64 Gy (range 54–71)	77% at 10 years (61% surgery alone—84% PORT)	64% at 5 years
Mendenhall et al. [11]	1966–2001	101	All sites	ACC	RT alone (42) PORT (59)	n.s.	72.4 Gy (range 61.3–79.2) 67.8 Gy (range 10.5–76.8) Conventional fractionation or hyperfractionation	69% at 10 years (43% RT alone—91% PORT)	49% at 10 years (42% RT alone—55% PORT)

(continued)

Table 11.1 (continued)

Author	Observation period	No. of patients	Site	Histology	Type of treatment (pts)	RT technique (pts)	Dose/fractionation	Local control	Overall survival
Silverman et al. [25]	1971–2001	75	All sites	ACC	Surgery alone (25) PORT (50)	n.s.	59.8 Gy (range 45–72) Conventional fractionation	79% at 10 years 71.6% at 10 years	67.9% at 10 years 60.5% at 10 years
Khan et al. [20]	1955–1999	68	All sites	ACC	Surgery alone (18) RT alone ± chemo (8) PORT (41)	n.s.	57.3 Gy (mean dose)	n.s.	44% at 10 years
Garden et al. [12]	1962–1991	198	All sites	ACC	PORT	Single-appositional (75) Parallel-opposed (52) Wedged pairs (29) 3-field (40)	60 Gy (range 50–69) Conventional fractionation	86% at 10 years	65% at 10 years

ACC adenoid cystic carcinoma, *RT* radiotherapy, *PORT* postoperative radiotherapy, *IMRT* intensity-modulated radiotherapy, *3D-CRT* three-dimensional conformal radiation therapy, *n.s.* not specified

11.2.3 Target Volumes, Doses, and Technique

Target volume delineation is based on preoperative imaging, preoperative physical exam, operative findings, and pathological findings. It is strongly recommended to map preoperative macroscopic disease onto the PORT planning CT scan using image registration with pre-surgical CT, and in general two target volumes can be defined. A high-risk target volume is commonly determined if microscopically affected margins are found. An intermediate-risk volume generally encompasses anatomical sites at risk of residual disease in addition to the original areas involved and the operative bed. These two RT volumes are usually planned to receive a total dose of 66–70 Gy and 54–63 Gy, respectively, with conventional fractionation [37, 47]. Garden et al. detected a trend toward improved LC with doses >56 Gy and suggested a minimum of 60 Gy to the original tumor volume and 66 Gy when multiple margins are positive or there is extensive soft tissue involvement [12]. Harrison et al. found a reduced 10-year LC rate of 53% in patients treated with lower doses compared to 72% in patients treated with more than 57.5 Gy [48]. Simpson et al. showed a statistically significant improvement in LC for patients receiving doses >60 Gy [49]. In the study by Chen et al., RT doses lower than 60 Gy were an independent predictor of local recurrence [14]. The extension of postoperative intermediate-risk volume varies according to primary site and occurrence of PNI. It is still doubtful whether an "elective perineural volume" (i.e., a prophylactic volume in the shape of nerves) should be drawn or not in case of microscopic PNI. Contouring can be performed according to indications reported in 1008 Radiation Therapy Oncology Group (RTOG) phase II trial [47]. In case of superficial parotidectomy, superficial lobe tumors should always encompass the deep lobe (to depth of styloid process). For deep lobe tumors or with a complete parotidectomy, this volume must also cover parapharyngeal space and temporal fossa. Finally, it should be delineated from the skull base up to the stylomastoid foramen if the VII nerve (facial nerve) is not grossly involved. When the facial nerve is hardly implicated, the contour should include the facial nerve canal through the petrous temporal bone [47]. If the tumor grossly involves one of the named large nerves in that area, such as the lingual nerve (branch of V3), the inferior alveolar nerve (branch of V3), or the hypoglossal nerve (cranial nerve XII), then the skull base needs to be included in this volume. In particular, it has to be up to the hypoglossal canal for hypoglossal nerve involvement or foramen ovale for V3 branch involvement. Moreover, if the inferior alveolar nerve (branch of V3) is involved near the skull base, intermediate-risk volume should include Meckel's cave [47]. When only focal perineural invasion is pathologically found, it can be questionable if it routinely includes nerve pathways to the base of the skull in treatment portals. For ACC of the palate or paranasal sinuses, the base of the skull is usually included because of its proximity to the tumor bed.

Contouring guidelines are available to guide radiation oncologists in the delineation of cranial nerve anatomy [50, 51].

In case of ACC involving sites with a rich lymphatic drainage or showing lymphovascular invasion, the neck has to be treated. If neck surgery has not been performed, ENI must be considered, and it should include at least the first echelon nodes. This low-risk volume usually receives 45–54 Gy.

The resultant target volumes are complex three-dimensional shapes, in particular for ACC arising from minor salivary gland of paranasal sinuses. Besides, several sensitive anatomical structures as the globes, lacrimal glands, optic nerves, chiasm, brainstem, and brain lie immediately adjacent or in close proximity to target volumes. Conventional RT has been associated either with incomplete target coverage or severe toxicity (e.g., radiation-induced blindness, retinopathy and neuropathy, dry syndrome) [19]. IMRT and VMAT, allowing steep dose gradients close to the target, turned out to be effective methods to optimize treatment planning of ACC and to deliver higher doses to the targets while minimizing the doses to the organs at risk [52–55]. Furthermore, the IMRT technique allows the simultaneous delivery of different dose levels to different target volumes within a single treatment fraction by using the "simultaneous integrated boost technique" or "SIB-IMRT" [56].

Target volume definition and RT dose distribution with postoperative VMAT in a case of ACC of submandibular gland are shown in Fig. 11.1.

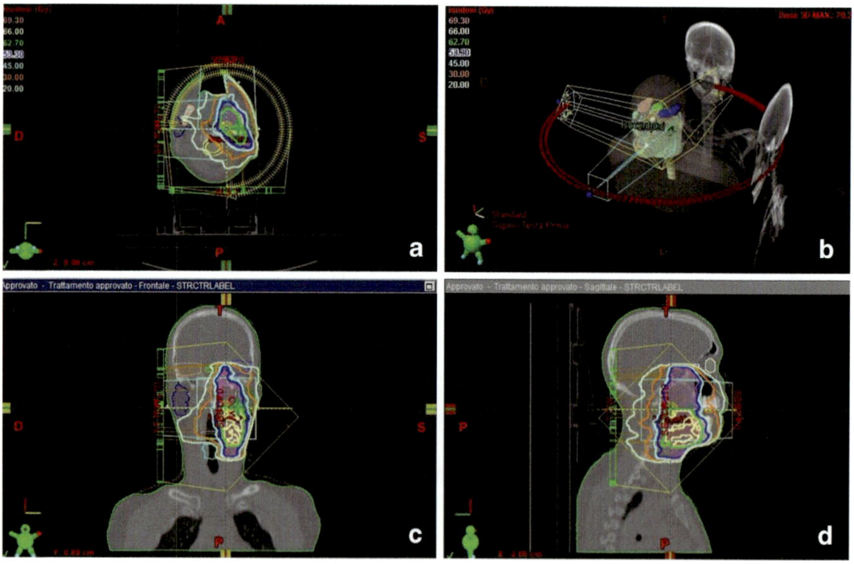

Fig. 11.1 ACC of the left submandibular gland (stage pT2R1, PNI, N0): treatment planning for postoperative VMAT 66 Gy. Figures (**a**, **c**, **d**) show axial, coronal, and sagittal, respectively, computed tomography (CT) simulation images. High-risk planning target volume (PTV) (66 Gy), in red, includes the surgical bed with wide margin along cranial direction due to the presence of R1; low-risk PTV (56.1 Gy) includes HR-PTV with margin and skull base up to the emergency of V cranial nerve. A three-dimensional view of VMAT plan with arches is reported in (**b**)

In the definitive non-operative setting, i.e., unresectable or inoperable cases, treatment volumes follow similar principles, but the total dose is usually carried to 70 Gy in 35 fractions to macroscopic disease, i.e., the high-risk volume [41, 57].

11.3 High-Grade Non-adenoid Cystic Carcinoma (Non-ACC)

11.3.1 Indications and Role of Postoperative Radiotherapy

Surgery is the preferred up-front treatment for high-grade non-ACC. The aim of surgery is complete excision of the tumor along with adequate margins, and incomplete gross tumor resection (R2) should be always avoided.

Whether radiotherapy should be considered for *all* as opposed to *selected* patients after resection is debated. Even if the (beneficial) role of PORT is supported only from retrospective studies, almost all studies consistently show an advantage mostly in terms of locoregional control (LRC) by adding PORT to surgery [38, 57–61]. One area of debate is represented by completely resected (R0) stage I (–II) disease without other risk factors, where some authors recommend observation rather than postoperative RT. For major SGTs, stage I would include T1N0 lesions or those confined to the parenchymal gland up to 2 cm in greatest dimension. In the matched pair analysis from Memorial Sloan Kettering Cancer Center, no benefit was found for PORT in stage I–II disease after complete resection [38]. In the Dutch series, completely resected T1–T2 lesions showed a 95% long-term control rate [57]. However, most authors would still support the adjunct of RT after R0 surgery for *all* high-grade lesions regardless of the stage.

There is little doubt that PORT is indicated for patients with extraglandular extension (T3–T4 tumors), incomplete or close resection, bone invasion, perineural invasion, and pathologically involved lymph nodes (pN+) [57].

Another issue is whether a "planned" R1 resection (a resection that ends up in microscopically positive margins) is acceptable under specific circumstances or surgery should always aim at achieving negative margins. This may happen when the tumor is close to the facial nerve, and thus complete resection with a margin would imply the sacrifice of the nerve. According to the experience of Shah et al. [62] at a median follow-up of 5 years, only 2 local failures were observed in a series of 50 parotid cancers operated mostly (82%) to close or positive margins and irradiated afterward up to 60 Gy. While the authors conclude that "facial nerve-sparing surgery" followed by RT (60 Gy) results in good LRC rates, it should be noted that only 20% of the patients in their series had high-grade tumors. Moreover, another 20% of local failures are to be expected with a longer follow-up [63]. PORT improves LC over surgery alone after R1 resection, but R1 resection remains a poor predictor of LC despite PORT [64]. Therefore, both the risk and amount of R1 resection should be minimized. Regarding facial nerve, if it is directly infiltrated and not functional, it should be sacrificed. However, if the nerve is functioning and not directly infiltrated, most authors would agree that conservative surgery ("tumor peel off") followed by PORT to 60–66 Gy is an acceptable strategy even if it may be associated with a slight increase in the risk of local failure.

Basically, all high-grade non-ACC are associated with a high risk of occult nodal spread. Squamous cell carcinoma, undifferentiated carcinoma, adenocarcinoma, and high-grade MEC have a remarkable (>30%) risk of occult nodal spread [59]. Besides pathology, another predictor of nodal spread is primary tumor stage [36, 65–68], while tumor location is somewhat controversial [57, 63]. Parotid tumors with facial paralysis are associated with a high percentage of occult lymph node metastases as well [69, 70]. ENI is highly effective to prevent regional failure [36]: 10-year regional control rates in cN0 patients treated without and with ENI between 1960 and 2004 at UCSF were 74% and 100%, respectively, $p = 0.0001$. Therefore, ENI is a reasonable alternative to neck dissection. The choice between ENI and surgery is related to the overall treatment strategy (including the treatment of the primary disease) and the benefits (if any) of surgical staging. One may argue that in case of a small (cT1N0) major SGT, a complete resection of the primary to negative margins (pT1, R0) along with pathological confirmation of negative lymph nodes (pN0) may lead to withhold PORT. In another scenario of a larger primary high-grade non-ACC for which the indication to PORT can be anticipated, the elective surgical treatment of the neck may be withheld provided that the neck is properly imaged and staged.

As previously mentioned, data on the outcome of high-grade non-ACC after combined therapy come from retrospective studies. Unfortunately, such retrospective series often include low-grade tumors and/or ACC as well. For instance, in the Dutch Head and Neck Oncology Cooperative Group report on 498 patients treated with surgery with ($N = 386$) or without ($N = 112$) PORT between 1984 and 1995, it is impossible to tease out the amount/percentage of patients with high- versus low-grade tumors (and thus their respective outcome) [57]. Anyhow, at a mean follow-up of 76 months, actuarial 5-year LC rate is 84% for surgery alone and 94% for combined surgery and RT ($p < 0.0005$). Independent prognostic factors for LC were treatment, with a relative risk for surgery alone compared with combined treatment, clinical tumor size, tumor location, status of the resection margins, and bone invasion [57]. A very similar outcome (5-year LRC: 89%) was reported in a subsequent group of patients treated for parotid carcinoma in Rotterdam between 1995 and 2010 [71]. Interestingly, in this series, more locoregional failures were reported in patients with squamous cell and high-grade MEC (21% and 19%, respectively) than in patients with other histological types ($p = 0.04$) and more distant metastases in patients with ACC and adenocarcinoma (20% and 19%, respectively) than in patients with other types ($p = 0.03$). Finally, in this analysis, more distant than locoregional failures were observed [71]. It should be noted that while most of failures occur within 5 years from initial surgery, another ≈10% and ≈20% of patients develop disease recurrence at 10 and 15 years, respectively, mostly at distant sites [36].

In the experience of the Danish Head and Neck Cancer Group (DAHANCA), out of 871 patients diagnosed with SGT between 1990 and 2005, 425 patients (49%) received a combination surgery and RT, while 350 (40%) were treated with surgery alone. Indications for PORT were incomplete tumor resection, perineural extension, high disease stages, lymph nodes with extracapsular spread, and high-grade tumors.

High-risk pathology included ACC, SCC, carcinoma ex pleomorphic adenoma, G2/3 adenocarcinoma, and G3 MEC. Another major difference to current standards is that the neck was rarely addressed electively. At a median follow-up of 78 months, 334 patients (38%) experienced recurrence. Interestingly, 23% of patients developed locoregional recurrence only (15% primary, 3% nodal, and 5% both), while 8% had also distant metastases and 8% developed only distant disease. In multivariable analysis, stage III/IV, lymphovascular invasion, involved or close microscopic margins, and high-risk pathology were all prognostic factors for both recurrence-free and overall survival. Unfortunately, the treatment approach (surgery vs combined surgery and radiotherapy) was not tested in the model [72].

In the recently published experience by the Princess Margaret Hospital, carcinomas of the major salivary glands treated with surgery and PORT between 2000 and 2012 were analyzed. High-risk pathology was defined, on central review, according to both histologic grade and WHO histologic subtype criteria, and included ACC, salivary duct carcinoma, squamous cell carcinoma, G2/3 adenocarcinoma, G2/3 MEC, G2/3 carcinoma ex pleomorphic adenoma, carcinosarcoma, undifferentiated (small-cell, large-cell, or lymphoepithelial) carcinoma, and G3 of other histologic subtypes. Out of a total of 304 eligible patients, 190 (62.5%) had high-risk pathology, including 55 patients with ACC. About 60% of the patients were treated with IMRT and the remaining ones with 3D CRT. At a median follow-up of 82 months, the estimated 5-(10-)year LC, RC, and DC were 96% (96%), 95% (94%), and 80% (77%), respectively. Only 13 patients developed local failure (LF); among these cases, 11 (85%) had positive resection margins ($p = 0.02$), and 10 (77%) had lymphovascular invasion ($p = 0.01$). During follow-up, diagnosis of DM was the most frequently observed treatment failure ($n = 62$) with a median DM-free interval of 21 months (range, 5–141); 74% (46/62) DM failures were with isolated DM [73].

Few studies focused on selected pathology types only. Resected MEC of the parotid gland treated with adjuvant radiotherapy for high-risk features was the topic of the paper of Chen et al. [74]. At multivariable analysis on 61 patients, high tumor grade (hazard ratio = 7.92) and T4 disease (HR = 3.35) were found to be independent predictors of decreased survival, with the former also predicting for distant metastasis and the latter predicting for local-regional recurrence. At a median follow-up of 45 months, the 5-year estimate of overall survival was 83% for patients with non-high-grade tumors, compared to 52% for those with high-grade histology ($p = 0.001$). In a similar paper by MDACC on 145 patients with MEC of the salivary glands treated primarily with surgery and (60%) PORT, grade and stage confirmed to be the major determinants of overall survival [75]. Patients with T3–4 and high-grade disease had a only 10% chance of long-term survival [75].

A couple of papers focused on carcinoma ex pleomorphic adenoma (CXPA) of the parotid gland that is a relatively rare malignancy that, as implied by its name, is believed to evolve from a preexisting benign adenoma [76]. In the first one [77], the authors retrospectively compared the outcome of high-grade tumors of the parotid gland (21 CPXA and 52 non-CXPA). Despite having similar stage of cancer and extent of surgical resection, patients with CXPA had a lower disease-specific survival compared to non-CXPA high-grade primary parotid cancer ($p = 0.02$). CXPA of the parotid gland seems a more aggressive cancer compared to non-CXPA high-grade primary parotid cancer. In the second one [76], 63 patients were treated with definitive surgery for carcinoma CXPA of the parotid gland, of whom 40 patients (63%) received also PORT to a median dose of 60 Gy (range, 45–71 Gy). Adenocarcinoma (29 patients), salivary duct carcinoma (16 patients), and ACC (9 patients) were the most common malignant subtypes. At a median follow-up of 50 months (range, 2–96 months), the use of PORT significantly improved 5-year LC from 49% to 75% ($p = 0.005$). At multivariate analysis, pathologic involvement of cervical lymph nodes was the only independent predictor of overall survival. In conclusion, surgery followed by PORT should be considered the standard of care for patients with carcinoma CXPA, which is an aggressive neoplasm.

11.3.2 Definitive RT

High-grade non-ACC includes a heterogeneous group of primary tumors that share the feature of being considered not particularly sensitive to ionizing radiations. Therefore, definitive RT is not considered an alternative to up-front resections and is usually reserved for unresectable lesions, for inoperable patients, and for those who refuse surgery. Definitive radiotherapy with photons has been associated in the past with dismal results. Two-dimensional photon-based RT was the control arm of a RTOG-MRC randomized study testing neutron therapy in inoperable or unresectable malignant SGTs [78]. The study was discontinued after enrollment of only 32 patients of which 25 were evaluable. Patients had remarkable advanced disease; median primary tumor size was 6 cm (range, 3–16 cm), and 1/3 of patients had clinically positive nodes. Moreover, pathology was not stratified by arms. As expected, at 10 years, the LRC in the control photon arm was only 17% [78]. Long-term LRC rates around 25% have been reported by others [79, 80].

In other series, 5-year LRC rates with photons have been reported around 50% [46, 57, 81], perhaps due to the higher dose of RT delivered (66–70 Gy). At UCSF, 45 patients with newly diagnosed SGTs were treated with definitive radiation to a median dose of 66 Gy (range, 57–74 Gy) between 1960 and 2004. Indications for primary radiation treatment were as follows: 17 surgically unresectable (38%), 13 with gross residual disease after subtotal resection or open biopsy (29%), 12 medically inoperable (27%), and 3 refusal of surgery (7%). The median tumor size, as determined by physical examination or radiographic imaging (or both), measured 3.4 cm (range, 1.2–9.2 cm) with six patients having tumors in excess of 7 cm. None of the patients had clinical or pathologic evidence of regional lymph node disease at the time of presentation, and only two patients received chemotherapy in addition to RT. The series includes both low- and high-grade SGTs. At a median follow-up of 101 months (range, 3–285 months), the 5-year and 10-year rate estimates of LC were 70% and 57%, respectively. A Cox proportional hazard model identified T3–4 disease ($p = 0.004$) and radiation dose lower than 66 Gy ($p < 0.001$) as independent predictors of local recurrence [46].

Results of contemporary photon-based series employing modern techniques (3D-CRT, IMRT, SBRT) are even better. From 1990 to 2009, 27 patients with unresectable SGC (63%, with HG tumors) underwent definitive photon radiotherapy at MSKCC. Nodal involvement was found in nine patients. Median primary tumor size was 5 cm (range, 3–12 cm). Median dose of radiotherapy was 70 Gy, with 9 patients receiving IMRT and 18 3D-CRT. Chemotherapy was given to 18 patients, most being platinum-based regimens. With a median follow-up of 52.4 months, the 5-year actuarial LC was 55% (±24.2%). High grade was significant for an increased rate of DM (intermediate grade vs low grade, $p = 0.04$, HR 7.93; high grade vs low grade, $p = 0.01$, HR 13.50) [82]. Karam et al. have reported encouraging results on a selected group of patients treated with hypofractionated SBRT boost [83].

In conclusion, surgery remains the treatment of choice for patients with HG non-ACC. For patients who have unresectable disease, are inoperable, or simply refuse surgery, definitive radiotherapy may offer a chance of cure. In this setting, heavy particles are usually preferred, but in their absence, photon-based IMRT may be a reasonable option as well.

11.3.3 Target Volumes, Doses, and Technique

In the postoperative setting, the tumor and involved lymph node bed constitute the target volume at intermediate risk. Electively treated uninvolved nodal regions represent the target volume at lower risk. Within a simultaneous integrated boost plan in 30 fractions, the former is usually planned to receive 60 Gy while the latter 54–56 Gy [73].

Regarding the intermediate-risk volume, preoperative imaging and examination findings, operative notes, and pathology findings should guide contouring to ensure that all areas originally involved by disease are targeted. For patients with partial removal of the involved gland (i.e., superficial parotidectomy), the whole remaining gland (i.e., the deep lobe of the gland) is part of the intermediate-risk target volume.

Another area of possible concern is the skull base, in the presence of "named" nerve perineural invasion, though this is more common for ACCs.

Regarding the nodal stations at risk of subclinical disease (low-risk volume), ipsilateral cervical lymph nodes are routinely targeted either with surgery or RT as previously discussed. Elective nodal irradiation to a dose of 54 Gy (in 30 fractions) is usually reserved for patients without clinical or pathologic lymph node involvement, while the areas originally involved and those with extracapsular extension are planned to receive 60 Gy and 64–66 Gy, respectively, in 30 fractions. The nodal regions to target depend on the location of the primary tumor and the nodal levels macroscopically involved. Periparotid and ipsilateral lymph nodes (level II) are most frequently involved in the tumors of parotid gland, although skip metastases to level III have been observed. In one study, for patients with three or fewer positive nodes at neck dissection, level IV and level V were positive in less than 10% of the cases [36, 59]. Therefore, in elective treatment of the neck, at least levels I, II, and III should be included [36, 65], while levels IV and V can be omitted in the cN0 neck. Level Ib nodes should be included when level II is involved, and levels IV and V nodes should be targeted when levels II and III are involved [36]. Submandibular gland cancers typically spread to levels I–III. Minor salivary gland cancers in the head and neck region can often be midline and may necessitate bilateral lymph node irradiation. Treatment of the contralateral neck should also be considered for patients who have multiple ipsilateral lymph nodes involved. In one recent paper on patients with resected major SGTs treated with PORT, regional failure occurred in 3 (2%) out of 171 patients treated with IMRT; interestingly, all patients failed outside the low-risk volume: ipsilateral level VI b ($N = 1$), ipsilateral level V ($N = 1$), and contralateral level V ($N = 1$) [73]. Other studies suggest that elective treatment of the neck is at least as effective as surgery in controlling subclinical disease [36].

Sometimes a third volume at higher risk is identified (CTC high risk). The Dutch study supports a higher than 60 Gy volume for incompletely resected regions [57]. This volume typically receives an additional boost of 6–10 Gy to areas considered at higher risk of microscopic/R1 disease, such as those corresponding to positive margins and extracapsular tumor extension. The boost is usually achieved by a simultaneous integrated boost to the nominal dose of 64–66 Gy in 30 fractions.

Treatment should start as soon as possible after surgery and possibly not longer than 6–8 weeks from surgery, though clinical evidence is controversial [57, 84].

Target volume definition and RT dose distribution with postoperative VMAT in a case of high-grade MEC of the parotid gland are shown in Fig. 11.2.

In the definitive non-operative setting, treatment volumes follow similar principles, but the total dose is usually carried to 70 Gy in 35 fractions to the gross tumor volume [57]. Wang et al. reported LC as high as 85% with accelerated hyperfractionated photon therapy. The follow-up was rather short, and the results have not been updated [85]. Regarding the technique, IMRT may help to limit both acute and late toxicity rates [86] besides the possibility to paint the dose to the various targets.

11.4 Toxicity

Radiation-induced side effects are the same observed in head and neck district. They can be acute (i.e., mucositis, xerostomia, loss of taste, dysphagia) or late (i.e., osteoradionecrosis, neck fibrosis, trismus), these latter in particular when cancer arises from major salivary gland. Previous surgery limits the amount of radiation dose prescribed and may increase the risk of late toxicity.

Garden et al. [84] reported complications of irradiation in 51 out of 160 patients receiving PORT for minor SGTs. The most relevant were decreased hearing, radiation-induced injury to the visual pathway, and bone necrosis or exposure. However, these complications have been hardly ever seen during the last decades with improved radiation therapy techniques [84].

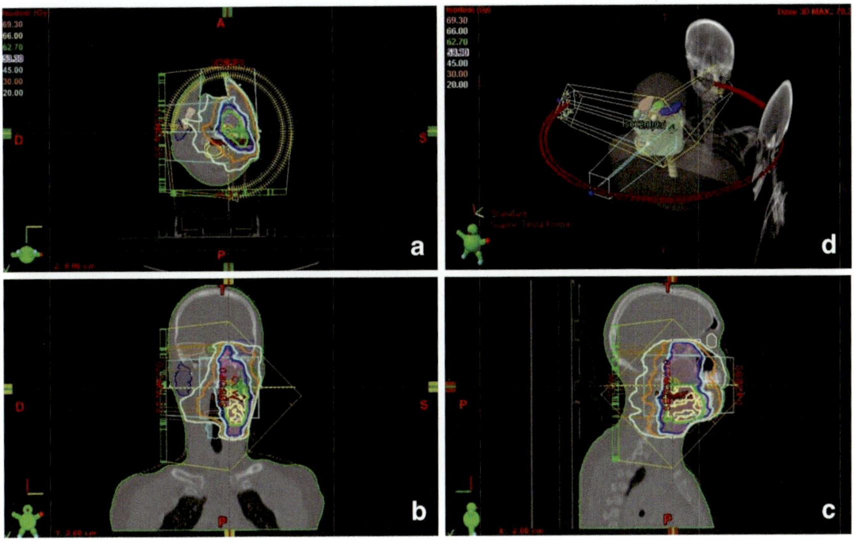

Fig. 11.2 High-grade MEC of the left parotid gland, stage pT4a R1 (multiple surgical positive margins), PNI, and N2b. This is a treatment plan for a postoperative RT VMAT dose 70 Gy. Pictures show axial (**a**), coronal (**b**), and sagittal (**c**) computed tomography simulation images. High-risk planning target volume (PTV) (70 Gy), in red, includes the surgical bed with wide margin along cranial direction due to the presence of R1; intermediate-risk PTV (60 Gy) includes HR-PTV all ipsilateral neck and skull base up to the emergency of VII cranial nerve; low-risk PTV (54 Gy) includes HR-PTV, IR-PTV, and the right neck. Figure (**d**) shows a three-dimensional view of PTVs and neurological organs at risk (OARS) eye (light green), left eye (yellow); left optic nerve (white) optic chiasm (lilac); brainstem (green)

In a series of patients treated after 2000 with either postoperative 3D-CRT or IMRT after a median follow-up of 82 months, the 5- and 10-year cumulative incidence of RTOG grade 3 late toxicity was both 3%. No grade 4 or 5 was reported [73]. In another study, the cumulative incidence of grade 2 toxicity at 5 years after surgery and PORT was 8% [71]. Concomitant chemotherapy may enhance the intensity of side effects. Therefore, nowadays, most of the patients develop minimal effects.

11.5 Reirradiation

There are no randomized trials or prospective studies specifically on reirradiation of SGTs. It can be assumed that most of the general considerations and recommendations may apply to recurrent SGTs. Retreatment usually involves additional surgery, if feasible, and PORT. In certain histological subtypes (e.g., ACC), retreatment of locally recurrent disease yields prolonged survival [49]. Reirradiation must always be considered for local recurrences not amenable to surgical therapy, and in ACC reirradiation should be taken into account even in the presence of distant metastasis.

Several photon techniques, such as IMRT, stereotactic RT, CyberKnife, and Gamma Knife radiosurgery, have been used with promising results in terms of acute and late toxicity [87–89]. Lee et al. reported on eight patients with skull base recurrences who underwent Gamma Knife radiosurgery. All patients experienced symptomatic response, usually pain resolution. The median local free from local progression and survival were 15.4 and 21.2 months, respectively [87]. In a paper by Karam, 18 patients diagnosed with recurrent, previously irradiated, SGTs were treated with SBRT reirradiation (CyberKnife) with a median dose of 30 Gy given in 5 fractions with a median cumulative dose of 91.1 Gy. The 2-year OS and LRC rates were 39% and 53%, respectively. However, long-term toxicity analysis revealed four patients in the reirradiated group with soft tissue necrosis, correlated with the cumulative dose [89].

11.6 Chemoradiotherapy (CRT)

There is no convincing evidence on the efficacy of CT in treating SGT patients with curative intent, both in postoperative and radical setting. Amini et al. retrospectively reviewed 2210 patients with resected major SGTs using data from the National Cancer Database. They found that OS was significantly inferior with adjuvant CRT ($n = 368$) compared with RT alone ($n = 1842$) ($p = 0.02$), and patients treated with multiagent chemotherapy appeared to have a worse OS, compared with single-agent chemotherapy ($P = 0.03$) [90]. In a paper by Mifsud, outcome of patients treated from 1998 to 2013 with postoperative CRT (37 patients) or RT (103 patients) was analyzed. A multivariate analysis showed a trend toward a benefit in PFS from CRT, but it was not statistically significant [91].

Therefore, the RTOG is conducting a phase II randomized trial (RTOG 1008) to explore the utility of a platinum-based adjuvant CRT in high-risk patients. High-risk factors are the following: histological types as salivary duct carcinoma, grade 2/3 MEC, grade 2/3 adenocarcinoma, grade 3 ACC, and grade 3 acinic cell carcinoma, pathologic stage III–IVB, and positive/close surgical margins [47]. Until the results of this trial will be available, the standard use of CRT for advanced SGTs is not recommended.

11.7 Low-Grade Non-adenoid Cystic Carcinoma (Non-ACC)

11.7.1 Radiotherapy: General Considerations

Low-grade (LG) SGTs are a constellation of different histologies [4]. While certain papers report on LGSGTs combining different histologic types, others are focused on specific subtypes (see the following sections).

Among the former, Walvekar et al. compared 34 patients with low-risk histology and grade, negative margins, and no ECE with 18 patients with low-risk histology and grade but with ECE and positive margins. Inclusion of ECE and margin status substantially improved the prediction of disease recurrence, supporting PORT for low-risk histologies with positive margins or ECS [92]. Richter et al. reported on a small series of 17 T1–3 patients operated for low-/intermediate-grade MEC and acinic cell carcinomas of the parotid with only one negative factor, close (≤5 mm) or positive margins. They coded as patients with positive margin also the cases in which the tumor was "peeled" off the VII nerve [93]. The operative (parotid) bed was treated with a modest margin; the neck was included in a few cases (policy no longer followed). Sixteen patients were treated with a wedged-pair technique or three-dimensional conformal radiation therapy (3DRT) using 6 mV photons, and one patient received 6 mV photons and 20 MeV electrons using a mixed-beam approach. The range of doses to the parotid was 45–66 Gy, with a median dose of 63 Gy mostly with daily fractions of 1.8–2 Gy; no disease failures were reported and acute and late toxicity were minimal [93].

Recently, Jae-Keun et al. from Korea reviewed the outcome of 179 LGSGTs. Various histologies were included, mainly LG MEC, ACC without solid component (tubular or cribriform subtypes), acinic cell carcinoma, and LG adenocarcinoma [94]. During the study period, radiation techniques were mainly 3D-CRT ($N = 98$) and IMRT ($N = 27$), with a median dose of nearly 60 Gy (range 50–66) by 1.8 or 2.0 Gy per fraction over 5.5–6 weeks. Recurrence-free survival (RFS) was chosen as primary endpoint because there were only two disease-specific deaths in their series. Nodal status (N1–3 vs N0) had significant impact on RFS (univariate and multivariate analysis). RFS was worse for patients with pathological risk factors, lymphovascular invasion being the strongest determinant (it was significant at univariate analysis). Only the presence of cancer cells at the margin of resection and not close margins (<5 mm) was significantly detrimental to RFS both at univariate and multivariate analyses. Contrary to common beliefs, less than total resection was equivalent to total resection (provided resection margins were not positive) [94].

Finally, the addition of PORT was highly significant in multivariate analysis in terms of improved RFS. They compared patients with N0 and negative pathological risk factors with patients with positive node/pathological risk factors. Results were equivalent in the first group with or without PORT, while in high-risk group among 13 patients without PORT, 6 experienced recurrence (46.2%; $p = 0.001$) versus 6.8% of the irradiated patients [94].

In conclusion, they stated that advanced T stage, nodal status, and pathological risk factors (positive margins, PNI and lymphovascular invasion, extraparenchymal extension) are an indication to PORT [94].

Therefore, PORT may be indicated in a substantial proportion of LGSGTs: actually, in the Jae-Keun series, only 10% of the patients had positive node, but approximately 50% of the patients had pathological risk factors [94].

11.7.2 Radiotherapy for LG and Intermediate-Grade (IG) MEC

Several grading systems have been reported for salivary MEC: AFIP, Brandwein, and Healey grading systems, all include LG (low-grade), IG (intermediate-grade), and HG (high-grade) MEC [95]. Not all authors report an IG group [96], but most studies have suggested that there is no statistically significant difference between patients with LG and IG MEC in OS or DFS [97–101].

The role of adjuvant radiation therapy for patients with MEC of the parotid gland is based on data from institution reviews and lacks data from randomized controlled trials.

However, in the Liu study, the LG tumors showed better survival outcomes compared to patients with IG tumors for whom a significantly worse outcome was found [102]. Furthermore, in the Mc Hugh series, IG MEC had more local, regional (nodal), and distant relapse vs LG MEC (8%, 4.4%, and 4.4% vs 0%) in spite of similar OS and DFS [99]. IG has more often aggressive features (such as positive or close surgical margins, perineural or lymphovascular invasion, and extraglandular extension) [98, 99]. This probably explains why, e.g., in the Chen study, PORT was applied in 25% of the LG cases, 37.2% of the IG, and 79.9% of the HG cases in MEC [101]. Finally, Ozawa et al. combined IG tumors with HG tumors in assessing OS and DFS [103].

The criteria for PORT in MEC (all grades) include multiple factors: patients with HG lesions, stage III/IV lesions, positive lymph node status, positive margins, incompletely excised tumors, perineural/lymphovascular invasion, extraglandular extension, and tumors of the deep lobe of the parotid [97, 99, 102]. Also the primary site (major vs minor salivary glands), age (>60 years), positive margins, tumor size (>2.5 cm), pattern of invasion (broad-pushing borders vs infiltrative permeation), and length of time that the tumor was present have been shown to be associated with prognosis in MEC [104].

Specific indications to PORT for LG/IG MEC can be found in few papers: 14 LG lesions had PORT in the series by Guzzo et al. due to microscopic residual and/or advanced stage [96] and 1 LG patient in another series because of close surgical margins [105]. Rapidis reported 6 cases with PORT; 3 out of 4 IG had positive margins [98]. In the largest available series of the 30 patients with LG tumors, 12 (41.4%) underwent PORT due to evidence of positive or close margins in 9 patients and PNI in 3 patients [99]. Advanced stage may represent an indication to PORT as well [99].

Finally, Olsen reported on two cases of LG MEC treated with PORT for positive surgical margins and PNI [106].

In summary, although evidences are weak, PORT may be considered in selected LG/IG patients that have a high risk of recurrence [99].

According to the update 2003 of the "Standards, Options, and Recommendations" (SOR) project, for completely resected patients, PORT should not be used in case of LG stage I and II tumors but should be used for LG stage III and IV tumors. For patients with incomplete macroscopic or microscopic residual disease, PORT must be delivered [107]. As for minor salivary glands, Vander Poorten [108] reported that most minor SGTs were treated with surgery and PORT, with the exception of completely resected LG, low-stage MEC, and well-resected PLGA [109]. Mean doses delivered in PORT range around 60 Gy in conventional fractionation ranging from 40 to 66 Gy [97, 98, 102, 105, 106]. According to Hosokawa, 5-year LC was worse with a dose lower than 55 Gy for patients with positive margins; however, the fraction of LG/IG cases in this subset analysis was not available [97].

The treatment volume includes generally the operative bed alone. Elective ND should be avoided in LG or IG tumors [95]. Actually, cervical lymph node metastases from MEC have been reported in tumors of all sites and grades, although lymphatic spread is considered overall very rare event for LG MEC, with a range reported between 0% and 2.5% [104]. Chen et al. reported a percentage of 3.3% of positive nodes at the levels I–III for LG tumors and 8.1 % for IG. Involvement of levels IV–V was more uncommon (0.4–0.6%). All patients with LG and IG MEC with positive lymph nodes in levels IV to V also had positive lymph nodes in levels I to III [101].

11.7.3 Radiotherapy for Acinic Cell Carcinoma

Acinic cell carcinoma (AciCC) is an uncommon low-grade (LG) malignant epithelial salivary gland cancer. Patients with well and moderately differentiated disease exhibited 20-year survivals of 97.79% and 83.33%, respectively, but despite being a predominantly LG cancer, it may have an aggressive behavior developing nodal and distant metastases, even many years after the initial diagnosis and treatment [108].

AciCC more often arise in parotid glands. Other sites, such as sinonasal cavities, are definitely less frequent [110]. Primary site may have an influence on survival. Biron et al., who compared patients with parotid AciCC to a matched cohort of AciCC of sinonasal cavities, found a higher 10-year OS for parotid tumor in comparison with paranasal sinus lesions (100% vs 52.3%); DFS was also higher, although not significantly different [110].

Primary radiotherapy should be restricted to patients not suitable for surgery or refusing surgery because AciCC is considered not particularly radiosensitive [111].

PORT is not frequently used in AciCC. Spafford et al. in 1991 proposed a series of indications for PORT in AciCC: recurrent tumor; equivocal or positive margins, or evidence of tumor spillage; tumor adjacent to the facial nerve; deep lobe involvement; lymph node metastases; extra-parotid extension PNI; and large tumors (e.g., greater than 4 cm) [112–114]. A total of 1241 cases of parotid AciCC in the Surveillance, Epidemiology, and End Results (SEER) Program database from 1988 to 2007 were identified and analyzed by Andreoli et al. [115]. Comparison groups were surgery and surgery plus RT. When comparing surgery alone with surgery plus RT, there was no statistical difference in OS when stratifying for stage. Similarly, adjuvant RT did not demonstrate a survival advantage when stratified by histologic grade of tumor. The authors concluded that PORT does not confer a survival advantage in low-grade and early-stage tumors and that RT can be spared for these patients, although the highest-grade and highest-stage tumors were fewer in number in this series. The most important limitation of this study is the lack of recurrence data available in the SEER database, which precludes the analysis of disease-free survival or local disease control. Similarly, surgical margin status is a key variable often used to determine the need for PORT, but this information was unavailable for these patients [115].

In the small study by Liu, no difference in survival rate was observed between 29 patients with surgery alone and 8 patients treated with surgery and adjuvant radiation. Patients older than 60 years with a fixed mass, high-grade tumor and nodal stage, perineural invasion, and angiolymphatic invasion had adverse OS and DFS ($P < 0.05$) [114].

Biron et al. [116] identified 2061 patients with AciCC 1973–2009 in the SEER database, although clinical information were available for 614 patients. Eighty-seven percent were grade I or II. Patients who received surgery alone had the highest 20-year DSS (92.4%), followed by those treated with surgery and RT (71.9%) or RT alone (62.3%).

This difference between treatment modality could not be accounted for by differences in grade, stage, sex, subsites, or other factors correlated with survival.

These data are difficult to interpret given that the basis for the decision to give adjuvant radiation therapy is unknown (e.g., the presence of positive margins). Authors concluded that despite the limitations in interpreting these data, histologic grade is a stronger predictor of survival than TNM classification [116].

According to Vander Poorten et al., caution should be, however, exerted as the SEER analysis does not correct for involved resection margins or initially inadequate treatment, which accounts for a substantial part of AciCC patients. Even after a "rough" correction for stage and grade, significant selection and information bias is still likely present in the retrospective SEER data [117].

11.7.4 Radiotherapy for Polymorphous Low-Grade Adenocarcinoma (PLGA)

The role of PORT in PLGA has not been proven so far.

Evidence for PORT is considered weak [118] due to the rarity of this tumor and its long natural history (requiring a long follow-up to establish the recurrence potential).

No relapse was reported in the review of Uemaetomari et al. [119] in cases of negative surgical margins. However, wide resections with clear margins of the parotid gland might be difficult to obtain without the sacrifice of the facial nerve in certain cases. Only one relapse (at 11 years) was reported in seven cases who underwent PORT, showing that PORT may have a role in selected cases of this indolent and slow-growing disease.

Verma et al. [120] suggest to refer patients with positive margins for PORT. PNI is not reported by the authors as a significant adverse prognostic factor for PLGA and is not considered a reason to administer PORT in patients with negative margins. Recommended RT doses are 66 Gy/33 fractions for microscopic residual disease and 70 Gy/35 fractions for gross residual disease [120].

From a literature search, Kimple et al. [121] reported that rates of recurrence after surgical excision without adjuvant radiation were 24.4% compared to 26.1% for surgical excision with adjuvant radiation therapy. However no information was available on selection criteria for PORT. The SEER database was queried for

HN-PLGA cases from 2001 to 2011 (460 cases) by Patel et al. [122]. Ten-year OS and disease-specific survival (DSS) were not significantly different for surgery alone and surgery plus PORT [122]. In a small group of patients treated with RT alone, DSS was 75%. Information were available only for 6 out of 11 patients; they were older and with advanced stage disease [122].

11.7.5 Radiotherapy for Epithelial-Myoepithelial Carcinoma

The SEER database (1973–2010) was queried for epithelial-myoepithelial carcinoma of the major salivary glands [123]. PORT was of no benefit, in terms of DSS, as compared to surgery alone in early stages (I–II); DSS was better after surgery plus RT vs surgery alone but not statistically significant in advanced stages (III–IV). However, stage was defined only in 93 out of 246 cases, and tumor size served as a proxy for clinical stage (tumor size of >4 cm had significant impact on survival). Furthermore, grading and margin status were not taken into account [123].

Therefore, no firm statement can be drawn on PORT indications.

11.7.6 Radiotherapy for Low-Grade Adenocarcinoma

A series of 51 patients with adenocarcinoma of the salivary gland, including 8 LG cases (unfortunately 15 patients had unknown grade), was reviewed [124].

Indications for PORT in low- to intermediate-risk adenocarcinoma of the salivary glands were aggressive features such as positive or close margins, PNI, angiolymphatic invasion, extensive extraglandular extension, or multiple lymph node involvement. Seventy-five percent and 62.5% of patients with IG and LG disease underwent PORT, respectively.

In general, treatment protocol at the authors' institution is to treat low- to intermediate-risk disease with surgery followed by radiation if aggressive features are determined. Although this treatment protocol is intuitive, adjuvant radiotherapy did not demonstrate a significant survival benefit; however, patients who received adjuvant therapy did reveal a trend toward better OS [124].

11.8 Benign Tumors: Pleomorphic Adenoma

11.8.1 Indications and Role of PORT

Pleomorphic adenomas account for 70–80% of benign SGTs and are especially common in the parotid gland [125].

Evidences of the role of PORT in pleomorphic adenoma after surgery come from various retrospective studies on institutional small series reporting on patients with primary disease [80, 126–129], recurrent disease [80, 130–136], or mixed cases [137, 138] and from a few review articles on the topic [139–143].

In Table 11.2 indications to RT, settings (primary treatment, recurrent tumor), treatments (surgery, surgery plus PORT), disease control, and follow-up duration are reported.

Primary RT is anecdotal; gross tumor is not irradiated primarily unless it is absolutely unresectable, since LC is relatively low in large tumor [138, 141].

Indications to PORT are controversial. Incomplete removal [128, 132]; gross residual disease [137]; tumor capsule rupture and spill [126, 128, 130, 132]; strict adherence and embedding of facial nerve [126, 132]; close [131], equivocal [137], or positive margins [126, 130, 131, 137]; and multiple [130] and multinodular [131] recurrences, all these features are reported as possible indications to RT after surgery.

The amount of disease left behind is of paramount importance to achieve LC both for primary and recurrent cases treated with surgery and PORT [135, 137, 138]. Hodge et al. analyzed LC in microscopic disease vs gross residual disease: the presence of macroscopic disease decreased LC of 37% [138]. This series was recently updated and a reduction of LC by 18% was observed [137].

The pattern of recurrence (uninodular vs multinodular) has been reported to influence LC after combined treatment as well. Renehan et al. found no difference in LC between surgery alone and surgery + RT for uninodular recurrences, while adjuvant RT improved results as compared to surgery alone for multinodular recurrences: authors concluded that uninodular recurrences per se should not be offered adjuvant RT [133]. In spite of the more aggressive disease pattern, LC for multinodular recurrences can be excellent: Renehan reported a 15-year LC of 96% [133], Leverstein observed recurrence in 16 patients with this pattern, and none developed a further recurrence after surgery plus RT [132].

Few retrospective series compared surgery alone vs surgery + RT. Improved LC for patients treated with adjuvant RT vs surgery alone in case of first treatment was reported by Robertson et al. [126].

Similarly, better LC for adjuvant RT vs surgery alone in recurrent cases was reported in other series [131, 133, 134].

In summary, if long natural history may favor wait and watch policy, the addition of PORT in selected cases can decrease the rate of locoregional recurrence (to less than 5%) and can reduce the chance of repeat surgery and damage to VII nerve [140].

11.8.2 Timing, Technique, Target Volume, and Schedules

Timing of radiotherapy is controversial. Whether to add RT after the first surgery rather after surgery for recurrence is a matter of debate.

Robertson et al. acknowledged the possible role of RT after primary surgery in reducing recurrence rates but emphasized the radio-induced toxicity and warned against delivering routinely RT [126].

On the contrary, Barton et al. stated that "patients having unsatisfactory surgery due to spill or residual tumor should have RT immediately and not delayed until local recurrence occurs because of the increased morbidity and the higher incidence of further recurrence" [128].

Table 11.2 Main characteristics and relative reported outcomes of studies on pleomorphic adenoma included in this chapter

Author	Year	Pri/ rec	N. pts	TMT	FU	% LC	Subsets	Indications to RT
Dawson	1985	Pri	311	S+RT	10 min	92	n.r.	
Dawson	1989	Rec	29	S+RT	8.5 mean	79	n.r.	
Ravasz	1990	Rec	16	S+RT	11 med	94	n.r.	
		Pri	62	S+RT		100	n.r.	
Samson	1991	Rec	21	S+RT	5.9 mean	81		
			17			94	Microscopic tumor	
			4			25	Gross tumor	
Barton	1992	Pri	115	S+RT	14 med	91	n.r.	Incomplete removal, T spill
		Rec	62	S+RT	14 med	87	n.r.	
Liu	1995	Rec	17	S	12.5 med	6	n.r.	
			16	S+RT		82	n.r.	
Renehan	1996	Rec	63	S	14 med	76	n.r.	
			51	S+RT		92	n.r.	
Leverstein	1997	Rec	16	S+RT	8.8 med	100	Multinodular	Embedded FN, incomplete removal, multinodular rec, T spill
Carew	1999	Rec	20	S	7.3 med	71	n.r.	
		Rec	11	S+RT		100	n.r.	Close or positive marg, multiple rec
Hodge	2005	Pri/ Rec	17	RT/ S+RT	9.6 med	61	n.r.	Equivocal or positive marg, gross residual, T spill
			2	RT		0	n.r.	
			10	S+RT		80	Microscopic tumor	
			7	S+RT		43	Gross tumor	
Chen	2006	Rec	34	S+RT	17.4 med	94	n.r.	Multiple rec, positive marg, T spill
Wallace	2013	Pri/ Rec	25	RT/ S+RT	10.5 med	72	n.r.	Equivocal or positive marg, gross residual, [multinodular rec]
			16			75	Subclinical disease	
			9			56	Gross disease	
Patel	2014	Pri	21	S+RT	7.6 med	90	n.r.	Close or positive marg
Robertson	2014	Pri	53	S	6.4 med	79	n.r.	
			25	S+RT		96	n.r.	Positive marg, T capsule rupture, adherence to FN

Abbreviations; *Rec* recurrent tumors, *Pri* primary tumors, *N.pts* number of patients, *TMT* treatment, *S* surgery, *S+RT* surgery plus postoperative radiotherapy, *FU* follow-up, *FN* facial nerve, *rec* recurrences, *T* tumor, *marg* margins, *mean* mean, *med* median

Multiple irradiation techniques have been developed over the years, from the conventional wedged-paired fields to the three-field techniques, 3D-CRT, and more recently IMRT in its various forms. Its highly conformal dose distributions and reduction in doses to the surrounding normal tissues are hoped to translate into a reduction in both acute (skin and mucosal) and late (functional and cosmetic) toxicities [144].

Bolus was routinely placed over the surgical scar by Chen et al. [130]. In the Carew series, more than half of the recurrences had multiple nodules, and in more than 40% of the cases, the recurrence involved the scar of the previous surgical incision, a fact attributed to tumor spillage that may explain the suggestion for bolus application [131].

The treatment volume, in case of parotid origin, must include the operative bed and the whole parotid space [130, 145]. Treatment of the neck in benign adenomas is not recommended [130, 145].

To delineate more accurately the treatment volume, a fusion of the CT CE simulation scan with the preoperative MRI is suggested [145]. A postoperative MRI is similarly helpful, namely, in case of residual disease. In case of multinodular recurrences, all the nodules even the tiniest have to be contoured [145].

As for treatment dose, Patel [127] delivered a median dose of 57.6 Gy (range 55.8–69.96) with fractions of 1.8–2 Gy/die; similarly, Robertson gave 60 Gy in 30 fractions [126].

A dose of 50–60 Gy with a boost of 10–20 Gy in case of gross residual disease is suggested by Jardel et al. [145] with conventional fractionation. In the Wallace [137] series, 17 patients received once-daily external beam RT to a median total dose of 64.8 Gy (range, 56.5–70 Gy) and a median dose per fraction of 1.8 Gy. For Chen the median radiation dose was 50 Gy (range, 45–59.40) with conventional fractionation [130].

Target volume definition and RT dose distribution with postoperative VMAT in a case of recurrent multinodular pleomorphic adenoma of parotid gland are shown in Fig. 11.3.

11.8.3 Toxicity

A first concern when adding PORT is the increase of morbidity [140].

Robertson emphasized the radio-induced toxicities. Of the 25 patients who received PORT, 22 developed complications from RT [126]. The majority were troubled with permanent erythema and skin discoloration (21 cases) at the treatment site. Cases of xerostomia (2 patients), dysphagia (2 patients), temporary hearing loss (1 patient), persisting aural discharge (1 patient), and altered taste (1 patient) were also reported [126].

On the contrary, in the series of Patel, acute morbidity was limited to RTOG grades 1–2, and no patients experienced RTOG grade 2–4 late toxicities [127]. Similarly no patients developed severe complications subsequent to RT in the series by Wallace. Dental caries and transient facial nerve deficits were the most common complications [137].

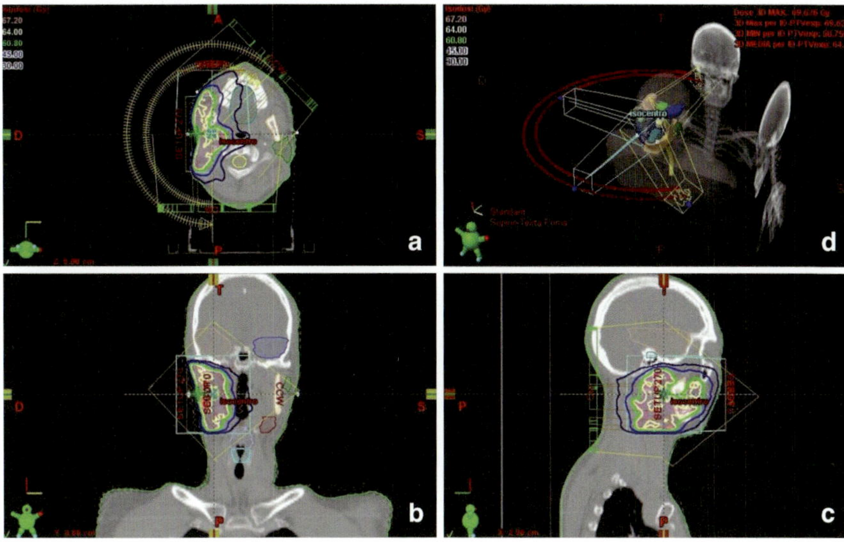

Fig. 11.3 Recurrent multinodular pleomorphic adenoma of the right parotid gland; treatment planning for postoperative VMAT dose 64 Gy. Figures (**a–c**), respectively, show axial (**a**), coronal (**b**), and sagittal (**c**) computed tomography (CT) simulation images. Planning target volume (PTV) (64 Gy), in red, includes the surgical bed with margins. Figure (**d**) shows a three-dimensional view of VMAT plan with arches

A second concern is the risk of radiation induced malignant changes [140], especially in younger patients.

Malignant degeneration into carcinoma ex pleomorphic adenoma occurring in recurrent pleomorphic adenomas is reported in the literature with varying rates (0–16%) [133]. Two cases of malignant change in 25 patients (0.5%) were reported by Wallace [137] and Leverstein series [132], and 1 case out of 62 patients was reported by Barton [128].

Pleomorphic adenomas rarely progress to carcinoma in the absence of previous RT, but it is difficult to say which is the exact contribution of RT. Olsen and Lewis reported on 73 patients treated at the Mayo Clinic (Rochester, MN) for carcinoma ex pleomorphic adenoma, and 70 patients (96%) had no history of prior RT to the site of the tumor [128].

Fourteen patients were observed at the Christie with three or more recurrences in the parotid gland; in 3 out of 14 cases (0.42%), carcinomatous changes were noted [133]. Previous RT was delivered in all three patients. Number of recurrences and time of follow-up may be correlated to malignant transformation in addition to previous RT [133].

The rate of malignant transformation may be lower with PORT, being reported in 3–4% of the cases [140]. Second malignancies of different and possibly radio-induced tumors have been also occasionally reported [140]. In the Chen series, one patient developed a second LG salivary gland malignancy at approximately 14 years after completion of therapy [130].

Rare cases of secondary adenocarcinoma have been reported, although adenocarcinomas were also observed after surgery alone [140]. Dawson reported one malignant tumor probably radiation-induced, while the other cases were compatible with spontaneous malignant transformation of benign pleomorphic adenoma, although radiation may have played a role [129].

References

1. Ciccolallo L, Licitra L, Cantú G, Gatta G, EUROCARE Working Group. Survival from salivary glands adenoid cystic carcinoma in European populations. Oral Oncol. 2009;45:669–74.
2. Adelstein DJ, Koyfman SA, El-Naggar AK, Hanna EY. Biology and management of salivary gland cancers. Semin Radiat Oncol. 2012;22:245–53.
3. Lopes ML, Barroso KM, Henriques ÁC, Dos Santos JN, Martins MD, de Souza LB. Pleomorphic adenomas of the salivary glands: retrospective multicentric study of 130 cases with emphasis on histopathological features. Eur Arch Otorhinolaryngol. 2017;274:543–51.
4. Seethala RR. An update on grading of salivary gland carcinomas. Head Neck Pathol. 2009;3:69–77.
5. Terhaard CH, Lubsen H, Van der Tweel I, Hilgers FJ, Eijkenboom WM, Marres HA, et al. Independent prognostic factors for locoregional control, distant metastases and overall survival: results of the Dutch Head and Neck Oncology Cooperative Group. Head Neck. 2004;26:681–92.
6. Purdy JA. From new frontiers to new standards of practice: advances in radiotherapy planning and delivery. Front Radiat Ther Oncol. 2007;40:18–39.
7. Bhide SA, Nutting CM. Advances in radiotherapy for head and neck cancer. Oral Oncol. 2010;46:439–41.
8. Mitin T, Zietman AL. Promise and pitfalls of heavy-particle therapy. J Clin Oncol. 2014;32:2855–63.
9. Grant SR, Grosshans DR, Bilton SD, Garcia JA, Amin M, Chambers MS, et al. Proton versus conventional radiotherapy for pediatric salivary gland tumors: acute toxicity and dosimetric characteristics. Radiother Oncol. 2015;116:309–15.
10. Balamucki CJ, Amdur RJ, Werning JW, Vaysberg M, Morris CG, Kirwan JM, et al. Adenoid cystic carcinoma of the head and neck. Am J Otolaryngol. 2012;33:510–8.
11. Mendenhall WM, Morris CG, Amdur RJ, Werning JW, Hinerman RW, Villaret DB. Radiotherapy alone or combined with surgery for adenoid cystic carcinoma of the head and neck. Head Neck. 2004;26:154–62.
12. Garden AS, Weber RS, Morrison WH, Ang KK, Peters LJ. The influence of positive margins and nerve invasion in adenoid cystic carcinoma of the head and neck treated with surgery and radiation. Int J Radiat Oncol Biol Phys. 1995;32:619–26.
13. van Weert S, Bloemena E, van der Waal I, de Bree R, Rietveld DH, Kuik JD, et al. Adenoid cystic carcinoma of the head and neck: a single-center analysis of 105 consecutive cases over a 30-year period. Oral Oncol. 2013;49:824–9.
14. Chen AM, Bucci MK, Weinberg V, Garcia J, Quivey JM, Schechter NR, et al. Adenoid cystic carcinoma of the head and neck treated by surgery with or without postoperative radiation therapy: prognostic features of recurrence. Int J Radiat Oncol Biol Phys. 2006;66:152–9.
15. Gomez DR, Hoppe BS, Wolden SL, Zhung JE, Patel SG, Kraus DH, et al. Outcomes and prognostic variables in adenoid cystic carcinoma of the head and neck: a recent experience. Int J Radiat Oncol Biol Phys. 2008;70:1365–72.
16. Kokemueller H, Eckardt A, Brachvogel P, Hausamen JE. Adenoid cystic carcinoma of the head and neck–a 20 years experience. Int J Oral Maxillofac Surg. 2004;33:25–31.

17. Oplatek A, Ozer E, Agrawal A, Bapna S, Schuller DE. Patterns of recurrence and survival of head and neck adenoid cystic carcinoma after definitive resection. Laryngoscope. 2010;120:65–70.
18. Spiro RH. Distant metastasis in adenoid cystic carcinoma of salivary origin. Am J Surg. 1997;174:195–8.
19. Katz TS, Mendenhall WM, Morris CG, Amdur RJ, Hinerman RW, Villaret DB. Malignant tumors of the nasal cavity and paranasal sinuses. Head Neck. 2002;24:821–9.
20. Khan AJ, DiGiovanna MP, Ross DA, Sasaki CT, Carter D, Son YH, et al. Adenoid cystic carcinoma: a retrospective clinical review. Int J Cancer. 2001;96:149–58.
21. Ellington CL, Goodman M, Kono SA, Grist W, Wadsworth T, Chen AY, et al. Adenoid cystic carcinoma of the head and neck: incidence and survival trends based on 1973-2007 surveillance, epidemiology, and end results data. Cancer. 2012;118:4444–51.
22. Lloyd S, Yu JB, Wilson LD, Decker RH. Determinants and patterns of survival in adenoid cystic carcinoma of the head and neck. Am J Clin Oncol. 2011;34:76–8.
23. Shen C, Xu T, Huang C, Hu C, He S. Treatment outcomes and prognostic features in adenoid cystic carcinoma originated from the head and neck. Oral Oncol. 2012;48:445–9.
24. Prokopakis EP, Snyderman CH, Hanna EY, Carrau RL, Johnson JT, D'Amico F. Risk factors for local recurrence of adenoid cystic carcinoma: the role of postoperative radiation therapy. Am J Otolaryngol. 1999;20:281–6.
25. Silverman DA, Carlson TP, Khuntia D, Bergstrom RT, Saxton J, Esclamado RM. Role for postoperative radiation therapy in adenoid cystic carcinoma of the head and neck. Laryngoscope. 2004;114:1194–9.
26. Ali S, Palmer FL, Katabi N, Lee N, Shah JP, Patel SG, Ganly I. Long-term local control rates of patients with adenoid cystic carcinoma of the head and neck managed by surgery and postoperative radiation. Laryngoscope. 2017;127:2265–9. https://doi.org/10.1002/lary.26565.
27. Vikram B, Strong EW, Shah JP, Spiro RH. Radiation therapy in adenoid-cystic carcinoma. Int J Radiat Oncol Biol Phys. 1984;10:221–3.
28. da Cruz Perez DE, de Abreu Alves F, Nobuko Nishimoto I, de Almeida OP, Kowalski LP. Prognostic factors in head and neck adenoid cystic carcinoma. Oral Oncol. 2006;42:139–46.
29. Barrett AW, Speight PM. Perineural invasion in adenoid cystic carcinoma of the salivary glands: a valid prognostic indicator? Oral Oncol. 2009;45:936–40.
30. Thompson LD, Penner C, Ho NJ, Foss RD, Miettinen M, Wieneke JA, et al. Sinonasal tract and nasopharyngeal adenoid cystic carcinoma: a clinicopathologic and immunophenotypic study of 86 cases. Head Neck Pathol. 2014;8:88–109.
31. Williams MD, Al-Zubidi N, Debnam JM, Shinder R, DeMonte F, Esmaeli B. Bone invasion by adenoid cystic carcinoma of the lacrimal gland: preoperative imaging assessment and surgical considerations. Ophthal Plast Reconstr Surg. 2010;26:403–8.
32. Suárez C, Barnes L, Silver CE, Rodrigo JP, Shah JP, Triantafyllou A, et al. Cervical lymph node metastasis in adenoid cystic carcinoma of oral cavity and oropharynx: a collective international review. Auris Nasus Larynx. 2016;43(5):477–84. https://doi.org/10.1016/j.anl.2016.02.013.
33. Min R, Siyi L, Wenjun Y, Ow A, Lizheng W, Minjun D, Chenping Z. Salivary gland adenoid cystic carcinoma with cervical lymph node metastasis: a preliminary study of 62 cases. Int J Oral Maxillofac Surg. 2012;41:952–7.
34. Lee SY, Shin HA, Rho KJ, Chung HJ, Kim SH, Choi EC. Characteristics, management of the neck and oncological outcomes of malignant minor salivary gland tumours in the oral and sinonasal regions. Br J Oral Maxillofac Surg. 2013;51:e142–7.
35. Lee SY, Kim BH, Choi EC. Nineteen-year oncologic outcomes and the benefit of elective neck dissection in salivary gland adenoid cystic carcinoma. Head Neck. 2014;36:1796–180.
36. Chen AM, Garcia J, Lee NY, Bucci MK, Eisele DW. Patterns of nodal relapse after surgery and postoperative radiation therapy for carcinomas of the major and minor salivary glands: what is the role of elective neck irradiation? Int J Radiat Oncol Biol Phys. 2007;67:988–94.
37. Orlandi E, Iacovelli NA, Bonora M, Cavallo A, Fossati P. Salivary Gland. Photon beam and particle radiotherapy: present and future. Oral Oncol. 2016;60:146–56.

38. Armstrong JG, Harrison LB, Spiro RH, Fass DE, Strong EW, Fuks ZY. Malignant tumors of major salivary gland origin. A matched-pair analysis of the role of combined surgery and postoperative radiotherapy. Arch Otolaryngol Head Neck Surg. 1990;116:290–3.
39. Regine WF, Mendenhall WM, Parsons JT, Stringer SP, Cassisi NJ, Million RR. Radiotherapy for adenoid cystic carcinoma of the palate. Head Neck. 1993;15:241–4.
40. Cowie VJ, Pointon RC. Adenoid cystic carcinoma of the salivary glands. Clin Radiol. 1984;35(4):331–3.
41. Spratt DE, Salgado LR, Riaz N, Doran MG, Tam M, Wolden S, et al. Results of photon radiotherapy for unresectable salivary gland tumors: is neutron radiotherapy's local control superior? Radiol Oncol. 2014;48:56.
42. Pommier P, Liebsch NJ, Deschler DG, Lin DT, McIntyre JF, Barker FG, et al. Proton beam radiation therapy for skull base adenoid cystic carcinoma. Arch Otolaryngol Head Neck Surg. 2006;132:1242–9.
43. Huber PE, Debus J, Latz D, Zierhut D, Bischof M, Wannenmacher M, et al. Radiotherapy for advanced adenoid cystic carcinoma: neutrons, photons or mixed beam? Radiother Oncol. 2001;59:161–7.
44. Laramore GE, Krall JM, Griffin TW, Duncan W, Richter MP, Saroja KR, et al. Neutron versus photon irradiation for unresectable salivary gland tumors: final report of an RTOG-MRC randomized clinical trial. Int J Radiat Oncol Biol Phys. 1993;27:235–40.
45. Jensen AD, Nikoghosyan AV, Lossner K, Haberer T, Jäkel O, Münter MW, et al. COSMIC: a regimen of intensity modulated radiation therapy plus dose escalated, raster-scanned carbon ion boost for malignant salivary gland tumors: results of the prospective phase 2 trial. Int J Radiat Oncol Biol Phys. 2015;93:37–46.
46. Chen AM, Bucci MK, Quivey JM, Garcia J, Eisele DW, Fu KK. Long-term outcome of patients treated by radiation therapy alone for salivary gland carcinomas. Int J Radiat Oncol Biol Phys. 2006;66:1044–50.
47. RTOG1008: a randomized phase II study of adjuvant concurrent radiation and chemotherapy vs. radiation alone in resected high-risk malignant salivary gland tumors, clinical trial registry: NCT01272037.
48. Harrison LB, Armstrong JG, Spiro RH, Fass DE, Strong EW. Postoperative radiation therapy for major salivary gland malignancies. J Surg Oncol. 1990;45(1):52–5.
49. Simpson JR, Thawley SE, Matsuba HM. Adenoid cystic salivary gland carcinoma: treatment with irradiation and surgery. Radiology. 1984;151:509.
50. Ko HC, Gupta V, Mourad WF, Hu KS, Harrison LB, Som PM, Bakst RL. A contouring guide for head and neck cancers with perineural invasion. Pract Radiat Oncol. 2014;4:e247–58.
51. Mourad WF, Hu KS, Shourbaji RA, Khorsandi A, Harrison LB. Cranial nerves contouring among patients treated with IMRT for base of skull, nasopharyngeal, and paranasal sinus cancer. Pract Radiat Oncol. 2013;3:S34.
52. Askoxylakis V, Hegenbarth P, Timke C, Saleh-Ebrahimi L, Debus J, Röder F, et al. Intensity modulated radiation therapy (IMRT) for sinonasal tumors: a single center long-term clinical analysis. Radiat Oncol. 2016;4:11–7.
53. Duprez F, Madani I, Morbée L, Bonte K, Deron P, Domján V, et al. IMRT for sinonasal tumors minimizes severe late ocular toxicity and preserves disease control and survival. Int J Radiat Oncol Biol Phys. 2012;83:252–9.
54. Daly ME, Chen AM, Bucci MK, El-Sayed I, Xia P, Kaplan MJ, Eisele DW. Intensity-modulated radiation therapy for malignancies of the nasal cavity and paranasal sinuses. Int J Radiat Oncol Biol Phys. 2007;67:151–7.
55. Orlandi E, Giandini T, Iannacone E, De Ponti E, Carrara M, Mongioj V, Stucchi C, Tana S, Bossi P, Licitra L, Fallai C, Pignoli E. Radiotherapy for unresectable sinonasal cancers: dosimetric comparison of intensity modulated radiation therapy with coplanar and non-coplanar volumetric modulated arc therapy. Radiother Oncol. 2014;113:260–6.
56. Orlandi E, Palazzi M, Pignoli E, Fallai C, Giostra A, Olmi P. Radiobiological basis and clinical results of the simultaneous integrated boost (SIB) in intensity modulated radiotherapy (IMRT) for head and neck cancer: a review. Crit Rev Hematol Oncol. 2010;73:111–25.

57. Terhaard CH, Lubsen H, Rasch CR, Levendag PC, Kaanders HH, Tjho-Heslinga RE, et al. The role of radiotherapy in the treatment of malignant salivary gland tumors. Int J Radiat Oncol Biol Phys. 2005;61:103–11.
58. Renehan A, Gleave EN, Hancock BD, Smith P, McGurk M. Long-term follow-up of over 1000 patients with salivary gland tumours treated in a single centre. Br J Surg. 1996;83:1750–4.
59. Chen AM, Granchi PJ, Garcia J, Bucci MK, Fu KK, Eisele DW. Local-regional recurrence after surgery without postoperative irradiation for carcinomas of the major salivary glands: implications for adjuvant therapy. Int J Radiat Oncol Biol Phys. 2007;67:982–7.
60. Therkildsen MH, Christensen M, Andersen LJ, Schiodt T, Hansen HS. Salivary gland carcinomas – prognostic factors. Acta Oncol. 1998;37:701–13.
61. Pohar S, Gay H, Rosenbaum P, Klish D, Bogart J, Sagerman R, et al. Malignant parotid tumors: presentation, clinical/pathologic prognostic factors, and treatment outcomes. Int J Radiat Oncol Biol Phys. 2005;61:112–8.
62. Shah K, Javed F, Alcock C, Shah KA, Pretorius P, Milford CA. Parotid cancer treatment with surgery followed by radiotherapy in Oxford over 15 years. Ann R Coll Surg Engl. 2011;93:218–22.
63. Chen AM, Garcia J, Granchi PJ, Johnson J, Eisele DW. Late recurrence from salivary gland cancer: when does "cure" mean cure? Cancer. 2008;112:340–4.
64. Storey MR, Garden AS, Morrison WH, Eicher SA, Schechter NR, Ang KK. Postoperative radiotherapy for malignant tumors of the submandibular gland. Int J Radiat Oncol Biol Phys. 2001;51:952–8.
65. Armstrong JG, Harrison LB, Thaler HT, Friedlander-Klar H, Fass DE, Zelefsky MJ, et al. The indications for elective treatment of the neck in cancer of the major salivary glands. Cancer. 1992;69:615–9.
66. McGuirt WF. Management of occult metastatic disease from salivary gland neoplasms. Arch Otolaryngol Head Neck Surg. 1989;115:322–5.
67. Regis De Brito Santos I, Kowalski LP, Cavalcante De Araujo V, Flavia Logullo A, Magrin J. Multivariate analysis of risk factors for neck metastases in surgically treated parotid carcinomas. Arch Otolaryngol Head Neck Surg. 2001;127:56–60.
68. Rodriguez-Cuevas S, Labastida S, Baena L, Gallegos F. Risk of nodal metastases from malignant salivary gland tumors related to tumor size and grade of malignancy. Eur Arch Otorhinolaryngol. 1995;252:139–42.
69. Frankenthaler RA, Byers RM, Luna MA, Callender DL, Wolf P, Goepfert H. Predicting occult lymph node metastasis in parotid cancer. Arch Otolaryngol Head Neck Surg. 1993;119: 517–20.
70. Medina JE. Neck dissection in the treatment of cancer of major salivary glands. Otolaryngol Clin N Am. 1998;31:815–22.
71. Al-Mamgani A, van Rooij P, Verduijn GM, Meeuwis CA, Levendag PC. Long-term outcomes and quality of life of 186 patients with primary parotid carcinoma treated with surgery and radiotherapy at the Daniel den Hoed Cancer Center. Int J Radiat Oncol Biol Phys. 2012;84: 189–95.
72. Bjorndal K, Krogdahl A, Therkildsen MH, Overgaard J, Johansen J, Kristensen CA, et al. Salivary gland carcinoma in Denmark 1990-2005: outcome and prognostic factors. Results of the Danish Head and Neck Cancer Group (DAHANCA). Oral Oncol. 2012;48:179–85.
73. Hosni A, Huang SH, Goldstein D, Xu W, Chan B, Hansen A, et al. Outcomes and prognostic factors for major salivary gland carcinoma following postoperative radiotherapy. Oral Oncol. 2016;54:75–80.
74. Chen AM, Lau VH, Farwell DG, Luu Q, Donald PJ. Mucoepidermoid carcinoma of the parotid gland treated by surgery and postoperative radiation therapy: clinicopathologic correlates of outcome. Laryngoscope. 2013;123:3049–55.
75. McHugh CH, Roberts DB, El-Naggar AK, Hanna EY, Garden AS, Kies MS, et al. Prognostic factors in mucoepidermoid carcinoma of the salivary glands. Cancer. 2012;118:3928–36.
76. Chen AM, Garcia J, Bucci MK, Quivey JM, Eisele DW. The role of postoperative radiation therapy in carcinoma ex pleomorphic adenoma of the parotid gland. Int J Radiat Oncol Biol Phys. 2007;67:138–43.

77. Lim CM, Hobson C, Kim S, Johnson JT. Clinical outcome of patients with carcinoma ex pleomorphic adenoma of the parotid gland: a comparative study from a single tertiary center. Head Neck. 2015;37:543–7.
78. Laramore GE, Krall JM, Griffin TW, Duncan W, Richter MP, Saroja KR, et al. Neutron versus photon irradiation for unresectable salivary gland tumors: final report of an RTOG-MRC randomized clinical trial. Radiation Therapy Oncology Group. Medical Research Council. Int J Radiat Oncol Biol Phys. 1993;27:235–40.
79. Borthne A, Kjellevold K, Kaalhus O, Vermund H. Salivary gland malignant neoplasms: treatment and prognosis. Int J Radiat Oncol Biol Phys. 1986;12:747–54.
80. Ravasz LA, Terhaard CH, Hordijk GJ. Radiotherapy in epithelial tumors of the parotid gland: case presentation and literature review. Int J Radiat Oncol Biol Phys. 1990;19:55–9.
81. Mendenhall WM, Morris CG, Amdur RJ, Werning JW, Villaret DB. Radiotherapy alone or combined with surgery for salivary gland carcinoma. Cancer. 2005;103:2544–50.
82. Spratt DE, Salgado LR, Riaz N, Doran MG, Tam M, Wolden S, et al. Results of photon radiotherapy for unresectable salivary gland tumors: is neutron radiotherapy's local control superior? Radiol Oncol. 2014;48:56–61.
83. Karam SD, Rashid A, Snider JW, Wooster M, Bhatia S, Jay AK, et al. IMRT with stereotactic body radiotherapy boost for high risk malignant salivary gland malignancies: a case series. Front Oncol. 2014;4:268.
84. Garden AS, Weber RS, Ang KK, Morrison WH, Matre J, Peters LJ. Postoperative radiation therapy for malignant tumors of minor salivary glands. Outcome and patterns of failure. Cancer. 1994;73:2563–9.
85. Wang CC, Goodman M. Photon irradiation of unresectable carcinomas of salivary glands. Int J Radiat Oncol Biol Phys. 1991;21:569–76.
86. Schoenfeld JD, Sher DJ, Norris CM Jr, Haddad RI, Posner MR, Balboni TA, et al. Salivary gland tumors treated with adjuvant intensity-modulated radiotherapy with or without concurrent chemotherapy. Int J Radiat Oncol Biol Phys. 2012;82:308–14.
87. Lee N, Millender LE, Larson DA, Wara WM, McDermott MW, Kapaln MJ, et al. Gamma knife radiosurgery for recurrent salivary gland malignancies involving the base of skull. Head Neck. 2003;25:210–6.
88. Zwicker F, Roeder F, Hauswald H, Thieke C, Timke C, Schlegel W, et al. Reirradiation with intensity-modulated radiotherapy in recurrent head and neck cancer. Head Neck. 2011;33:1695–702.
89. Karam SD, Snider JW, Wang H, Wooster M, Lominska C, Deeken J, et al. Reirradiation of recurrent salivary gland malignancies with fractionated stereotactic body radiation therapy. Int J Radiat Oncol Biol Phys. 2012;1:147–53.
90. Amini A, Waxweiler TV, Brower JV, Jones BL, McDermott JD, Raben D, et al. Association of adjuvant chemoradiotherapy *vs* radiotherapy alone with survival in patients with resected major salivary gland carcinoma: data from the national cancer data base. JAMA Otolaryngol Head Neck Surg. 2016;142:1100–10.
91. Mifsud MJ, Tanvetyanon T, Mccaffrey JC, Otto KJ, Padhya TA, Kish J, et al. Adjuvant radiotherapy versus concurrent chemoradiotherapy for the management of high-risk salivary gland carcinomas. Head Neck. 2016;38:1628–33.
92. Walvekar RR, Andrade Filho PA, Seethala RR, Gooding WE, Heron DE, Johnson JT, et al. Clinicopathologic features as stronger prognostic factors than histology or grade in risk stratification of primary parotid malignancies. Head Neck. 2011;33:225–31.
93. Richter SM, Friedmann P, Mourad WF, Hu KS, Persky MS, Harrison LB. Postoperative radiation therapy for small, low-/intermediate-grade parotid tumors with close and/or positive surgical margins. Head Neck. 2012;34:953–5.
94. Cho JK, Lim BW, Kim EH, Ko YH, Oh D, Noh JM, et al. Low-grade salivary gland cancers: treatment outcomes, extent of surgery and indications for postoperative adjuvant radiation therapy. Ann Surg Oncol. 2016;23:4368–75.
95. Coca-Pelaz A, Rodrigo JP, Triantafyllou A, Hunt JL, Rinaldo A, Strojan P, Haigentz MA, et al. Salivary mucoepidermoid carcinoma revisited. Eur Ann Otorhinolaryngol. 2015;272: 799–819.

96. Guzzo M, Andreola S, Sirizzotti G, Cantù G. Mucoepidermoid carcinoma of the salivary glands: clinicopathologic review of 108 patients treated at the National Cancer Institute of Milan. Ann Surg Oncol. 2002;9:688–95.
97. Hosokawa Y, Shirato H, Kagei K, Hashimoto S, Nishioka T, Tei K, et al. Role of radiotherapy for mucoepidermoid carcinoma of salivary gland. Oral Oncol. 1999;35:105–11.
98. Rapidis AD, Givalos N, Gakiopoulou H, Stavrianos SD, Faratzis G, Lagogiannis G. Mucoepidermoid carcinoma of the salivary glands. Review of the literature and clinicopathological analysis of 18 patients. Oral Oncol. 2007;43(2):130–6.
99. McHugh CH, Roberts DB, El-Naggar AK, Hanna EY, Garden AS, Kies MS. Prognostic factors in mucoepidermoid carcinoma of the salivary glands. Cancer. 2012;118:3928–36.
100. HistoKatabi N, Ghossein R, Ali S, Dogan S, Klimstra D, Ganly I. Prognostic features in mucoepidermoid carcinoma of major salivary glands with emphasis on tumour histologic grading. Histopathology. 2014;65:793–804.
101. Chen MM, Roman SA, Sosa JA, Judson BL. Histologic grade as prognostic indicator for mucoepidermoid carcinoma: a population-level analysis of 2400 patients. Head Neck. 2014;36:158–63.
102. Liu S, Ow A, Ruan M, Yang W, Zhang C, Wang L, et al. Prognostic factors in primary salivary gland mucoepidermoid carcinoma: an analysis of 376 cases in an Eastern Chinese population. Int J Oral Maxillofac Surg. 2014;43:667–73.
103. Ozawa H, Tomita T, Sakamoto K, Tagawa T, Fujii R, Kanzaki S. Mucoepidermoid carcinoma of the head and neck: clinical analysis of 43 patients. Jpn J Clin Oncol. 2008;38:414–8.
104. Kolokythas A, Connor S, Kimgsoo D, Fernandes RP, Ord RA. Low-grade mucoepidermoid carcinoma of the intraoral minor salivary glands with cervical metastasis: report of 2 cases and review of the literature. J Oral Maxillofac Surg. 2010;68:1396–9.
105. Boahene DKO, Olsen KD, Lewis JE, Pinheiro AD, Pankratz VS, Bagniewski SM. Mucoepidermoid carcinoma of the parotid gland the Mayo clinic experience. Arch Otolaryngol Head Neck Surg. 2004;130:849–56.
106. Olsen MP, Mitchell AO, Miles EF. Postoperative radiation therapy for parotid mucoepidermoid carcinoma. Case Rep Oncol Med. 2014;2014:345128.
107. Bensadoun RJ, Allavena C, Chauvela P, Dassonville O, Demard F, Dieu-Bosquet L, et al. Standards, options et recommandations 2003 pour la radiothérapie des patients atteints de tumeurs malignes des glandes salivaires (lymphomes, sarcomes et mélanomes exclus), mise à jour. Cancer Radiother. 2003;7:280–95.
108. Patel NR, Sanghvi S, Khan MN, Husain Q, Baredes S, Eloy JA. Demographic trends and disease-specific survival in salivary acinic cell carcinoma: an analysis of 1129 cases. Laryngoscope. 2014;124:172–8.
109. Vander Poorten V, Hunt J, Bradley PJ, Haigentz M Jr, Rinaldo A, Mendenhall WM, et al. Recent trends in the management of minor salivary gland carcinoma. Head Neck. 2014;36:444–55.
110. Biron VL, Lentsch EJ, Gerry DR, Bewley AF. Case-control analysis of survival outcomes in sinonasal acinic cell carcinoma. Int Forum Allergy Rhinol. 2014;4:507–11.
111. Cha W, Kim MS, Ahn JC, et al. Clinical analysis of acinic cell carcinoma in parotid gland. Clin Exp Otorhinolaryngol. 2011;4:188–92.
112. Spafford PD, Mintz DR, Hay J. Acinic cell carcinoma of the parotid gland: review and management. J Otolaryngol. 1991;20:262–6.
113. Greig SR, Chaplin JM, McIvor NP, et al. Acinic cell carcinoma of the parotid gland: Auckland experience and literature review. ANZ J Surg. 2008;78:754–8.
114. Liu Y, Su M, Yang Y, et al. Prognostic factors associated with decreased survival in patients with acinic cell carcinoma of the parotid gland. J Oral Maxillofac Surg. 2016;75(2): 416–22.
115. Andreoli MT, Andreoli SM, Shrime MG, et al. Radiotherapy in parotid acinic cell carcinoma does it have an impact on survival? Arch Otolaryngol Head Neck Surg. 2012;138:463–6.
116. Biron VL, Lentsch EJ, Gerry DR, et al. Factors influencing survival in acinic cell carcinoma: a retrospective survival analysis of 2061 patients. Head Neck. 2015;37:870–7.

117. Vander Poorten V, Triantafyllou A, Thompson LDR, et al. Salivary acinic cell carcinoma: reappraisal and update. Eur Arch Otorhinolaryngol. 2015;273(11):3511–31.
118. Paleri V, Max Robinson M, Bradley P. Polymorphous low-grade adenocarcinoma of the head and neck. Curr Opin Otolaryngol Head Neck Surg. 2008;16:163–9.
119. Uematomari I, Tabuchi K, Tobita T, et al. The importance of postoperative radiotherapy against polymorphous low-grade adenocarcinoma of the parotid gland: case report and review of the literature. Tohoku J Exp Med. 2007;2111:297–302.
120. Verma V, Mendenhall WM, Werning JW. Polymorphous low-grade adenocarcinoma of the head and neck. Am J Clin Oncol. 2014;37:624–6.
121. Kimple AJ, Austin GK, Shah RN, et al. Polymorphous low-grade adenocarcinoma: a case series and determination of recurrence. Laryngoscope. 2014;124:2714–9.
122. Patel TD, Vazquez A, Marchiano E, et al. Polymorphous low-grade adenocarcinoma of the head and neck: a population-based study of 460 cases. Laryngoscope. 2015;125:1644–9.
123. Vazquez A, Patel TD, D'Aguillo CM, et al. Epithelial-myoepithelial carcinoma of the salivary glands: an analysis of 246 cases. Otolaryngol Head Neck Surg. 2015;153:569–74.
124. Huang AT, Tang C, Diana Bell D, et al. Prognostic factors in adenocarcinoma of the salivary glands. Oral Oncol. 2015;51:610–5.
125. Ascani G, Pieramici T, Messi M, et al. Salivary glands tumours: a retrospective study of 454 patients. Minerva Stomatol. 2006;55:209–14.
126. Robertson BF, Robertson GA, Shoaib T, et al. Pleomorphic adenomas: post-operative radiotherapy is unnecessary following primary incomplete excision: a retrospective review. J Plast Reconstr Aesthet Surg. 2014;67:e297–302.
127. Patel S, Mourad WF, Wang C, et al. Postoperative radiation therapy for parotid pleomorphic adenoma with close or positive margins: treatment outcomes and toxicities. Anticancer Res. 2014;34:4247–51.
128. Barton J, Slevin NJ, Gleave EN. Radiotherapy for pleomorphic adenoma of the parotid gland. Int J Radiat Oncol Biol Phys. 1992;22:925–8.
129. Dawson AK, Orr JA. Long term results of local excision and radiotherapy in pleomorphic adenoma of the parotid. Int J Radiat Oncol Biol Phys. 1985;11:451–5.
130. Chen AM, Garcia J, Bucci MK, et al. Recurrent pleomorphic adenoma of the parotid gland: long-term outcome of patients treated with radiation therapy. Int J Radiat Oncol Biol Phys. 2006;66:1031–5.
131. Carew JF, Spiro RH, Singh B, et al. Treatment of recurrent pleomorphic adenomas of the parotid gland. Otolaryngol Head Neck Surg. 1999;121:539–42.
132. Leverstein H, Tiwari RM, Snow GB, et al. The surgical management of recurrent or residual pleomorphic adenomas of the parotid gland. Analysis and results in 40 patients. Eur Arch Otorhinolaryngol. 1997;254:313–7.
133. Renehan A, Gleave EN, McGurk M. An analysis of the treatment of 114 patients with recurrent pleomorphic adenomas of the parotid gland. Am J Surg. 1996;172:710–4.
134. Liu FF, Rotstein L, Davison AJ, et al. Benign parotid adenomas: a review of the Princess Margaret Hospital experience. Head Neck. 1995;17:177–83.
135. Samson MJ, Metson R, Wang CC, et al. Preservation of the facial nerve in the management of recurrent pleomorphic adenoma. Laryngoscope. 1991;101:1060–2.
136. Dawson AK. Radiation therapy in recurrent pleomorphic adenoma of the parotid. Int J Radiat Oncol Biol Phys. 1989;16:819–21.
137. Wallace AS, Morris CG, Kirwan JM, et al. Radiotherapy for pleomorphic adenoma. Am J Otolaryngol – Head Neck Med Surg. 2013;34:36–40.
138. Hodge CW, Morris CG, Werning JW, et al. Role of radiotherapy for pleomorphic adenoma. Am J Clin Oncol. 2005;28:148–51.
139. Witt RL, Nicolai P. Recurrent benign salivary gland neoplasms. Adv Otorhinolaryngol. 2016;78:63–70.
140. Thomson DJ, Slevin NJ, Mendenhall WM. Indications for salivary glands radiotherapy. Adv Otorhinolaryngol. 2016;78:141–7.

141. Witt RL, Eisele DW, Morton RP. Etiology and management of recurrent parotid pleomorphic adenoma. Laryngoscope. 2015;125:888–93.
142. Jardel P, Fakhryb N, Makeieffc M, et al. Adénomes pléomorphes parotidiens récidivants: place de la radiothérapie Radiation therapy for pleomorphic adenoma of the parotid. Cancer Radiother. 2014;18:68–76.
143. Mendenhall WM, Mendenhall CM, Werning JW, et al. Salivary gland pleomorphic adenoma. Am J Clin Oncol. 2008;31:95–9.
144. Dunne JA, Matteucci PL, Foote M, et al. Pleomorphic adenomas: post-operative radiotherapy is unnecessary following primary incomplete excision: a retrospective review. J Plast Reconstr Aesthet Surg. 2015;67(12):e297–302.
145. Jardel P, Fakhry N, Makeieff M, Ferrie JC, Milin S, Righini C, et al. Radiation therapy for pleomorphic adenoma of the parotid. Cancer Radiother. 2014;18:68–76.

Protons and Heavy Ions

12

A. D. Jensen and P. Fossati

Abbreviations

ACC	Adenoid cystic carcinoma
ART	Adaptive radiotherapy
BED	Biological effective dose
C12	Carbon ions
CTCAE	Common Terminology Criteria for Adverse Events
EORTC	European Organisation for Research and Treatment of Cancer
ICRU	International Commission on Radiation Units and Measurements
IGRT	Image-guided radiotherapy
IMRT	Intensity-modulated radiotherapy
LEM	Local effects model
LET	Linear energy transfer
MKM	Microdosimetric kinetic model
MRC	Medical Research Council
MSGT	Malignant salivary gland tumour
NTCP	Normal tissue complication probability
OAR	Organ at risk
RBE	Relative biological effectiveness
RTOG	Radiation Therapy Oncology Group
SOBP	Spread-out Bragg peak
VMAT	Volumetric arc therapy

A. D. Jensen (✉)
Department of Radiation Oncology Gießen,
University Hospital Gießen and Marburg (UKGM), Marburg, Germany
e-mail: AlexDJensen@gmx.de

P. Fossati
Fondazione CNAO, Pavia, Italy

EBG MedAustron GmbH, Wiener Neustadt, Austria

© Springer Nature Switzerland AG 2019
L. Licitra, L. D. Locati (eds.), *Salivary Gland Cancer*,
https://doi.org/10.1007/978-3-030-02958-6_12

12.1 Introduction

Radiotherapy is always a compromise: as pointed out by Hermann Holthusen already in the 1930s, radiation oncologists act within a narrow therapeutic window. While tumour control improves as dose to the tumour increases, toxicity also does. The trade-off therefore is between tumour control and acceptable toxicity (Fig. 12.1: Holthusen curve).

Technical developments in radiation oncology in the past decades such as 3D conformal therapy, stereotactic radiotherapy, intensity-modulated radiotherapy (IMRT), as well as image-guided and adaptive radiotherapy (IGRT and ART) have always worked towards increasing this therapeutic window by producing more conformal dose distributions and reducing margins.

Treatment of malignant salivary gland tumours of the head and neck is complex. For example, minor salivary gland carcinomas involve most commonly the paranasal sinuses, and unfortunately they are also comparatively radioresistant. Doses in excess of 60 Gy are needed to achieve long-term local control in this disease [1–4]. In order to give high radiation dose to these complex anatomical sites without simultaneously increasing toxicity, sophisticated radiotherapeutic techniques are needed.

Generally, there are three strategies to increase therapeutic effects of radiation: the addition of radiosensitizing agents (chemoradiation), dose escalation or the use of heavy particles to enhance the radiobiological effectiveness of radiation.

Data on radiosensitization in malignant salivary gland tumours (MSGTs) and especially adenoid cystic carcinoma (ACC) is clearly limited. Only a few groups have reported their experiences with platinum-based chemoradiation [5–10] or bioradiation [11, 12]. Reports are mostly retrospective and patient numbers are small. However, chemoradiation in MSGTs is a topic of increasing interest. RTOG is currently conducting and recruiting patients into a multicentric randomized

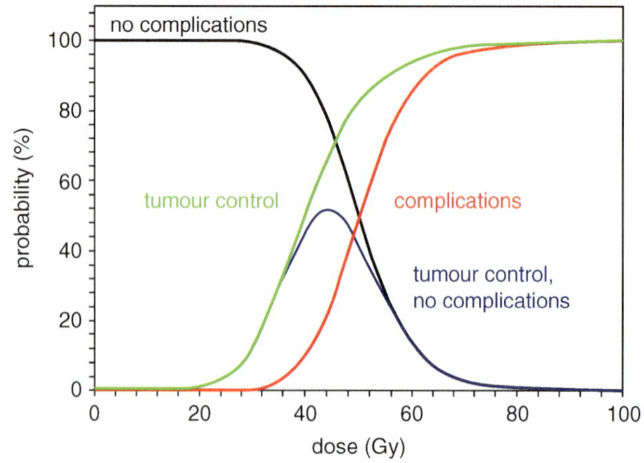

Fig. 12.1 According to Hermann Holthusen (1936)

phase II/phase III trial to investigate this issue further in adjuvant setting for high-risk cases (NCT01220583) [13]. Chemoradiation is currently not the standard treatment approach.

12.2 Dose Escalation with Charged Particles

Dose escalation can be achieved by alternative radiation modalities such as radiotherapy with charged particles. As opposed to photons and neutrons, charged particles lose most of their energy towards the end of their path. Their penetration depth is characterized by their specific mass and charge as well as their kinetic energy on entering tissue. The point of the particle's maximum energy deposition in tissue is called "Bragg peak". Beyond the Bragg peak, dose drops to almost zero. Carbon ions do exhibit a so-called fragmentation tail corresponding to nuclear reactions and energy deposited beyond the Bragg peak; however, this effect is less pronounced in helium or neon.

Due to their dosimetric properties, charged particles offer the advantage of extremely sharp dose gradients. Critical structures even in close proximity to the target volume can therefore be spared while still applying high doses to the tumour. In order to use charged particles for clinical treatments and cover the complete extent of the tumour, multiple Bragg peaks need to be superposed ("spread-out Bragg peak", SOBP) (Fig. 12.2). This can be achieved by either prefixing material with different thicknesses (modulator wheel or range modulator)

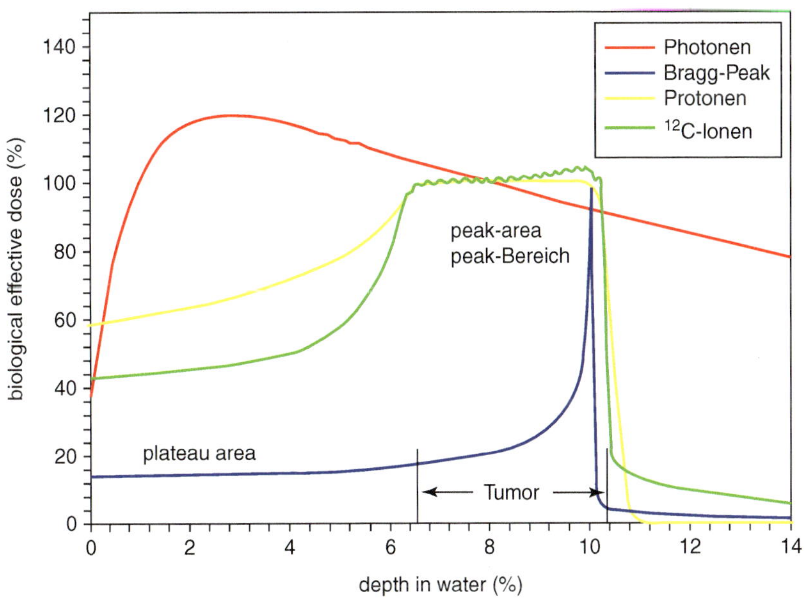

Fig. 12.2 Bragg peak and SOBP, ©Springer: Praxis der Viszeralchirurgie: Kapitel Partikeltherapie [14]

into a homogenous particle beam with constant energy (passive beam application) or by modulating particle energy in the accelerator system (active beam application) [15].

Compared to proton beams, heavy charged particles have the additional benefit of a very small lateral dose penumbra (Fig. 12.3, [14]).

In view of their physical properties, charged particle beams are therefore ideally suited for dose escalation in complex anatomical sites such as paranasal sinuses or the base of the skull where tumours are located close to critical and radiosensitive organs at risk. The use of this highly conformal radiation technique allows treatment with high radiation doses without increasing dose and consequently toxicity to critical structures such as brain stem, optic nerves, optic chiasm, etc. Figures 12.4 and 12.5 show the dose distribution of carbon ions in patients with advanced MSGT of the paranasal sinus both at first diagnosis and for re-irradiation of tumour recurrence. As can be seen, organs at risk (OARs) can be spared in an optimal way, achieving adequate target coverage and obtaining early metabolic response and durable local control (Figs. 12.4 and 12.5).

Particle beams with high linear energy transfer (high-LET) beams such as ion or neutron beams show an increased relative biological effectiveness (RBE). The RBE though changes with the position within the particle track. As energy deposition increases (increased linear energy transfer, LET), the RBE also increases. Particle beams therefore reach their maximum RBE with the Bragg peak towards the end of their penetration depth.

The RBE, however, not only depends on the position within the beam but also on particle charge, energy and absorbed dose in the tissue. In scanned particle beams and especially with multiple irradiation fields and dose contributions by different particle tracks, the RBE can no longer be calculated intuitively. In Europe all carbon

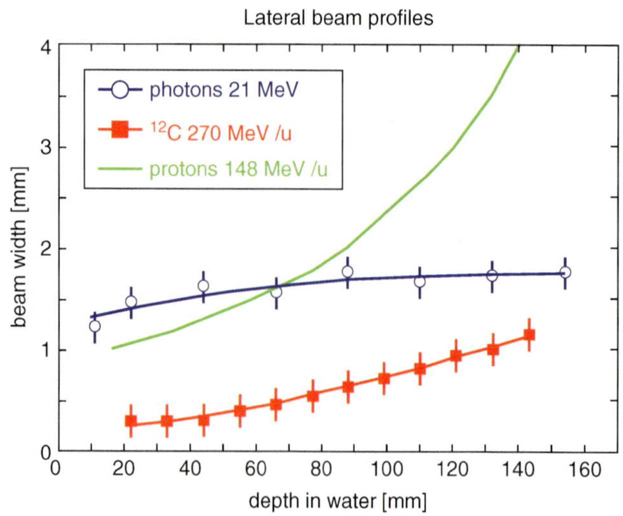

Fig. 12.3 Lateral penumbra of charged particle beams

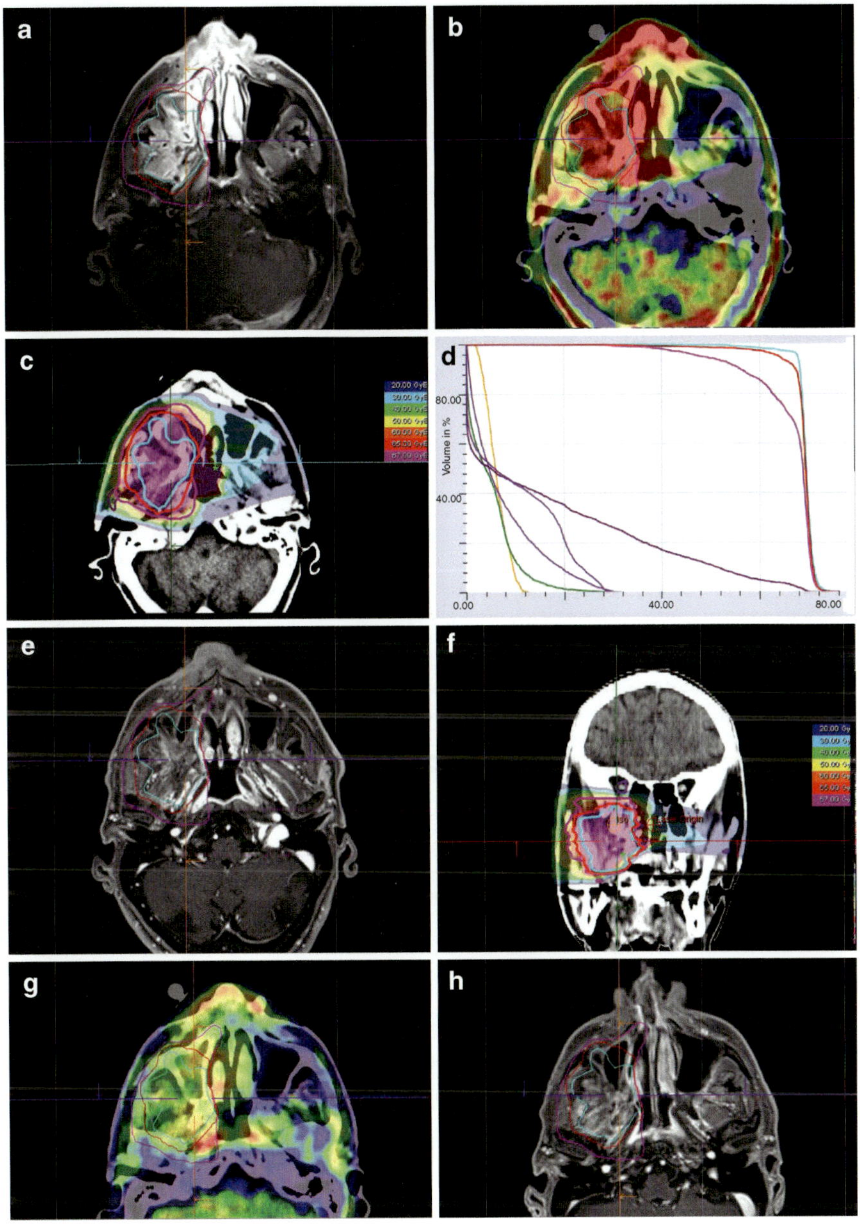

Fig. 12.4 Maxillary sinus adenoid cystic carcinoma pT4 pN0 R2 (intracranial extension and macroscopic disease after surgical resection) treated with carbon ion radiotherapy with radical intent at CNAO. Prescription dose 68.8 Gy RBE in 16 fractions of 4.3 Gy RBE. Low-dose CTV including perineural spread 38.7 Gy RBE. (**a**) Pretreatment MR: light blue GTV, red CTV high dose, purple CTV low dose. (**b**) Pretreatment C11 methionine PET. (**c**) Dose distribution in axial plane. (**d**) DVH: light blue GTV, red CTV high dose, purple CTV low dose, violet from right to left right side parotid, left side parotid and right side optic nerve, green right side eyeball, yellow right side cochlea; other OARs received negligible dose. (**e**) MR response at 3 months. (**f**) Dose distribution in coronal plane. (**g**) B C11 methionine PET response at 1 month. (**h**) MR response at 2 years

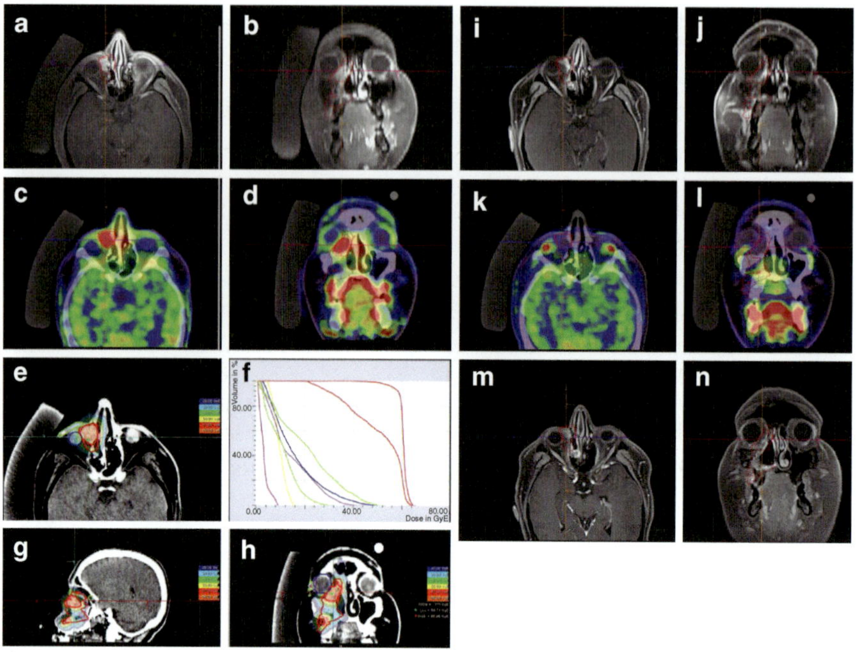

Fig. 12.5 Local recurrence of maxillary sinus adenoid cystic carcinoma treated with surgery and IMRT 50 Gy in 25 fraction 7 years before treated at CNAO with radical intent (intracranial extension and macroscopic disease after surgical resection) treated with carbon ion radiotherapy with radical intent at CNAO. Prescription dose 60 Gy RBE in 15 fractions of 4.0 Gy RBE. (**a**, **b**) Pretreatment MR, the orbital nodule and maxillary nodule are contoured and are joined in a single CTV with small margins. (**c**, **d**) Pretreatment C11 methionine PET. (**e**) Dose distribution in the axial plane. (**f**) DVH; from right to left: red GTV, red CTV, green right eyelid, blue right eyeball, violet right cornea, green right optic nerve, yellow, right lens, purple right lacrimal gland; other OARs received negligible dose. (**g**, **h**) Dose distribution in coronal and sagittal planes. (**i**, **j**) MR response at 6 months. (**k**, **l**) PET response at 1 month. (**m**, **n**) MR response at 3 years

ion facilities employ the local effects model (LEM) [16–19]. In Japan, a semiempirical model was used (the so-called Kanai model), and more recently the microdosimetric kinetic model (MKM) has been introduced [20–23]. Sophisticated calculation models are therefore an integral part of the respective treatment planning system.

Particle beams have further biological properties: while the effects of photon irradiation depend on the presence of oxygen in cells, the mechanism of action in particle radiotherapy is less dependent on oxygen. Hence, particle therapy may be especially advantageous in hypoxic tumours. In addition, there is less variation in radiosensitivity in particle radiotherapy related to position in the cell cycle. Due to massive energy depositions by single-particle tracks, cell repair phenomena tend to be less prominent; therefore fractionation effects are much smaller in ion RT.

Also, as particle radiation allows less cell repair, it is selectively more efficient against tumour cells with high repair capacities such as chordomas, chondrosarcomas, prostate carcinomas, etc.

The (almost) negligible dependence of the dose-response relationship on tumour differentiation for carbon ions has been recently elegantly shown in an in vivo model: rat prostatic carcinomas displayed wide variations in their response to photons RT according to their grade, but only limited differences were detectable for well-differentiated, hormone-resistant or anaplastic tumours when carbon ions were employed [24].

While both charged ions and neutrons show similar biological properties which have been exploited in neutron radiotherapy already decades ago, heavy ion beams have several advantages over neutron and even proton radiotherapy: due to the physical properties of heavy ions and protons, dose distributions are significantly more conformal and dose gradients steeper than with neutrons. However, due to their higher mass, Coulomb scatter and therefore lateral penumbra are lower in heavy ions as compared to protons.

12.3 Biological Properties of Particle Beams: Proton and Carbon Ions

The idea to use particle beams for cancer treatment is not new. Barely 27 years after the proton had been discovered by Lord Rutherford, the physicist Robert R Wilson was the first to propose treatment with protons and heavy ions for malignant tumours as early as 1946. The first patients received particle therapy at the Berkeley Radiation Laboratory in 1954. More than 2500 patients with various indications were treated with both protons and heavy ions at this institution until closure of its clinical project in 1992.

Due to biological properties of neutron beams, these were investigated for relatively radioresistant tumours such as MSGTs and especially ACC already in the 1980s. To date, the majority of our experience with particle therapy in the treatment of MSGTs stems from these neutron studies.

Griffin and Laramore reported results of the randomized RTOG-MRC trial comparing radiotherapy with photons and neutrons in head and neck malignancies. Patients were treated with either 70 Gy standard fractionated or 55 Gy hypofractionated photons vs. 16.5–22 Gy neutrons in 12 fractions over 4 weeks. Trial recruitment was terminated early as locoregional control was significantly higher in the neutron arm as compared to the photon arm (67% vs. 17% at 2 years). Overall survival did show a trend towards improvement in the neutron arm at 2 years (62% vs. 25%); however, this trend was not statistically significant [25] and disappeared at 5- and 10-year follow-up [26]. The Seattle group updated their prior neutron experience [27, 28] in 2000 and reported outcomes of a large patient cohort with ACC (159 pts) who were treated between 1985 and 1997 with a median dose of 19.2 neutron Gy (1.05–1.7 neutron Gy/fraction; the total dose corresponds to approximately 60 Gy for normal tissues and approximately 150 Gy for salivary gland malignancies [29]). Ninety-five percent of these patients had gross residual or unresectable disease; 48% of patients had T4 disease. Local control in patients with gross residual disease was 57% at 5 years. However, local control showed considerable variations for various subsites in the head and neck with between 21% for nasopharynx to 67% and 68% for parotid and oral cavity, respectively [28]. Also, Douglas et al. reported a local control rate of 80% for ACCs of the lacrimal gland [28]. These results have recently been updated by Gensheimer et al. with a median follow-up of 75 months. Local control in these 11 patients was 80% at 3 and 5 years and an estimated 55% at 10 years [30]. Overall survival at 5 years is estimated to 71% in the complete cohort [28] and 90% in lacrimal gland ACC [30].

The European neutron centres have also shared their expertise from the 1980s and early 1990s. Patient numbers range from 8 to 72 with a follow-up between 36 and 52 months [31–33]. Patients with mostly gross residual or unresectable disease received between 13.7 and 19 nGy in 3–4 fractions per week. Local control rates in these cohorts range from 73% at 3 years to 64% at 5 years [31–33].

Stannard and colleagues recently reported outcomes of patients treated with neutrons at iThemba Labs in Cape Town. Among the 335 patients treated between 1989 and 2008, 5-year local control rates in the 108 patients were 55% in ACC and 47% in various high-grade histologies and 32% in squamous cell carcinoma (SCC) and 77% in patients with low-grade histologies [34].

Mixed-beam regimens with a combination of neutrons and photon techniques were also investigated. As Huber et al. demonstrated, the local control rates in patients with advanced tumour stages (T3/4: 86–90%) and gross residual or unresectable disease (up to 40%) treated with mixed-beam regimens or only photons were inferior (mixed, 40% at 5 years; photons, 34% at 5 years) to neutrons (75% at 5 years) [35].

Especially considering the risk profile of patients treated with neutrons (advanced T-stages, gross residual or unresectable disease), neutron-based treatments consistently showed very good control rates. Unfortunately though, these were bought at the expense of considerably higher late toxicities. The final report of the randomized RTOG-MRC trial described significantly more severe late toxicities in the neutron arm as compared to photons [25, 26]. These findings are consistent with published experience in other centres reporting higher-grade late toxicities (RTOG/EORTC ≥grade III) of around 14% (9%–23%) [27, 28, 30–33, 36]. Only Stannard and co-workers achieved comparatively low complication rates with less than 9% ≥grade III (CTCAE) [34].

Positive effects on local tumour control using high-LET radiation modalities in these early neutron studies led to the investigation of charged particle therapy for these tumours. In addition to their dosimetric advantages with steep dose gradients beyond the Bragg peak, steering of charged particle beams is much more convenient than for neutrons. In addition, heavy charged particles show a very narrow lateral penumbra and also increased RBE as compared to either photons or protons.

The initial experience with carbon ions for head and neck cancer of the group in HIMAC, Chiba (Japan), was very promising. In a prospective pilot trial, patients mostly suffering from advanced tumour stages (T4: 44%) were treated with either 52.8–64 GyE carbon ions (C12) in 16 fractions (4 weeks) or 70.2 GyE C12 in 18 fractions (6 weeks). Despite their unfavourable risk profiles, carbon ions led to a 5-year local control rate of 50% in ACCs and 35% in SCC. No grade III toxicity or higher was observed [37]. The group's prospective follow-up protocol prescribed either 57.6 GyE C12 or 64 GyE C12 (both in 16 fractions). With a median follow-up of 54 months, local control in all included patients ($N = 236$ pts) was 68%, 73% in ACC, 61–73% in adenocarcinoma and 61% in SCC. Corresponding 5-year overall survival was 47% in all series, 68% in ACC, 31–56% in adenocarcinoma and 17% in SCC. The Chiba group observed one case of grade IV late toxicity (ipsilateral loss of vision, 0.5%) but no other higher-grade late effects [38]. The recent update on results of the same treatment regimen in patients receiving carbon ions for ACC of the tongue base ($n = 18$) showed a 5-year local control rate of 92% albeit accompanied by the observation of three grade III late toxicities (17%: osteoradionecrosis, 2 pts; vascular haemorrhage, 1 pt) [39].

In the late 1990s, the Heidelberg/GSI group started treatment with a mixed-beam regimen of intensity-modulated radiotherapy (IMRT) plus carbon ion boost. Initial analyses on 29 patients showed very promising local control rates (77.5% at 4 years) as compared to IMRT alone (24.6% at 4 years). Overall survival did show a trend in favour of the mixed-beam regimen, although differences were not statistically significant at that time. All of these patients had gross residual or unresectable disease [40]. Updated results of these patient cohorts including 94% patients with T4 tumours confirmed the initial findings: with a median follow-up of 63 months, 5-year local control in the photon group is 40% vs. 60% in the mixed beam regi men. Also, 5-year overall survival in the mixed-beam group is superior to photons (79% vs. 60%). Higher-grade late toxicities remained consistently low (grade III: 5%) [41]. While most investigations support the combination of radical resection followed by high-dose radiotherapy in ACC both in the photon and in the particle world, ACCs with gross residual/inoperable disease seem to benefit from dose escalation to approximately 76–80 Gy BED: no significant differences could be detected in local control between patients following radical resection with gross residual tumour and patients with inoperable disease [41]. Prospective data from the COSMIC trial evaluating a combination of IMRT and dose-escalated carbon ion boost also showed promising local control rates with a consistently low toxicity profile [42–44]. However, comparison of toxicity in patients after resections vs. patients after biopsy-only suggests a more favourable toxicity profile in patients who underwent only biopsy and treated with definitive radiation. Local control does not seem to be compromised by definitive particle therapy [43]. Retrospective analysis of more than 300 patients with ACC treated with a mixed-beam regimen of IMRT plus carbon ion boost supports these findings. Moreover, there is no significant difference in control rates even in patients after macroscopically complete resections in this analysis. Looking at T4 tumours, no significant differences were found regarding control and survival rates between patients undergoing surgery (any margin status) followed by combined IMRT and C12 vs. patients undergoing radiotherapy (IMRT+C12) only. However, follow-up of the patients with macroscopically complete resections (R1) treated by combination radiotherapy is still short; hence these results need to be viewed with caution [45].

ACCs differ significantly from other MSGTs in their propensity to perineural spread, local recurrence and development of distant disease. The benefit of dose escalation in non-ACC histologies was subject of investigation in a retrospective analysis of 40 patients treated with a combination of carbon ions and IMRT between 2009 and 2013. In addition to a very high proportion of advanced tumour stages (T3/T4, 33%/46%) and a 58% of patients with gross residual disease, 40% of patients had also positive neck nodes. At a median follow-up of 26 months, 3-year local control was 82% in all series and 100% both for adenocarcinoma and acinic cell carcinoma, whereas local control was significantly lower (69%) in mucoepidermoid carcinoma (MEC). Overall survival at 3 years was 100% for acinic cell carcinoma, 88% for adenocarcinoma and 64% for MECs. One high-grade late toxicity (tissue necrosis) in a patient receiving concomitant chemoradiation was observed which did not result in long-term sequelae. Otherwise, no grade III and up to 13% grade II late toxicities, most commonly xerostomia grade I and hearing impairment grades I–II, were recorded [45].

With a regimen of either protons or carbon ions, the group at HIBMC (Hyogo) reported a 3-year local control rate and 3-year overall survival of 63% and 80% in their patient cohort with unresectable ACCs of the head and neck. Patients received either protons (65 Gy in 26 fractions or 70 Gy in 28 fractions) or carbon ions to 57.6 GyE (16 fractions) [46]. The update by Takagi and co-workers confirmed these results with a 3-year and 5-year local control of 84% and 75%, respectively, while the proportion of patients with T4 tumours was as high as 61% [47]. Late toxicities in this patient cohort were moderate, although 2 patients developed CNS necrosis grade 3, 3 patients loss of vision (grade 3), 11 patients osteoradionecrosis and 2 patients trismus [47].

Radiobiological properties of carbon ions are not constant over their penetration path. In a clinical scenario, target volumes for SGCs have typical dimensions of several centimetres, and they are treated with multiple beams from different angles. In consequence the tumour receives dose contributions from different beams, beam angles and intensities. Since the RBE in scanned carbon ions varies along the path and reaches its maximum around the Bragg peak, the overall relative biological effectiveness is not easily predictable and no longer intuitively calculable. To achieve a clinical effect which resembles that of a constant dose of photons (or of a constant dose of neutrons), complex mathematical models are used to calculate RBE at the millimetric (voxel) scale and increase absorbed dose where RBE is lower.

RBE models used in Japan and in Europe differ considerably; therefore the same nominal RBE-weighted dose may correspond to rather different treatments with different probabilities of local control and toxicity in different institutions. Patients with salivary gland malignancies treated with carbon ions in Germany have received a mix of photons to (1) the macroscopic tumours; (2) the area at risk of microscopic spread (including wide volumes for perineural invasion for ACC); and (3) macroscopically negative laterocervical lymph node level II (elective nodal irradiation, ENI) plus a boost of carbon ions to the macroscopic disease or tumour bed. Carbon ions were delivered at 3 Gy RBE per fraction with 5–6 fractions per week to a total dose of 18–24 Gy RBE. Patients treated in Japan have exclusively received carbon ions without ENI. Fraction size was either 3.6 Gy RBE or 4 Gy RBE to a total dose 57.6–64 Gy RBE in 16 fractions at 4 fractions per week. No case of isolated neck recurrence has been reported in Japanese series.

At CNAO (Pavia) Italy, carbon ion radiotherapy is performed since 2012, and 159 patients with ACC have been treated so far. Results have not yet been reported. The Japanese fractionation schedule was selected, but the nominal prescription dose was decided, analysing in silico plans delivered in Japan and optimized with the Kanai RBE models and recalculating them with the LEM model [48, 49]. Fraction size was 4.3 Gy RBE to a total dose 68.8 RBE in 16 fractions at 4 fractions per week. This nominal RBE-weighted dose is nominally higher than the highest dose employed at NIRS, however simulations correcting for different RBE models showed that it was intermediate between the 3.6 and 4 Gy RBE doses used in Japan.

At CNAO, ENI was employed only for selected cases of salivary gland malignancies in which the risk of microscopic lymphatic infiltration was considered high.

The uncertainty in the beneficial effect of ENI is not unusual in radiation oncology even for very common diseases (e.g. high-risk prostate cancer) and has no aspect that is peculiar to carbon ions; on the other hand, the existence of several RBE models introduces a degree of complexity that has to be taken into account. In the attempt to reproduce the results obtained by different institutions and in designing multicentric trials, it should be never forgotten that RBE-weighted doses cannot be trusted at nominal value if different RBE models are employed. At present, a large cooperative effort involving European and Japanese facilities is ongoing to standardize conversion of prescription doses and OAR dose constraints. A report from the International Commission on Radiation Units and Measurements (ICRU) on this issue is under development and is expected in the next months.

While carbon ion facilities are scarce, protons are still more easily available. Pommier and Linton reported outcomes of 23 and 26 patients treated with standard fractionated protons to 76 Gy (Boston) and 72 Gy (Indianapolis). Despite very advanced tumour stages (T4, 77% [50]) and high proportions of gross residual disease (87% [51]), the 2-year and 5-year local control rates were promising with 92% [50] and 93% [51], respectively. One has to bear in mind though that these control rates need to be confirmed in larger cohorts.

12.4 Re-Irradiation

While treatment of head and neck ACCs at the first diagnosis can be a challenge even using charged particle therapy, this is even more true in case of recurrent tumours and for patients already treated with a prior radiotherapy. In cases where radical resection is not an option, patients face the choice between palliative chemotherapy with response rates of up to 25% [52, 53] and undergoing another course of radiotherapy. In the past radiation oncologists were generally reluctant to use high-dose re-irradiation for fear of considerable early and late toxicity. In addition, recurrent tumours seemed to be more radiation-resistant than their initial clone [54]. Neutron and charged particle therapy produced encouraging local control rates albeit at considerable side-effects [55, 56]. In head and neck SCC, there is an emerging evidence that re-irradiation can lead to long-term local control in a carefully selected subset of patients [57–60] although the local control remains strongly dependent on the re-irradiation dose [57, 58, 61].

Early neutron data by Saroja on 40 patients treated for locally recurrent tumours at Fermilab after initial radiotherapy showed an impressive overall and complete remission rates (78% and 50%). Patients were treated with 18–27 nGy which led to an actuarial 2-year local control rate of 44% with a median overall survival of 9.3 months. Patients with complete remissions lived significantly longer (14.5 months) than patients with partial remissions (7.5 months). While acute toxicities were described as mild, significant severe late toxicities (grade III or higher) were observed in 25% of the patients: fistula, ulcer, tissue necrosis, osteoradionecrosis and severe fibrosis [56]. The UK neutron group achieved a complete response rate of 82% in the 28 patients treated with 15.6 nGy corresponding to a median local control of 29 months and median overall survival of 18 months [55].

More recent data on re-irradiation of heavily pretreated patients with recurrent MSGTs were also able to demonstrate a high objective response rates up to 57% [62, 63]. Median applied dose was 51 GyE (3 GyE/fraction) C12 corresponding to 63 Gy BED with a median interval of 61 months from the prior RT treatment. Median cumulative dose was 128 Gy BED. Despite high re-irradiation and cumulative doses, acute and late toxicities were tolerable [62, 63]. Two out of 52 treated patients developed central nervous system (CNS) necrosis grade III (CTCAE), and a corneal ulceration was described in one patient. Two patients experienced tissue necrosis, one of them developed a grade IV haemorrhage that was interventionally controlled and did not lead to any neurological sequelae. Both patients had received cumulative doses in excess of 128 Gy BED [63]. While local control is dose-dependent also in re-irradiation, so is the risk of late effects [56]. High-dose re-irradiation produced a 1-year local control rate of about 70% for a median time of 19 months. However, most of the local relapses after re-irradiation still occurred within the high-dose area. In view of these two cases mentioned above, further dose escalation should be used with caution, even with particle therapy [63].

12.5 Conclusion

Based on the existing published data, particle radiotherapy can be considered the best radiation modality for radical treatment of inoperable or macroscopically residual MSGTs. There is at present no reason to recommend debulking surgery as a routine procedure in ACC. The possibility of radical carbon ion therapy to achieve results identical to surgery in resectable tumours has to be considered as a hypothesis to be tested in clinical trials, ideally beginning with tumours in which the expected sequelae of surgery may impact severely on quality of life. The possibility to achieve the same results with proton therapy as with carbon ions has to be validated in larger cohorts. At present, proton therapy can be considered for radical treatment of macroscopic diseases if carbon ion RT is not available. Tumours resected with microscopically positive margins (R1) should also be treated with carbon ions. There are no data to support the use of carbon ions after a radical resection (R0), whereas the use of proton therapy may be adequate in order to spare toxicity to noninvolved OARs on the basis of dosimetric evaluation and normal tissue complication probability (NTCP) model predictions. Significant uncertainties remain on the optimal dose and fractionation as well as on the tolerance dose of OARs for radical carbon ion RT of MSGTs. There is no major disagreement on target volume with the one significant exception of the need of ENI. A consensus-guided contouring atlas by experienced institutions could be a valuable tool especially for new facilities. There is the need to strengthen international cooperation both for the pooled analysis of already delivered treatments and their outcomes and for prospective cooperative trial design.

References

1. Harrison LB, Armstrong JG, Spiro RH, Fass DE, Strong EW. Postoperative radiation therapy for major salivary gland malignancies. J Surg Oncol. 1990;45:52–5.
2. Choi Y, Kim SB, Yoon DH, Kim JY, Lee SW, Cho KJ. Clinical characteristics and prognostic factors of adenoid cystic carcinoma of the head and neck. Laryngoscope. 2013;123(6): 1430–8.
3. Chen AM, Bucci MK, Weinberg V, Garcia J, Quivey JM, Schechter NR, Phillips TL, Fu KK, Eisele DW. Adenoid cystic carcinoma of the head and neck treated by surgery with or without postoperative radiation therapy: prognostic features of recurrence. Int J Radiat Oncol Biol Phys. 2006;66(1):152–9.
4. Terhaard CH, Lubsen H, Rasch CR, Levendag PC, Kaanders HH, Tjho-Heslinga RE, van Den Ende PL, Burlage F, Dutch Head and Neck Oncology Cooperative Group. The role of radiotherapy in the treatment of malignant salivary gland tumors. Int J Radiat Oncol Biol Phys. 2005;61(1):103–11.
5. Choi KN, Rotman M, Aziz H, Potters L, Stark R, Rosenthal JC. Locally advanced paranasal sinus and nasopharynx tumors treated with hyperfractionated radiation and concomitant infusion cisplatin. Cancer. 1991;67(11):2748–52.
6. Hsieh CE, Lin CY, Lee LY, Yang LY, Wang CC, Wang HM, Chang JT, Fan KH, Liao CT, Yen TC, Fang KH, Tsang YM. Adding concurrent chemotherapy to postoperative radiotherapy improves locoregional control but Not overall survival in patients with salivary gland adenoid cystic carcinoma-a propensity score matched study. Radiat Oncol. 2016;11:47.
7. Samant S, van den Brekel MW, Kies MS, Wan J, Robbins KT, Rosenthal DI, Rasch C, Weber RS. Concurrent chemoradiation for adenoid cystic carcinoma of the head and neck. Head Neck. 2012;34(9):1263–8.
8. Haddad RI, Posner MR, Busse PM, Norris CM Jr, Goguen LA, Wirth LJ, Blinder R, Krane JF, Tishler RB. Chemoradiotherapy for adenoid cystic carcinoma: preliminary results of an organ sparing approach. Am J Clin Oncol. 2006;29(2):153–7.

9. Jensen AD, Poulakis M, Vanoni V, Uhl M, Chaudhri N, Federspil PA, Freier K, Krauss J, Debus J. Carbon ion therapy (C12) for high-grade malignant salivary gland tumors (MSGTs) of the head and neck: do non-ACCs profit from dose escalation? Radiat Oncol. 2016;11(1):90.
10. Adachi M, Mitsudo K, Yamamoto N, Hagiwara S, Shigetomi T, Fujimoto Y, Lai SY, Tohnai I. Chemoradiotherapy for maxillary sinus adenoid cystic carcinoma using superselective intra-arterial infusion via a superficial temporal artery. Head Neck. 2013;35(3):E89–93.
11. Hitre E, Budai B, Takácsi-Nagy Z, Rubovszky G, Tóth E, Remenár É, Polgár C, Láng I. Cetuximab and platinum-based chemoradio- or chemotherapy of patients with epidermal growth factor receptor expressing adenoid cystic carcinoma: a phase II trial. Br J Cancer. 2013;109(5):1117–22.
12. Jensen AD, Krauss J, Weichert W, Debus J, Münter MW. RadioImmunotherapy for adenoid cystic carcinoma: a single-institution series of combined treatment with cetuximab. Radiat Oncol. 2010;5:102.
13. RTOG 1008: a randomized phase II/phase III study of adjuvant concurrent radiation and chemotherapy versus radiation alone in resected high-risk malignant salivary gland tumors. Protocol information via https://www.rtog.org/ClinicalTrials/ProtocolTable/StudyDetails.aspx?study=1008. Accessed 25 July 2016.
14. Jensen A, Münter MW, Debus J. Partikeltherapie. In: Siewert JR, Rothmund M, Schumpelick V, editors. Praxis der Viszeralchirurgie. Onkologische Chirurgie. 3rd ed. Berlin: Springer; 2010.
15. Kanai T, Endo M, Minohara S, Miyahara N, Koyama-Ito H, Tomura H, Matsufuji N, Futami Y, Fukumura A, Hiraoka T, Furusawa Y, Ando K, Suzuki M, Soga F, Kawachi K. Biophysical characteristics of HIMAC clinical irradiation system for heavy-ion radiation therapy. Int J Radiat Oncol Biol Phys. 1999;44(1):201–10.
16. Krämer M, Scholz M. Treatment planning for heavy-ion radiotherapy: calculation and optimization of biologically effective dose. Phys Med Biol. 2000;45(11):3319–30.
17. Krämer M, Scholz M. Rapid calculation of biological effects in ion radiotherapy. Phys Med Biol. 2006;51(8):1959–70.
18. Gemmel A, Hasch B, Ellerbrock M, Weyrather WK, Krämer M. Biological dose optimization with multiple ion fields. Phys Med Biol. 2008;53(23):6991–7012.
19. Jäkel O, Krämer M, Karger CP, Debus J. Treatment planning for heavy ion radiotherapy: clinical implementation and application. Phys Med Biol. 2001;46(4):1101–16.
20. Inaniwa T, Kanematsu N, Matsufuji N, Kanai T, Shirai T, Noda K, Tsuji H, Kamada T, Tsujii H. Reformulation of a clinical-dose system for carbon-ion radiotherapy treatment planning at the National Institute of Radiological Sciences, Japan. Phys Med Biol. 2015;60(8):3271–86.
21. Kase Y, Kanai T, Matsufuji N, Furusawa Y, Elsässer T, Scholz M. Biophysical calculation of cell survival probabilities using amorphous track structure models for heavy-ion irradiation. Phys Med Biol. 2008;53(1):37–59.
22. Inaniwa T, Furukawa T, Kase Y, Matsufuji N, Toshito T, Matsumoto Y, Furusawa Y, Noda K. Treatment planning for a scanned carbon beam with a modified microdosimetric kinetic model. Phys Med Biol. 2010;55(22):6721–37.
23. Kanai T, Matsufuji N, Miyamoto T, Mizoe J, Kamada T, Tsuji H, Kato H, Baba M, Tsujii H. Examination of GyE system for HIMAC carbon therapy. Int J Radiat Oncol Biol Phys. 2006;64(2):650–6.
24. Glowa C, Karger CP, Brons S, Zhao D, Mason RP, Huber PE, Debus J, Peschke P. Carbon ion radiotherapy decreases the impact of tumor heterogeneity on radiation response in experimental prostate tumors. Cancer Lett. 2016;378(2):97–103.
25. Griffin TW, Pajak TF, Laramore GE, Duncan W, Richter MP, Hendrickson FR, Maor MH. Neutron vs photon irradiation of inoperable salivary gland tumors: results of an RTOG-MRC Cooperative Randomized Study. Int J Radiat Oncol Biol Phys. 1988;15(5):1085–90.
26. Laramore GE, Krall JM, Griffin TW, Duncan W, Richter MP, Saroja KR, Maor MH, Davis LW. Neutron versus photon irradiation for unresectable salivary gland tumors: final report of an RTOG-MRC randomized clinical trial. Radiation Therapy Oncology Group. Medical Research Council. Int J Radiat Oncol Biol Phys. 1993;27(2):235–40.

27. Buchholz TA, Shimotakahara SG, Weymuller EA Jr, Laramore GE, Griffin TW. Neutron radiotherapy for adenoid cystic carcinoma of the head and neck. Arch Otolaryngol Head Neck Surg. 1993;119(7):747–52.
28. Douglas JG, Laramore GE, Austin-Seymour M, Koh W, Stelzer K, Griffin TW. Treatment of locally advanced adenoid cystic carcinoma of the head and neck with neutron radiotherapy. Int J Radiat Oncol Biol Phys. 2000;46(3):551–7.
29. Rockhill JK, Laramore GE. Neutron radiotherapy. In: Gunderson LL, Tepper JE, editors. Clinical radiation oncology. 4th ed. Oxford: Elsevier; 2015. Chapter 20.
30. Gensheimer MF, Rainey D, Douglas JG, Liao JJ, Laramore GE, Jian-Amadi A, Chow LQ, Koh WJ, Parvathaneni U. Neutron radiotherapy for adenoid cystic carcinoma of the lacrimal gland. Ophthal Plast Reconstr Surg. 2013;29(4):256–60.
31. Duncan W, Orr JA, Arnott SJ, Jack WJ. Neutron therapy for malignant tumours of the salivary glands. A report of the Edinburgh experience. Radiother Oncol. 1987;8(2):97–104.
32. Pötter R, Prott FJ, Micke O, Haverkamp U, Wagner W, Willich N. Results of fast neutron therapy of adenoid cystic carcinoma of the salivary glands. Strahlenther Onkol. 1999;175(Suppl. 2):65–8.
33. Brackrock S, Krüll A, Röser K, Schwarz R, Riethdorf L, Alberti W. Neutron therapy, prognostic factors and dedifferentiation of adenoid cystic carcinomas (ACC) of salivary glands. Anticancer Res. 2005;25(2B):1321–6.
34. Stannard C, Vernimmen F, Carrara H, Jones D, Fredericks S, Hille J, de Kock E. Malignant salivary gland tumours: can fast neutron therapy results point the way to carbon ion therapy? Radiother Oncol. 2013;109(2):262–8.
35. Huber PE, Debus J, Latz D, Zierhut D, Bischof M, Wannenmacher M, Engenhart-Cabillic R. Radiotherapy for advanced adenoid cystic carcinoma: neutrons, photons or mixed beam? Radiother Oncol. 2001;59(2):161–7.
36. Douglas JG, Laramore GE, Austin-Seymour M, Koh WJ, Lindsley KL, Cho P, Griffin TW. Neutron radiotherapy for adenoid cystic carcinoma of minor salivary glands. Int J Radiat Oncol Biol Phys. 1996;36(1):87–93.
37. Mizoe JE, Tsujii H, Kamada T, Matsuoka Y, Tsuji H, Osaka Y, Hasegawa A, Yamamoto N, Ebihara S, Konno A, Organizing Committee for the Working Group for Head-And-Neck Cancer. Dose escalation study of carbon ion radiotherapy for locally advanced head-and-neck cancer. Int J Radiat Oncol Biol Phys. 2004;60(2):358–64.
38. Mizoe JE, Hasegawa A, Jingu K, Takagi R, Bessyo H, Morikawa T, Tonoki M, Tsuji H, Kamada T, Tsujii H, Okamoto Y, Organizing Committee for the Working Group for Head Neck Cancer. Results of carbon ion radiotherapy for head and neck cancer. Radiother Oncol. 2012;103(1):32–7.
39. Koto M, Hasegawa A, Takagi R, Ikawa H, Naganawa K, Mizoe JE, Jingu K, Tsujii H, Tsuji H, Kamada T, Okamoto Y, Organizing Committee for the Working Group for Head and Neck Cancer. Evaluation of the safety and efficacy of carbon ion radiotherapy for locally advanced adenoid cystic carcinoma of the tongue base. Head Neck. 2016;38(Suppl. 1):E2122–6.
40. Schulz-Ertner D, Nikoghosyan A, Didinger B, Münter M, Jäkel O, Karger CP, Debus J. Therapy strategies for locally advanced adenoid cystic carcinomas using modern radiation therapy techniques. Cancer. 2005;104(2):338–44.
41. Jensen AD, Nikoghosyan AV, Poulakis M, Höss A, Haberer T, Jäkel O, Münter MW, Schulz-Ertner D, Huber PE, Debus J. Combined intensity-modulated radiotherapy plus raster-scanned carbon ion boost for advanced adenoid cystic carcinoma of the head and neck results in superior locoregional control and overall survival. Cancer. 2015;121(17):3001–9.
42. Jensen AD, Nikoghosyan AV, Lossner K, Haberer T, Jäkel O, Münter MW, Debus J. COSMIC: a regimen of intensity modulated radiation therapy plus dose-escalated, raster-scanned carbon ion boost for malignant salivary gland tumors: results of the prospective phase 2 trial. Int J Radiat Oncol Biol Phys. 2015;93(1):37–46.
43. Jensen AD, Nikoghosyan A, Windemuth-Kieselbach C, Debus J, Münter MW. Combined treatment of malignant salivary gland tumours with intensity-modulated radiation therapy (IMRT) and carbon ions: COSMIC. BMC Cancer. 2010;10:546.

44. Jensen AD, Nikoghosyan AV, Lossner K, Herfarth KK, Debus J, Münter MW. IMRT and carbon ion boost for malignant salivary gland tumors: interim analysis of the COSMIC trial. BMC Cancer. 2012;12:163.
45. Jensen AD, Poulakis M, Nikoghosyan AV, Welzel T, Uhl M, Federspil PA, Freier K, Krauss J, Höss A, Haberer T, Jäkel O, Münter MW, Schulz-Ertner D, Huber PE, Debus J. High-LET radiotherapy for adenoid cystic carcinoma of the head and neck: 15 years' experience with raster-scanned carbon ion therapy. Radiother Oncol. 2016;118(2):272–80.
46. Morimoto K, Demizu Y, Hashimoto N, Mima M, Terashima K, Fujii O, Otsuki N, Murakami M, Fuwa N, Nibu K. Particle radiotherapy using protons or carbon ions for unresectable locally advanced head and neck cancers with skull base invasion. Jpn J Clin Oncol. 2014;44(5):428–34.
47. Takagi M, Demizu Y, Hashimoto N, Mima M, Terashima K, Fujii O, Jin D, Niwa Y, Morimoto K, Akagi T, Daimon T, Sasaki R, Hishikawa Y, Abe M, Murakami M, Fuwa N. Treatment outcomes of particle radiotherapy using protons or carbon ions as a single-modality therapy for adenoid cystic carcinoma of the head and neck. Radiother Oncol. 2014;113(3):364–70.
48. Molinelli S, Magro G, Mairani A, Matsufuji N, Kanematsu N, Inaniwa T, Mirandola A, Russo S, Mastella E, Hasegawa A, Tsuji H, Yamada S, Vischioni B, Vitolo V, Ferrari A, Ciocca M, Kamada T, Tsujii H, Orecchia R, Fossati P. Dose prescription in carbon ion radiotherapy: how to compare two different RBE-weighted dose calculation systems. Radiother Oncol. 2016;120(2):307–12.
49. Fossati P, Molinelli S, Matsufuji N, Ciocca M, Mirandola A, Mairani A, Mizoe J, Hasegawa A, Imai R, Kamada T, Orecchia R, Tsujii H. Dose prescription in carbon ion radiotherapy: a planning study to compare NIRS and LEM approaches with a clinically-oriented strategy. Phys Med Biol. 2012;57:7543–54.
50. Linton OR, Moore MG, Brigance JS, Summerlin DJ, McDonald MW. Proton therapy for head and neck adenoid cystic carcinoma: initial clinical outcomes. Head Neck. 2015;37(1):117–24.
51. Pommier P, Liebsch NJ, Deschler DG, Lin DT, McIntyre JF, Barker FG 2nd, Adams JA, Lopes VV, Varvares M, Loeffler JS, Chan AW. Proton beam radiation therapy for skull base adenoid cystic carcinoma. Arch Otolaryngol Head Neck Surg. 2006;132(11):1242–9.
52. Dreyfuss AI, Clark JR, Fallon BG, Posner MR, Norris CM Jr, Miller D. Cyclophosphamide, doxorubicin, and cisplatin combination chemotherapy for advanced carcinomas of salivary gland origin. Cancer. 1987;60(12):2869–72.
53. Laurie SA, Ho AL, Fury MG, Sherman E, Pfister DG. Systemic therapy in the management of metastatic or locally recurrent adenoid cystic carcinoma of the salivary glands: a systematic review. Lancet Oncol. 2011;12(8):815–24.
54. Weichselbaum RR, Beckett MA, Schwartz JL, Dritschilo A. Radioresistant tumor cells are present in head and neck carcinomas that recur after radiotherapy. Int J Radiat Oncol Biol Phys. 1988;15(3):575–9.
55. Errington RD, Catterall M. Re-irradiation of advanced tumors of the head and neck with fast neutrons. Int J Radiat Oncol Biol Phys. 1986;12(2):191–5.
56. Saroja KR, Hendrickson FR, Cohen L, Mansell J, Lennox A. Re-irradiation of locally recurrent tumors with fast neutrons. Int J Radiat Oncol Biol Phys. 1988;15(1):115–21.
57. Salama JK, Vokes EE, Chmura SJ, Milano MT, Kao J, Stenson KM, Witt ME, Haraf DJ. Long-term outcome of concurrent chemotherapy and reirradiation for recurrent and second primary head-and-neck squamous cell carcinoma. Int J Radiat Oncol Biol Phys. 2006;64(2):382–91.
58. Lee N, Chan K, Bekelman JE, Zhung J, Mechalakos J, Narayana A, Wolden S, Venkatraman ES, Pfister D, Kraus D, Shah J, Zelefsky MJ. Salvage re-irradiation for recurrent head and neck cancer. Int J Radiat Oncol Biol Phys. 2007;68(3):731–40.
59. Tanvetyanon T, Padhya T, McCaffrey J, Zhu W, Boulware D, Deconti R, Trotti A. Prognostic factors for survival after salvage reirradiation of head and neck cancer. J Clin Oncol. 2009;27(12):1983–91.
60. Janot F, de Raucourt D, Benhamou E, Ferron C, Dolivet G, Bensadoun RJ, Hamoir M, Géry B, Julieron M, Castaing M, Bardet E, Grégoire V, Bourhis J. Randomized trial of postoperative reirradiation combined with chemotherapy after salvage surgery compared with salvage surgery alone in head and neck carcinoma. J Clin Oncol. 2008;26(34):5518–23.

61. Haraf DJ, Weichselbaum RR, Vokes EE. Re-irradiation with concomitant chemotherapy of unresectable recurrent head and neck cancer: a potentially curable disease. Ann Oncol. 1996;7(9):913–8.
62. Jensen AD, Nikoghosyan A, Ellerbrock M, Ecker S, Debus J, Münter MW. Re-irradiation with scanned charged particle beams in recurrent tumours of the head and neck: acute toxicity and feasibility. Radiother Oncol. 2011;101(3):383–7.
63. Jensen AD, Poulakis M, Nikoghosyan AV, Chaudhri N, Uhl M, Münter MW, Herfarth KK, Debus J. Re-irradiation of adenoid cystic carcinoma: analysis and evaluation of outcome in 52 consecutive patients treated with raster-scanned carbon ion therapy. Radiother Oncol. 2015;114(2):182–8.

Systemic Therapy in Salivary Gland Carcinoma

13

Laura D. Locati, S. Alfieri, and Lisa Licitra

Abbreviations

ACC	Adenoid cystic carcinoma
ADT	Androgen deprivation therapy
AR	Androgen receptor
CAB	Combined androgen blockade
CDDP	Cisplatin
CI	Confidence interval
DFI	Disease-free interval
ECOG	Eastern Cooperative Oncology Group
EGFR	Epidermal growth factor receptor
EORTC	European Organisation for Research and Treatment of Cancer
FGFR	Fibroblast growth factor receptor
FISH	Fluorescent in situ hybridization
HDAC	Histone deacetylase
IGFR	Insulin growth factor receptor
IHC	Immunohistochemistry
IL2R	Interleukin-2 receptor
LHRH	Luteinizing hormone-releasing hormone
MEC	Mucoepidermoid carcinoma

L. D. Locati (✉) · S. Alfieri
Head and Neck Cancer Medical Oncology Department,
Fondazione IRCCS Istituto Nazionale dei Tumori of Milan, Milan, Italy
e-mail: Laura.Locati@istitutotumori.mi.it

L. Licitra
Head and Neck Cancer Medical Oncology Department,
Fondazione IRCCS Istituto Nazionale dei Tumori of Milan, Milan, Italy

University of Milan, Milan, Italy

© Springer Nature Switzerland AG 2019

L. Licitra, L. D. Locati (eds.), *Salivary Gland Cancer*,
https://doi.org/10.1007/978-3-030-02958-6_13

NOS	Not other specified
ORR	Overall response rate
OS	Overall survival
PCa	Prostate cancer
PD-1	Programmed death-1
PDGFR	Platelet-derived growth factor receptor
PD-L1	Programmed death-ligand 1
PFS	Progression-free survival
RFA	Radiofrequency ablation
RT	Radiotherapy
SDC	Salivary duct carcinoma
SGC	Salivary gland cancer
TACE	Trans-arterial chemoembolization
TGF-β	transforming growth factor-β
TKI	Tyrosine kinase inhibitor
VEGF	Vascular endothelial growth factor
VEGFR	Vascular endothelial growth factor receptor

13.1 Introduction

As reported in Chap. 1, the classification of SGC is complex, including more than 20 histotype variants, almost each one characterized by peculiar molecular profile as well as a different clinical behavior. In the clinical practice, metastatic ACC is the most common form of SGCs with medical oncologist deal. Distant metastasis from other histotypes (here defined as non-ACC) as SDC; adenocarcinoma, NOS; MEC; etc. is less frequent, and data on systemic treatments are generally few. Moreover, ACC and non-ACC tumors have a different clinical behavior in most of the cases. ACC is usually a slow-growing disease, having patients a prolonged survival, while non-ACC cases could be very aggressive with a rapid dismal outcome. These differences in the natural history pave the way to different clinical issues in the management and potentially diverse clinical approaches. For all these reasons, we have decided to separate the description of systemic treatments in ACC patients versus non-ACC patients.

13.2 ACC

The most important question to be addressed with regard to relapsed and/or metastatic ACC patients is if a prompt management of disease may be worthwhile or not. This is because ACC is characterized by a typically slow-growing and indolent evolution in the majority of cases, and, moreover, effective treatments are completely lacking. Recent biological and clinical evidences seem to have identified two "groups" of ACC patients: one group with lung metastasis (plus or minus local relapse) with a better prognosis and the other group with liver, bone, and distant metastasis in atypical sites (e.g., skin, brain) with an aggressive disease with worse outcome [1]. The solid variant (or with solid component as the most represented part of the tumor) of ACCs has a worse prognosis in respect to the other histotype variants such as cribriform and tubular. These latter seem to be a completely different tumor either from a genetic and phenotypic point of view. Notably, cribriform and tubular variants have mutations mostly in the *MYB* oncogene pathway, while the solid variant is strongly associated with *NOTCH-1*-activating mutations [2]. This dichotomous genetic situation is mirroring in a corresponding, totally different, clinical phenotype: solid ACCs have worse prognosis with higher stage at diagnosis, higher probability of relapse, and shorter survival and propensity to spread in the liver and bone; on the other hand, patients with no solid ACCs have better outcomes with primary diffusion in the lung and longer survival. Considering that the most common presentation of advanced ACCs is just with lung metastases, it could be reasonable to provide a "wait and see" strategy, reserving active therapy only to patients with symptomatic and/or rapidly progressing disease [3] or those with worse prognosis. In this context, the role of locoregional treatments (e.g., lung metastasectomy) is still to be defined, especially in terms of final outcome due to few available data and lack of clinical trials. Lung metastasectomy could have a role in very selected patients with a disease-free interval (DFI) longer than 36 months between the diagnosis of primary tumor and the appearance of distant metastases. Indeed, the 5-year and the 10-year overall survival (OS) for patients with DFI less than 36 months was 47.7 (95% CI 29.1–64.2%) and 21.9% (95% CI 8.4–39.5%) versus 76.5% (95% CI 63.3–85.4%) and 51.1% (95% CI 35–65.1%) in those patients with DFI more than 36 months ($p = 0.007$). Complete resection is another important factor that could potentially influence the outcome of patients (5-year and 10-year OS was 69.5% and 46.1% in case of complete resection versus 51.3% and no survivors, respectively, in presence of residual disease, $p = 0.004$) [4]. The number of metastatic nodes is not an absolute limit to metastasectomy albeit it does not compromise the feasibility of a complete resection. It is not clear whether an incomplete resection could result in a relief in case of symptomatic patients although in these cases other locoregional approaches, as RT or RFA, could also take into account. No data are available about the long-term effects of these locoregional therapies on the rest of healthy lung tissue. Long life expectancy of our patients should always be taken into consideration before clinical decision since treatment-induced fibrosis could compromise the respiratory reserve, possibly worsening the quality of life of long-living survivors. The employ of other locoregional treatments, as TACE or RFA or RT, could be reserved for local disease control (e.g., symptoms, selective growth of the lesions) or symptom palliation.

13.3 Chemotherapy

13.3.1 Monochemotherapy

ACC is "historically" judged as a chemo-refractory tumor. Table 13.1 summarizes all trials conducted with monochemotherapy in ACC patients. It is quite clear as the ORR is globally ranging from 0 to 15.4% [3, 5]. The result of ORR at 70%, reached in one study with CDDP, does not reflect the real outcome of CDDP in this setting at all. In fact, another study with the same drug demonstrated that ORR of CDDP was 15.4% (two partial responses out of 13 ACC patients) that was much more "realistic" and similar to what is observed with all other monochemotherapy-based regimens. The most important message to be extrapolated by Table 13.1 is that some drugs as CDDP and doxorubicin are active, and their use is supported by clinical evidence, although weak; other compounds, such as paclitaxel and gemcitabine, have no activity, and therefore their use should not be advised in oncologists' daily clinical practice. Recently a phase II trial with eribulin 1.4 mg/m^2 i.v. on days 1 and 8 q3 weeks was published. Twenty nine patients, 11 of whom with ACC, were enrolled. Objective responses were reported in three cases, two ACC patients and one case of carcinoma ex pleomorphic adenoma. Activity was described both in chemo-naive and pretreated patients [6].

13.3.2 Polichemotherapy

Table 13.2 reported five trials in which few ACC patients (45 in total) were treated with polichemotherapy-based regimens. CDDP, anthracyclines, 5-fluorouracil, cyclophosphamide, vincristine, vinorelbine, and bleomycin resulted as moderately active and well-tolerated drugs when used in different combinations within this

Table 13.1 All clinical trials conducted in ACC patients with a single-agent chemotherapy-based regimen

Drug	Study population	Drug dose and schedule	ORR% (Nb responders patients/Nb total patients)
Mitoxantrone	18	12 mg/sm q21 days	5.5 (1/18)
Gemcitabine	21	1250 mg/sm (days 1 and 8) q21 days	0
Epirubicin	20	30 mg/sm weekly	10 (2/20)
Mitoxantrone	32	14 mg/sm q21 days	12.5 (4/32)
Cisplatin	10	80–100 mg/sm q4–6 weeks	70 (7/10)
Cisplatin	13	100 mg/sm q21 days	15.4 (2/13)
Paclitaxel	14	200 mg/sm q21 days	0
Vinorelbine	13	30 mg/sm weekly	15.4 (2/13)

ORR overall response rate, *Nb* number, *sm* square meter

tumor setting. In literature, it is possible to extrapolate information regarding the use of polichemotherapy in ACCs from other 13 trials conducted in unselected histotypes of SGCs whose 107 patients were ACCs. All data confirmed cisplatin and doxorubicin as those agents with better activity and acceptable safety [3]. It seems that a polichemotherapy leads to a higher activity. Indeed, it showed higher ORR in comparison to monochemotherapy regimens (Table 13.2). This was also confirmed in other studies which tested a triple agent-based chemotherapy [cyclophosphamide, doxorubicin, CDDP, q3–4 weeks, in a combination known as CAP regimen] with a response rate ranging from 18.1 to 62.5% at maximum [3]. Laurie et al. [3] reported an ORR of 25% (95% CI 11–39%) (9 responders out of the 36 included ACCs) for studies using CAP regimen in ACCs. This concept found confirmation even when four drugs (cyclophosphamide, doxorubicin, cisplatin, 5-fluorouracil) were administered concomitantly in seven ACC patients obtaining a 42.8% (3/7) of ORR without any advantage in survival outcomes. On the other hand, this study showed a great side effect rate with two drug-related deaths: one due to neutropenia and sepsis after the first chemotherapy cycle and one because of doxorubicin cardiotoxicity (after two chemo cycles). In this scenario, there is no consensus about which and how many drugs have to be considered as the best option for systemic treatment in ACC patients. Therefore in routinary clinical practice, based on this complex risk/benefit balance, the choice between a single agent versus a combined chemo regimen is simply driven by the general clinical condition and patients' performance status, reserving a polichemotherapy to those patients in better status.

Table 13.2 All clinical trials conducted in ACC patients with a polichemotherapy-based regimen

Drug	Study population	Drug dose and schedule	ORR % (Nb responders/Nb total patients)
CDDP vs CDDP Bleomycin Doxorubicin	10 vs 9	*CDDP*: 50–120 mg/sm (q28 days) vs *CDDP*: 20 mg/sm (days 1 → 5) *Bleomycin*: 30 mg (days 1 → 5) *Doxorubicin*: 50 mg/sm (day 1) q21 days	0 vs 33 (3/9)
CDDP 5-fluorouracil	11	*CDDP*: 100 mg/sm (day 1) *5FU*: 1 g/sm/day (days 1 → 4)	0
Epirubicin CDDP 5-fluorouracil	8	*Epirubicin*: 50 mg/sm *CDDP*: 60 mg/sm *5FU*: 200 mg/sm/day q21 days	12.5 (1/8)
Cyclophosphamide Vincristine 5-fluorouracil	8	*Cyclophosphamide*: 1000 mg/sm (day 1) *Vincristine*: 1 mg (days 1 and 4) *5FU*: 750 mg/sm (days 1 → 4) q28 days	25 (2/8)
Vinorelbine CDDP	9	*VNB*: 25 mg/sm (days 1and 8) *CDDP*: 80 mg/sm (day 1) q21 days	44.4 (4/9)

ACC adenoid cystic carcinoma, *ORR* overall response rate, *Nb* number, *sm* square meter, *CDDP* cisplatin, *5FU* 5-fluorouracil, *VNB* vinorelbine

The most used chemotherapy combination is a double-based regimen including CDDP and doxorubicin. Starting from this unsatisfactory context, the selection of ACC patients eligible to chemotherapy remains a mainstay in the clinical decision-making process. In all chemo combinations, CDDP (if feasible) should be preferred to carboplatin considering that all studies with carboplatin have showed a lower response rate [3]. In the lack of any objective response, no more than four courses of chemotherapy should be administered since the probability to have a late response after six cycles is practically null.

Starting from this unsatisfactory context, the selection of ACC patients eligible to chemotherapy remains a mainstay to bearing in mind in the clinical decision-making process. Good performance status (ECOG scale of 0–1), no significant comorbidities, and a symptomatic/rapidly progressive disease more advice physicians to start with active treatment. If feasible, CDDP plus doxorubicin is a good option as first line; there are not enough evidence to support the use of a second-line chemotherapy. Enrollment of patients in clinical trials is strongly recommended.

13.3.3 Tyrosine Kinase Inhibitors and New Agents

Low rate of DNA mutations (0.3 mutations/megabase) characterizes ACCs, and, therefore, potentially druggable targets are still lacking [5]. The most recurrent gene alteration of ACCs (50–60% of cases) regards *MYB* oncogene where t(6:9) *MYB-NFIB* translocation is the most frequent one. *MYB-NFIB* regulates genes involved in cell cycle control, DNA replication/repair, and RNA processing. The *MYB-NFIB* fusion is regulated through *AKT*-dependent signaling induced by *IGF1R* overexpression, and it is downregulated upon *IGF1R* inhibition. The *MYB-NFIB*-induced transcriptional program affects critical oncogenic mediators that are normally controlled by *MYC* and is reversed by pharmacological inhibition of *IGF1R*. This is very intriguing in the hypothesis of a tailored approach [7]. To date, there are no drugs active on *MYB* even if two trials (NCT00002592 and NCT00780052) are testing *MYB* antisense oligonucleotides in hematologic malignancies. In the last few years, many target therapies have been studied in this cancer setting. *KIT* and *EGFR* are frequently overexpressed but rarely mutated or amplified. Imatinib was tested but failed to show any activity. Indeed, the lack of *KIT* somatic mutations in ACCs could justify the lack of activity of imatinib. All of the anti-EGFR family members (lapatinib, gefitinib, cetuximab, and trastuzumab) failed to detect any responses in ACCs. Dasatinib, a small molecule of SRC-family protein tyrosine kinase inhibitors (TKIs), combined with multi-TKIs including *KIT*, showed a low response rate (2.5%) with disease control in half of the cases. Dovitinib is a TKI anti-fibroblast growth factor receptor-1 (FGFR-1). This receptor is commonly highly expressed and activated in ACCs. Despite the biological premises, dovitinib showed a very modest response rate (4.5%). The unsatisfactory results of tailored agents have led to focusing on new compounds characterized by a completely different action profile. Literature evidences [5] suggest a linkage between the VEGF and a worse outcome in SGCs, supporting the possible use of anti-angiogenic drugs in ACCs. From now on, sunitinib, sorafenib, and axitinib have been studied in ACC population, unfortunately with lower results than what is expected: 0%, 11, and 9% in terms of ORR, respectively. In the trial with axitinib, the tumor samples of two responding patients harbored both *MYB/NFIB* fusions as well as the 4q12 amplification. This latter increases the gene copy number for three molecular targets of axitinib: PDGFR-A, VEGFR2, and KIT. This evidence supports the hypothesis of oncogenic dependence upon *PDGFR-A/KDR/KIT* signaling and susceptibility to axitinib by a subset of ACC. The first randomized trial comparing axitinib to placebo has been recently completed, but preliminary data are not available yet. Disappointing results have been also reported for nintedanib, regorafenib, and pazopanib [5].

Many other targeted agents (e.g., bortezomib, everolimus, nelfinavir, MK-2206, and vorinostat) have been studied in ACCs [5]. Among them, vorinostat, a histone deacetylase (HDAC) inhibitor, has to be cited because of its activity in 7% of cases and its promising role in upregulating PD-1 or PD-L1 expression (targets of the most recent immune modulators). In fact, a trial (NCT02538510) with combination of vorinostat and pembrolizumab is currently ongoing in advanced SGCs (ACCs included).

Combining multiple agents has been revealed as a successful strategy. In fact, tailored drugs with conventional chemotherapies resulted in higher ORR: CDDP + imatinib (vs imatinib alone), doxorubicin + bortezomib (vs bortezomib alone), and cetuximab + CDDP-based chemoradiotherapy vs chemotherapy alone. In all of these cases, the benefit was given by the addition of traditional chemotherapies based on the absent (or very low) activity of targeted agents when used alone [5].

Several progresses have been made in the recent years in the therapeutic modulation of the tumor-immune system especially in lung cancer, melanoma, and renal cancer. PD-L1 expression is very low in ACC, about 2%. A retrospective analysis on 21 patients did not show any PD-L1 expression on tumor cells. On the other hand, 60% of primary tumor samples and 72% of distant metastases demonstrated a PD-L2 expression. Intratumoral lymphocyte infiltrate was present in 42% of patients both in primary and metastatic lesions. In this context, PD-L1 expression has been reported in 86% and 80% of immune cells in primary and distant metastases, respectively. The presence of intratumoral lymphocyte infiltrate correlates with the expression of some genes such as *SyK* ($p = 0.04$), *IL2RB* ($p = 0.02$), and *TGFbeta* ($p = 0.02$). From these data the employ of an anti-PD-1 seems to be more rationale than anti-PD-L1 [8]. PD-1 inhibitors, as pembrolizumab, are currently under evaluation in several malignant diseases, including SGCs. In a phase 1b trial KEYNOTE-028, the use of pembrolizumab did not lead to any response in ACC cases [5].

13.4 Systemic Chemotherapy in Non-ACC Histotypes

Unlike ACC, the watchful waiting is rarely considered in this group of tumors, and systemic chemotherapy is generally started at diagnosis. Locoregional treatments could be employed for symptom control since disease progression is rapid in most of the cases, and systemic therapy is advisable, although a clear evidence of benefit is still lacking also in this context. Several trials including different histotypes have been conducted, so data on single tumor type could be extrapolated from these studies. MEC, adenocarcinoma, NOS, and SDC are the histotypes numerically more consistent included in these studies. Data on chemotherapy activity from other histotypes, such as acinic cell carcinoma, clear cell carcinoma, etc., are anecdotal. CDDP alone or in combination with other agents is the most common drug used also for non-ACC histotypes. Two responses (ORR 17%) in 12 non-ACC subjects were reported in a phase II trial with CDDP 100 mg/mq q21 days. In a phase II study with CAP, six partial responses were reported (ORR 27%, 95% CI 27%–50%) among 22 enrolled patients, including 1 patient with MEC [5]. Three responses (two complete and one partial) were observed among five patients with adenocarcinoma enrolled in another trial and treated with CAP. The addition of 5FU (500 mg/mq day 1 and 2) to CAP (cyclophosphamide 500 mg/mq; doxorubicin 50 mg/mq; cisplatin 40 mg/mq) every 3–4 weeks was tested in 17 patients of whom 16 are evaluable for toxicity and response. Nine out of 16 patients had an adenocarcinoma, NOS. The ORR was 44% including four responders out of nine patients with adenocarcinoma, NOS. Although the ORR was higher in comparison to other regimens, toxicities were consistent, and two toxic deaths were reported. The use of this regimen did not proceed further in the clinical practice. More recently, new combinations with CDDP or carboplatin have been tested. The regimen with gemcitabine 1000 mg/mq day 1–8 plus CDDP 70 mg/mq q21 tested in 30 evaluable patients with mixed histologies showed one complete remission and seven partial responses (ORR 24%, 95% CI 11%–42%). Although the study did not meet the predefined criteria for being declared an active regimen, an interesting activity emerged for the eight patients with adenocarcinoma, NOS, for whom one complete response and two partial responses were reported. A response rate of 47% with a median OS of 13.6 months was reported with CDDP 80 mg/mq plus vinorelbine 25 mg/mq days 1–8 q3 weeks [5]. More recently, the same regimen was studied as first-line therapy in 40 patients with different histologies with an ORR of 35% and a median OS of 16.9 months. Looking at specific histotypes as adenocarcinoma, NOS (ten patients), and MEC (six patients), ORR was 40% and 33%, respectively, supporting the activity of this combination in these histotypes [9]. The combination of carboplatin AUC 6 plus paclitaxel 200 mg/mq q3 weeks has been also evaluated. Response rate was 39% in 18 patients with SDC out of 38 patients treated. This study includes the largest number of patients with SDC ever enrolled, so this combination should be preferable in this subgroup of patients. Data on the activity of paclitaxel as monotherapy 200 mg/mq were available in 45 patients. Responses were observed in 3 out of 14 MEC patients (21%) and in 5 out of 17 patients (29%) with adenocarcinoma, NOS, supporting the use of paclitaxel in these histotypes [5].

13.4.1 New Treatments

Multiple targets potentially useful for a tailored approach have been identified in the last few years. Androgen receptor (AR) is one of the most studied marker, and we will extensively talk about it in Sect. 13.5. *HER2* is another largely investigated target. It is overexpressed in about 44% and amplified in about 35–50% of the SDCs

[10]. HER2 overexpression and amplification have been reported also in other histotypes, although rarely. *RAS*, *EGFR*, *MET*, *FGFR*, *BRAF*, *RET*, *ALK*, and others are potentially druggable targets studied. Interestingly, within the *RAS* family, only mutations in the exon 2 and 3 of the *H-RAS* gene have been reported (20–25% of the cases), while no mutation has been identified in *K*- and *N-RAS*. The mutation rate for the other genes reported above is very low being less than 10% of the cases [11].

Trastuzumab is an anti-HER2 monoclonal antibody, approved for HER2-positive breast cancer as well as for stomach and gastroesophageal junction adenocarcinoma. Trastuzumab was investigated within a phase II trial in 14 subjects. HER2 was overexpressed in 10 out of 14 cases; only one long-lasting partial response was described in a case of MEC with HER2 overexpression, and no data on HER2 amplification status was reported. Seven patients with a progressive SDC were retrospectively reviewed. HER2 overexpression and amplification were present in 100% and in 43% of the cases, respectively. There was a complete response lasting for 3 years in one patient out of the three patients who had been treated with trastuzumab. The *HER2* gene status of the responding patient was unknown. Activity of trastuzumab has been reported in five patients with metastatic SDC, HER2 3+ and amplified by FISH in all cases: one patient had a complete remission lasting 52 months during treatment with trastuzumab, two patients experienced a partial response, and progression was reported in other two cases. Trastuzumab was also employed as adjuvant treatment in eight patients with stage IVA disease: with a median follow-up of 27 months (range 8–48 months), five out of eight patients were alive and with no evidence of disease after more than 2 years of treatment, while in other three cases, there had been a disease relapse [5].

Recently, the activity of targeted drugs, such as entrectinib and crizotinib [12] and cabozantinib and regorafenib [5], was reported in the presence of specific genetic, fusion- or duplication-based, alterations (e.g., *ETV-NTRK3* for entrectinib and crizotinib, *NCOA4-RET* for cabozantinib, BRAF kinase domain duplication for regorafenib).

Anti-angiogenic agents exert some activity in non-ACC tumors. VEGF expression has been reported in SGCs, particularly in MEC and in squamous cell carcinomas, and it seems to correlate with a worse outcome, representing a potential target for therapy. Recently, a phase II trial with sorafenib 800 mg daily has been carried out in 37 subjects (19 ACC and 18 non-ACC) with recurrent and/or metastatic SGCs. A higher ORR was reported in the non-ACC population in comparison with the ACC group (22% vs 11%). Partial remission was reported in one SDC, one adenocarcinoma, NOS, one high-grade MEC, and one poorly differentiated carcinoma. The anti-angiogenic activity seems to be the main mechanism of action, supported by the lack of correlation between the activity of sorafenib and the expression of its targets as well as the overexpression of PDGFR-β in the stromal component of responding cases. However, results with more potent anti-angiogenic compounds, such as pazopanib, were not satisfactory. Indeed, pazopanib was tested at 800 mg daily in a phase II trial with 49 ACC and 20 non-ACC patients (including 11 adenocarcinomas). Pazopanib showed 1 partial response (6%) and 13 stable diseases (72%) in the non-ACC group with 6-months progression-free survival (PFS) > 40% [5].

PD-L1 is upregulated in high-grade SGCs, being expressed in 36% of carcinomas ex pleomorphic adenoma, in 30% of SDCs, in 10% of large cell carcinomas, and in 8% of adenocarcinoma, NOS [13]. Pembrolizumab, an anti-PD1 antibody, was tested in a phase 1b trial, KEYNOTE-028 [5]. In this trial, the patient population was enriched for PD-L1 expression, and the objective responses were observed in histotypes with a high PD-L1 expression [13] and a higher mutational load [14]. Three partial responses (11.5%) were reported, two in cases of adenocarcinoma and one in high-grade serous carcinoma. Stable disease was the best response in 12 cases (46.2%, 95% CI 26.6–66.6). Six-months survival was 70.4% and PFS was 20.7%. Drug-related adverse events were common in 84.6% of cases: diarrhea, reduced appetite, pruritus, and fatigue were the most common events (≥15% of the cases). Three patients experienced a toxicity higher than grade 3 with one case evolved in a toxic death due to lung inflammatory complications. The evaluation of pembrolizumab activity is currently ongoing within the phase II basket trial KEYNOTE-158 (NCT02628067). Several trials testing the activity of a single agent or combination of more immune modulators are ongoing. The efficacy of nivolumab (monoclonal antibody anti-PD1) alone (NCT031332038) or combined with ipilimumab (NCT 03146650) is the object of two trials. The primary endpoint of the first trial is to test the activity of nivolumab in 92 patients including SGC patients. Median PFS is the primary objective of the second study in which 63 subjects have been planned. The evaluation of PD-L1 expression is not mandatory as inclusion criteria in both trials: patients with progressing metastatic SGCs could be enrolled. The activity of pembrolizumab plus vorinostat is under evaluation in another trial (NCT02538510), as mentioned above (Sect. 13.3.3).

13.5 Androgen Deprivation Therapy

SDC is characterized by the AR expression, which is reported in 75–99% of cases. AR is also reported in about 21–33% of adenocarcinomas, NOS, being AR the hallmark of these two histotypes. The prevalence of AR expression varies substantially among different subtypes of SGCs, except for SDC and adenocarcinoma, NOS, where the expression is generally strong. In MEC, acinic cell carcinoma and ACCs, the AR expression is ranging from 0 to 20% [15]. Nuclear AR expression based on immunohistochemistry (IHC) is the most widely used marker of active AR signaling. Although a minimum of 1% of immunoreactive tumor cell nuclei was required to consider a sample as AR positive, the amount of immunoreactive cells seems to correlate with response to androgen deprivation therapy (ADT), similarly to prostate cancer (PCa). For this reason, we have proposed a combined score to assess the AR expression (Table 13.3) [16]. The staining intensity and the percentage of positive nuclei were evaluated, with a final score deriving from the sum of these latter. Only patients with a high score of AR expression are the best candidate to ADT. Activity of ADT has been largely investigated in the last few years. In 2011, a Dutch group presented their series of ten SDC patients treated with bicalutamide 150 mg daily [only one patient received both bicalutamide and luteinizing hormone-releasing hormone (LHRH) analog]: the results were two partial responses and

Table 13.3 Combined score proposed to assess the androgen receptor (AR) expresson

Staining intensity		Staining extent in nuclei		Combined score	
Negative	0	<10%	0	Negative	0
Weak	1	≥10% to <30%	1	Low	<6
Moderate	2	≥30% to <70%	2	High	=6
Strong	3	≥70%	3		

Modified from Locati LD [16]

three stable diseases. The median PFS was 12 months and the treatment was overall well tolerated. In 2012, a Japanese group retrospectively analyzed their series of eight SDC patients treated with LHRH analog, reporting two partial responses and three stable diseases; treatment was also well tolerated in this case. A retrospective work on 17 patients confirmed the activity of CAB (combined androgen blockade) with bicalutamide 50 mg plus LHRH analog with ORR of 64.7% [95% CI, 38.3–85.8%] along with a 3-year PFS and 5-year OS of 11.8% and 19.3%, respectively [16]. The results obtained by CAB have been recently confirmed by a prospective phase II trial on 36 patients [17]. Objective response rate was 41.7% including four complete remissions, with a median PFS of 8.8 months (range 6.3–12.3 months) and a median OS of 30.5 months (range 16.8 not reached). The lower response rate could be potentially explained by the enrolment of six patients with AR expression lower than 70% hypothesizing in this group of patients a lower activity of CAB. A prospective proof-of-concept randomized clinical trial held by the EORTC is currently ongoing to demonstrate the efficacy and safety of ADT versus chemotherapy in patients with recurrent and/or metastatic, AR-positive SGCs (NCT01969578).

Following PCa treatment approaches, we firstly used abiraterone (1000 mg daily plus prednisone 5 mg q12 h), an inhibitor of androgen synthesis, in AR-expressing SGCs which had failed to respond to ADT. Abiraterone has been approved as a second-line treatment in hormone-resistant PCa patients. Two patients with recurrent/metastatic adenocarcinoma, NOS, progressive to ADT have been treated with abiraterone, obtaining a clinical response in both cases [5]. A phase II trial is currently ongoing to test the activity of abiraterone in a larger cohort of patients with hormone-resistant, AR-expressing SGCs (NCT02867852). Another phase II trial with enzalutamide is currently recruiting in the same patient setting (NCT02749903).

13.6 Conclusions

First-line treatment is still to be defined in advanced SGCs. To date, evidences would suggest cisplatin alone or combined with other agents as the preferable option as systemic therapy both in ACC and non-ACC groups. Considering the novel agents, promising results are coming from ADT in AR-expressing SDC and adenocarcinoma, NOS. Multinational cooperation is crucial to improve research and clinical results in this cancer setting. For these rare cancers, a comprehensive understanding of genetics and biology could be the backbone to identify further and more active treatments. Enrollment in clinical trials is strongly advised for all patients with incurable SGCs.

References

1. Gao M, Hao Y, Huang MX, et al. Clinicopathological study of distant metastases of salivary adenoid cystic carcinoma. Int J Oral Maxillofac Surg. 2013;42(8):923–8.
2. Ferrarotto R, Mitani Y, Diao L, et al. Activating NOTCH1 mutations define a distinct subgroup of patients with adenoid cystic carcinoma who have poor prognosis, propensity to bone and liver metastasis, and potential responsiveness to Notch1 inhibitors. J Clin Oncol. 2017;35(3):352–60.
3. Laurie SA, Ho AL, Fury MG, et al. Systemic therapy in the management of metastatic or locally recurrent adenoid cystic carcinoma of the salivary glands: a systematic review. Lancet Oncol. 2011;12(8):815–24.
4. Girelli L, Locati L, Galeone C, et al. Lung metastasectomy in adenoid cystic cancer: is it worth it? Oral Oncol. 2017;65:114–8.
5. Alfieri S, Granata R, Bergamini C, et al. Systemic therapy in metastatic salivary gland carcinomas: a pathology-driven paradigm? Oral Oncol. 2017;66:58–63.
6. Rodriguez CP, Martins RG, Baik C, et al. Phase II trial of eribulin mesylate in recurrent or metastatic salivary gland malignancies. Head Neck. 2018;40(3):584–9.
7. Andersson MK, Afshari MK, Andrén Y, et al. Targeting the oncogenic transcriptional regulator MYB in adenoid cystic carcinoma by inhibition of IGF1R/AKT signaling. J Natl Cancer Inst. 2017;109(9). https://doi.org/10.1093/jnci/djx017.
8. Sridharan V, Gjini E, Liao X, et al. Immune profiling of adenoid cystic carcinoma: PD-L2 expression and associations with tumor-infiltrating lymphocytes. Cancer Immunol Res. 2016;4(8):679–87.
9. Hong MH, Kim CG, Koh YW, et al. Efficacy and safety of vinorelbine plus cisplatin chemotherapy for patients with recurrent and/or metastatic salivary gland cancer of the head and neck. Head Neck. 2018;40(1):55–62.
10. Locati LD, Perrone F, Losa M, et al. Treatment relevant target immunophenotyping of 139 salivary gland carcinomas (SGCs). Oral Oncol. 2009;45(11):986–90.
11. Keller G, Steinmann D, Quaas A, et al. New concepts of personalized therapy in salivary gland carcinomas. Oral Oncol. 2017;68:103–13.
12. Cipriani NA, Blair EA, Finkle J, et al. Salivary gland secretory carcinoma with high-grade transformation, CDKN2A/B loss, distant metastasis, and lack of sustained response to crizotinib. Int J Surg Pathol. 2017;25(7):613–8.
13. Mukaigawa T, Hayashi R, Hashimoto K, et al. Programmed death ligand-1 expression is associated with poor disease free survival in salivary gland carcinomas. J Surg Oncol. 2016;114(1):36–43.
14. Cros J, Sbidian E, Hans S, et al. Expression and mutational status of treatment-relevant targets and key oncogenes in 123 malignant salivary gland tumours. Ann Oncol. 2013;24(10):2624–9.
15. Dalin MG, Watson PA, Ho AL, et al. Androgen receptor signaling in salivary gland cancer. Cancers (Basel). 2017;9(2):17.
16. Locati LD, Perrone F, Cortelazzi B, et al. Clinical activity of androgen deprivation therapy in patients with metastatic/relapsed androgen receptor-positive salivary gland cancers. Head Neck. 2016;38(5):724–31.
17. Fushimi C, Tada Y, Takahashi H, et al. A prospective phase II study of combined androgen blockade in patients with androgen receptor-positive metastatic or locally advanced unresectable salivary gland carcinoma. Ann Oncol. 2018;29(4):979–84.

Printed by Printforce, the Netherlands